Additive Manufacturing with Medical Applications

Edited by
Harish Kumar Banga
Rajesh Kumar
Parveen Kalra
Rajendra M. Belokar

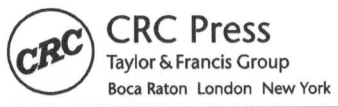

CRC Press
Taylor & Francis Group
Boca Raton London New York

CRC Press is an imprint of the
Taylor & Francis Group, an **Informa** business

First edition published 2022
by CRC Press
6000 Broken Sound Parkway NW, Suite 300, Boca Raton, FL 33487-2742

and by CRC Press
4 Park Square, Milton Park, Abingdon, Oxon, OX14 4RN

CRC Press is an imprint of Taylor & Francis Group, LLC

© 2023 selection and editorial matter, Harish Kumar Banga, Rajesh Kumar, Parveen Kalra Rajendra M. Belokar; individual chapters, the contributors

Library of Congress Cataloging-in-Publication Data
Names: Kumar Banga, Harish, editor.
Title: Additive manufacturing with medical applications / edited by Harish Kumar Banga, Rajesh Kumar, Parveen Kalra, Rajendra M. Belokar.
Description: First edition. | Boca Raton : CRC Press, [2023] | Includes bibliographical references and index.
Identifiers: LCCN 2022003826 (print) | LCCN 2022003827 (ebook) | ISBN 9781032110776 (hbk) | ISBN 9781032293257 (pbk) | ISBN 9781003301066 (ebk)
Subjects: LCSH: Medical instruments and apparatus. | Additive manufacturing.
Classification: LCC R856 .A625 2023 (print) | LCC R856 (ebook) | DDC 610.28/4--dc23/eng/20220401
LC record available at https://lccn.loc.gov/2022003826
LC ebook record available at https://lccn.loc.gov/2022003827

ISBN: 978-1-032-11077-6 (hbk)
ISBN: 978-1-032-29325-7 (pbk)
ISBN: 978-1-003-30106-6 (ebk)

DOI: 10.1201/9781003301066

Typeset in Times
by SPi Technologies India Pvt Ltd (Straive)

Additive Manufacturing with Medical Applications

This text discusses integrated approaches to improve the objectives of additive manufacturing in medical applications.

It covers case studies related to product design and development and discusses biomaterials, artificial intelligence applications and machine learning, using additive manufacturing techniques. It focuses on important topics, including 3D-printing technology, materials for 3D printing in medicine, rapid prototyping in clinical applications, and additive manufacturing in customized bone tissue engineering scaffolds.

Features:

- discusses additive manufacturing techniques and their utilization in medical applications
- covers important applications of additive manufacturing in the fields of medicine, education and the space industry
- explores regulatory challenges associated with the emergence of additive manufacturing
- examines the use of rapid prototyping in clinical applications

This book will serve as a useful reference guide for graduate students and academic researchers in the fields of industrial engineering, manufacturing science, mechanical engineering and aerospace engineering.

Contents

Preface

The book entitled *Additive Manufacturing with Medical Applications* presents various practical outbreaks of 3D-printing technologies in the medical field associated with recent innovations: creating tissues and organoids, surgical tools, patient-specific surgical models and custom-made prosthetics.

This book presents multidisciplinary aspects of the evolutionary growth of this exceptional technology, including social, medical, administrative and scientific. This book presents the medical industry's requirements for the error-free exact anatomy of the patient for diagnosis, surgical planning, surgical guides, implants, etc. Since every patient has a unique anatomy, additive manufacturing (AM) suits as best fit for the medical industry. The AM medical model provides the advantage of customising each model according to the patient's specific requirement, which is not easy in a conventional way. Overall, it is believed that the combined efforts of the editorial team members and contributing authors will provide this book with enormous attention across R&D, manufacturing, medical and academic platforms.

Harish Kumar Banga

Rajesh Kumar

Parveen Kalra

Rajendra M. Belokar

Editors

Dr Harish Kumar Banga is currently working as an Assistant Professor, Department of Fashion & Life Style Accessories Design, National Institute of Fashion Technology, Mumbai and completed his PhD in Production & Industrial Engineering. He is honored as 'Fellow' by the Indian Pharma Educational Society. He has one year of industry experience and seven years of teaching as well as research experience. His areas of interest are Additive Manufacturing, CAD/CAM. Human Factor Engineering and Robotics. He has taught courses including CAD/CAM, Modern Manufacturing Systems, Additive Manufacturing, Thermal Engineering, and Industrial Engineering at undergraduate levels. He has more than 75 research publications in national and international conferences and journals of repute. He is a Life Member of IIIE, HKSME, IAENG, and PUNJ Robotics. He has participated in and organised many workshops, seminars and FDPs and delivered numerous expert lectures. He has published 7 books and 22 book chapters in the additive manufacturing and product design area. He is a certified Six Sigma Green Belt.

Dr Rajesh Kumar is working as an Assistant Professor in the Department of Mechanical Engineering, UIET, Panjab University, Chandigarh. He published more than 80 research papers in national and international journals. He graduated from Punjab Engineering College, Chandigarh, in 1999. He did post-graduation and PhD from PEC University of Technology, Chandigarh, in 2004 and 2012, respectively. His areas of interest are Finite Element Analysis, Additive Manufacturing, CAD/CAM and Robotics. He has more than 15 years of teaching and research experience. He has taught courses including Finite Element Analysis, Thermal Engineering and CAD/CAM at undergraduate levels. He has participated in and organised many workshops, seminars and FDPs and delivered numerous expert lectures.

Dr Parveen Kalra graduated in Mechanical Engineering from PEC University of Technology, Chandigarh, in 1987 and post-graduation in Industrial Robotics from Memorial University, Canada, in 1989. He obtained his PhD in Mechanical Engineering from Panjab University, Chandigarh in 1995. Currently, he is a Professor in the Department of Production & Industrial Engineering at Punjab Engineering College, Chandigarh. His area of specialisation is Human Engineering, Industrial & Product Design, CAD/CAM and Robotics. He has more than 25 years of teaching and research experience. He has taught courses including Product Design & Development, Advanced Robotics, and CAD/CAM at postgraduate levels. He has published more than 95 research papers in international and national journals. He is a member of ISTE. He established the Centre of Excellence (Industrial & Product Design) by the DST project at PEC Chandigarh.

Dr Rajendra M. Belokar graduated in Production Engineering from Amravati University, Amravati, in 1987. He did post-graduation and PhD from Panjab University, Chandigarh, in 1999 and 2010, respectively. Presently, he is a Professor in the Department of Production & Industrial Engineering, Punjab Engineering College, Chandigarh. He published more than 85 research papers in national and international journals. He has more than 25 years of teaching and research experience. He has taught SCM, TQM, Industrial Metrology and Technology Management courses at undergraduate and postgraduate levels. He has published three books and two book chapters with international publishers. He is a Senior Member SME (USA), M.I.E, C. Eng (I), LM-IS TE, Member-INVEST, and Member APICS (USA). He established a Centre of Excellence in collaboration with SIEMENS in PEC Chandigarh. He is a certified Six Sigma Black, Green & Black Belt.

Contributors

Sangita Agarwal
Department of Applied Science
RCC Institute of Information
  Technology
Beliaghata, India

Ashish Aggarwal
Associate Professor of Radiodiagnosis
  & Imaging (Neuroimaging and
  Interventional Radiology)
PGIMER
Chandigarh, India

Chirag Ahuja
Associate Professor of Radiodiagnosis
  & Imaging (Neuroimaging and
  Interventional Radiology)
Centre of Excellence in Industrial and
  Product Design, Punjab Engineering
  College
Chandigarh, India

Sümeyra Ayan
Department of Bioengineering, Faculty
  of Chemical and Metallurgical
  Engineering
Yildiz Technical University
Istanbul, Turkey

Harish Kumar Banga
Department of Fashion & Life Style
  Accessories Design
National Institute of Fashion
  Technology
Mumbai, India

R. M. Belokar
Department of Production and Industrial
  Engineering
Punjab Engineering College (Deemed to
  Be University)
Chandigarh, India.

Najla Bentrad
Department of Biology and Physiology
  of Organisms
University of Sciences and Technology
  Houari Boumediene (USTHB)
Algiers, Algeria

Muhammet Emin Cam
Department of Mechanical Engineering
University College London
London, UK

Harpreet Kaur Channi
Department of Electrical Engineering
Chandigarh University
Mohali, India

Fatih Ciftci
Department of Bioengineering, Faculty
  of Chemical and Metallurgical
  Engineering
Yildiz Technical University
Istanbul, Turkey

Soumendra Darbar
Department of Pharmaceutical
  Technology
Jadavpur University
Kolkata, India

Parneet Kaur Deol
Department of Pharmaceutics
G.H.G. Khalsa College of Pharmacy
  Gurusar Sadhar
Ludhiana, India

Himanshu Deswal
Dental Officer
Department of Ex-servicemen
  Contributory Health Scheme
  (ECHS), Polyclinic Sonipat
Haryana, India

Nazmi Ekren
Electrical and Electronics Engineering,
  Faculty of Technology
Marmara University
Istanbul, Turkey

Amoljit Singh Gill
Department of Mechanical Engineering
I.K. Gujral Punjab Technical University
Kapurthala, India

Dr Vishakha Grover
Department of Periodontology
Dr. H.S.J. Institute of Dental Sciences
Panjab University Chandigarh
Chandigarh, India

Dr Shipra Gupta
Unit of Periodontics
Oral Health Sciences Centre
Post Graduate Institute of Medical
  Education & Research (PGIMER)
Chandigarh, India

Oguzhan Gündüz
Department of Metallurgical and
  Materials Engineering, Faculty of
  Technology
Marmara University
Istanbul, Turkey

Asma Hamida-Ferhat
Pierre and Marie Curie Center (CPMC),
  Pharmacy Department
University Hospital Center Mustapha
Algiers, Algeria

Ganesh S. Jadhav
Department of Design
Dr VK MIT World Peace University
Pune, India

Atul Kadam
Department of Pharmaceutics
Shri Santkrupa College of Pharmacy
Ghogaon, India

Parveen Kalra
Department of Production and Industrial
  Engineering
Punjab Engineering College (Deemed to
  Be University)
Chandigarh, India

Anoop Kapoor
Department of Periodontology
Sri Sukhmani Dental College and
  Hospital
Dera Bassi (Punjab), India

Indu Pal Kaur
Department of Pharmaceutics
University Institute of Pharmaceutical
  Sciences, Panjab University
  Chandigarh
Chandigarh, India

Prachi Khamkar
Department of Research &
  Development
Next Big Innovation Labs
Bangalore

Kamal Kishore
Department of Mechanical
  Engineering
National Institute of Technology
  Hamirpur
Hamirpur (H.P.), India

Raj Kumar
Department of Production and Industrial
  Engineering
Punjab Engineering College (Deemed to
  Be University)
Chandigarh, India

Rajender Kumar
Department of Mechanical
  Engineering
Manav Rachna International Institute of
  Research & Studies
Faridabad, India

Rajesh Kumar
Department of Mechanical Engineering,
    UIET
Panjab University
Chandigarh, India

Rakesh Kumar
Department of Regulatory Affairs
Auxein Medical Private Limited
Sonipat, India

Raman Kumar
Department of Mechanical &
    Production Engineering
Guru Nanak Dev Engineering College
Ludhiana
Punjab, India

Santosh Kumar
Department of Mechanical Engineering
Chandigarh Group of Colleges, Landran.
Mohali, Punjab, India

Parth K. Patel
Department of Pharmaceutical Sciences,
    Jefferson College of Pharmacy
Thomas Jefferson University
Philadelphia, PA, USA

Jagjit Singh Randhawa
Centre of Excellence in Industrial and
    Product Design
Punjab Engineering College
Chandigarh, India

Ranbir Singh Rooprai
Department of Mechanical Engineering
Chitkara University Institute of
    Engineering and Technology
Chitkara University
Punjab, India

Srimoyee Saha
Department of Life Science and
    Biotechnology
Jadavpur University
Kolkata, India

Vaibhav Sahni
Unit of Periodontics,
Oral Health Sciences Centre,
Post Graduate Institute of Medical
    Education & Research (PGIMER),
Chandigarh, India

Kritik Saxena
Department of Mechanical Engineering
National Institute of Technology Calicut
Kerala, India

Komal Sehgal
Department of Prosthodontics
Dr. H.S.J. Institute of Dental Sciences
Panjab University Chandigarh
Chandigarh, India

Mustafa Sengor
Center for Nanotechnology &
    Biomaterials Application and
    Research (NBUAM)
Marmara University
Istanbul, Turkey

Shagun Sharma
Centre of Excellence in Industrial and
    Product Design
Punjab Engineering College
Chandigarh, India

Parnika Shrivastava
Department of Mechanical Engineering
National Institute of Technology Hamirpur
Hamirpur, India

Jaswinder Singh
Department of Mechanical Engineering
Chitkara University Institute of
    Engineering and Technology
Chitkara University
Punjab, India

Manarshhjot Singh
Department of Robotics & Automation
University Lille, CNRS, Centrale Lille
Lille, France

Mandeep Singh
Department of Pharmaceutics
University Institute of Pharmaceutical
    Sciences, Panjab University
    Chandigarh
Chandigarh, India

Navdeep Singh
Department of Mechanical Engineering
National Institute of Technology
    Hamirpur
Hamirpur, India

Param Singh
Department of Mechanical Engineering
National Institute of Technology
    Hamirpur
Hamirpur, India

Manoj Kumar Sinha
Department of Mechanical Engineering
National Institute of Technology
    Hamirpur
Hamirpur, India

Cem Bülent Üstündag
Department of Bioengineering, Faculty
    of Chemical and Metallurgical
    Engineering
Yildiz Technical University
Istanbul, Turkey

Roopak Varshney
Department of Mechanical Engineering
National Institute of Technology
    Hamirpur
Hamirpur, India

1 Introduction and Need for Additive Manufacturing in the Medical Industry

Prachi Khamkar

Next Big Innovation Labs, Bengaluru, India

Ashokrao Mane College of Pharmacy, Peth Vadgaon, India

Atul Kadam

Shree Santkrupa College of Pharmacy, Karad, India

Ashokrao Mane College of Pharmacy, Peth Vadgaon, India

CONTENTS

DOI: 10.1201/9781003301066-1

1

1.1 INTRODUCTION

Industrial Revolution 4.0 is on the brink. Outstanding innovative technological developments in the twenty-first century are of an age turning towards digitalisation. Additive manufacturing (AM) is an overarching term for a variety of technologies [1]. Advances in AM in endless fields of application have come about in the last three decades [2]. AM technologies are also described as layered manufacturing, 3D printing, computer-automated manufacturing, rapid prototyping, or solid free-form technology [3]. This technology has been widely used in various engineering and biomedical fields [4,5]. AM has previously been used mostly to create scientific prototypes, but is now making inroads into the healthcare sector. This technique has opened the door to a modern era in precision medicine, and modern developments in molecular biology and gene profiling. Application of 3D printers for the production of customised pharmaceutical products and manufacture of personalised medicine enables stability and release profiles of multiple drugs. AM aims to exhibit the future of technology by manufacturing tailored products as a one-stop solution. With AM technologies pharmaceutical products are developed using computer-aided design (CAD) tools [7]. The object to be printed is rendered using CAD programming that transforms a drawn picture into a standard tessellation language (STL) file format suitable for 3D printers. A structure can be drawn in a layer-by-layer manner with the assistance of CAD drawing software. For example, some drugs have been found to be more effective in patients with hereditary differences, while some have been shown to have harmful effects on certain ethnic groups. Advances in the area of pharmacogenomics, according to how individual's genetic profile influences their unique drug reaction, offer more detailed dose and drug selection details that can better support a single person depending on their genetic makeup. AM can be implemented in the healthcare sector on request to deliver medicine on demand [8]. Healthcare currently works on the principle in recent therapies of 'one size fits all'. The setting forward of customised therapy, generally requiring the tailoring of treatments of a patient depending on their specific attributes, desires and expectations at all stages of care, has formulated the extraordinary area of personalised medicine. AM technology has been used to manufacture numerous formulations in pharmaceuticals, such as floating tablets, sustained release, patches and microneedles, that simplify the process of manufacturing complex dosage forms [9]. The conventional manufacturing process cannot be manipulated according to patient needs. 3D printing can strengthen the healthcare system, further enhancing medical compliance by tailoring the prescription to the patient. 3D printing is an AM process that enables the production of flexible and patient-specific scaffolds with high structural sophistication and design versatility. Recently, 3D printing has encountered a broad variety of uses in medicine, including craniofacial braces, dental moulds, crowns and implants. Recent advances in mechanical devices and software have greatly enhanced the precision, quality, speed and versatility of 3D printing methods. 3D printed items have often seen success clinically.

Developments in the field of AM have enabled researchers to explore technology within the medical field and its usage. The application of AM in various fields is contributing to the revolution of modern medicine and its development. Traditional manufacturing preferred large-scale processes which, although cost-effective, are time-consuming and involve manual labour [10]. A recent rise in multiple diseases is reflected in a sharp increase in surgical procedures of internal organs and tissues, AM technology helps surgeons to preplan the surgery with the help of 3D models [11]. With the help of AM, objects were able to be planned and placed for manufacturing instantly and used for developing patient-specific biomedical devices. The biomedical instruments and implants suitable to the patient's anatomical profile can be modified in AM technology, which was an obstacle in traditional manufacturing technology. In AM technology, each medical device or implant is uniquely configured according to the patient. Intermediate processing steps such as production line assembly and mould construction can be eliminated and medical devices can be printed without a hitch. AM would be the preferred technique in the biomedical field because of its high precision and revolution. This review aims to summarise the recent advances within medical development by AM drug delivery systems, devices and organs, along with technological regulative challenges and opportunities. In recent years, AM has developed in the media. These AM processes are far from being a completely new technique. AM printers now hold an increasingly important role in the mainstream, largely because of the opening up of this technology to the general public [12].

1.2 HISTORICAL ASPECTS

Charles Hull was the father of 3D printing and developed the stereolithography technique in the mid-1980s. Later, Hull established the organisation of a 3D system that built up primary 3D printers called 'stereolithography' [13]. Many organisations have created 3D printers for business applications [14]. In 1988, Charles Deckard filed a selective laser sintering patent in which laser light was projected over a pulver bed in order to heat the powder on a pulver bed [15]. In 1989, utilising this methodology, the Scott Crump file on fused deposition modelling (FDM) and the object was constructed by the sequential layering of solidified materials until the form of the part was obtained. The developers of Stratasys also created and patented FDM. Luken Massella received the first 3D-printed bladder in 1999 which was a 3D cell amalgamation. The United States Food and Drug Administration (USFDA) was licensed for the first 3D-printed pill in 2015 [16].

1.3 CUTTING-EDGE TECHNOLOGY

All the cutting-edge technologies like artificial intelligence (AI), Internet of Things (IoT) and machine learning (ML), data analytics or data scientists changing the world have an impact on the healthcare revolution. Hospitals generate a large amount of data, of course. The patient records' details are developed by visual data in X-rays and CT scans by doctors and engineers. This can be very important information, often when companies have access and the tools to evaluate it in a situation at the right moment. This detail is open to doctors as much as possible from modern AI and the medical IoT [17]. As a consequence, the way hospitals are working is transformed.

The identification of so-called 'edge cases' also means that it may be rare or hard to measure diseases. Since ML systems of this kind consist of huge databases containing digital files of these diseases (and different transformations), they are also more accurate for this kind of detection than humans. All these technologies, including AM printing, are going to transform everything which has a huge impact on human lives and indirectly on the whole globe. So we should be ready to handle these technologies like doubled-edged swords [18].

1.4   THE PROCEDURE OF 3D PRINTING

Three-dimensional (3D) bioprinting begins with a model of a framework that is recreated layer by layer using a bio-ink that is either blended with live cells or seeded with cells after the print is final. These initial models may originate from any source – a CT or MRI scan, a CAD application, or an internet file. This 3D model file is then fed into a slicer – a specialised type of computer program that analyses the model's geometry and produces a series of thin layers, or slices that, when stacked vertically, form the shape of the initial model. Examples of slicers widely used for 3D printing are Cura and Slic3r. After slicing a model, the slices are converted into path data and saved as a g-code file that can be submitted to a 3D bioprinter for printing. The bioprinter follows the g-code file's instructions in sequence, including instructions for controlling extruder temperature, extrusion strength, bedplate temperature, cross-linking strength and frequency, and, of course, the slicer's 3D movement direction. After completing all of the g-code instructions, the print is final and can be cultured or seeded with cells as part of a biostudy. The designs are usually converted into a computer-readable suitable format (STL) file which explains the arrangement and framework of the 3D model (see Figure 1.1). Materials like API and excipients are transformed into preferred substances like granules, hot melt, filaments or binder ink, based on their printing use. Add-on materials are used in a layered manner to shape a finished product like tablets or capsules. Unless the printing process is finished, the resultant dosage type may be dried, sintered, polished or hardened as needed.

1.5   NEED FOR ADDITIVE MANUFACTURING PRINTING
IN THE MEDICAL INDUSTRY

Every year, additive manufacturing brings far more applications in the medical field to preserve and enrich lives in forms that have never been thought of before.

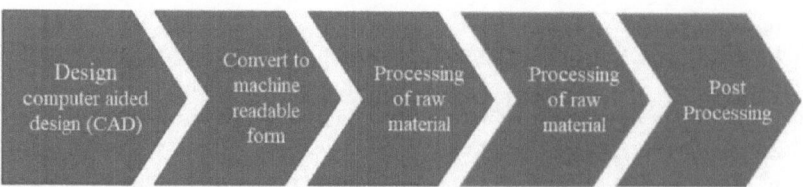

FIGURE 1.1   Process of 3D printing.

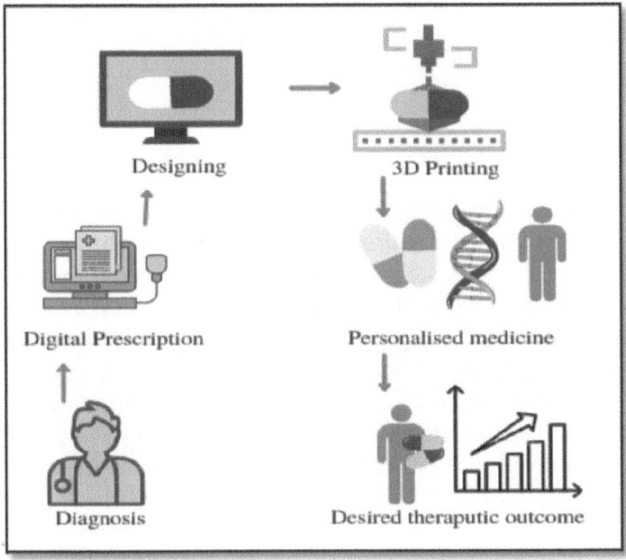

FIGURE 1.2   Tailoring of dose by additive manufacturing.

1.5.1 TAILORING OF DOSE

AM has the potential to emerge in the pharmaceutical industry by its ability to create tailor-made dosage formulations for patients, as depicted in Figure 1.2. It aims to enhance patient services, to promote diagnostic testing and research, therapy, and the detection of human illness or disorder predispositions [19]. Therefore, doctors should use the gene mutation history of a patient that helps to choose medications and treatment solutions that minimise the adverse effects that yield good results. In addition, before the outbreak, the vulnerability of persons to such diseases can be detected and AM can be applied as drug therapy for the prevention of susceptible diseases in humans [20]. AM also enables the printing of pills in a complex layer, built by using a mixture of medicine to treat different diseases simultaneously. The technology provides healthcare professionals with a standard for the treatment of patients with multiple diseases.

1.5.2 PATIENT COMPLIANCE IMPROVED

From numerous studies performed, it is clear that the process of 3D printing is feasible in producing a dosage type that may contain more than one active ingredient. such as a polypill or a multi-layer pill [21]. Dose variety configuration can encourage consistency with treatment, as elderly people will have to take the medication less often. If a patient has a chronic health condition, individuals might only take a single pill, with the necessary modifications according to their genetic composition [22]. For example, producing pills with a mixture of more than one active pharmaceutical compound or dispensed as multi-reservoir printed tablets is another key potential in AM. Therefore, people who suffer from more than one disease can have multi-dose forms, providing the patient with a better, or better customized, and reliable dosage [23].

1.5.3 New Design in Medicine

Because varieties of medication are prepared by using AM printing methods and are focused on design by the information fed into the computer program, various possibilities are afforded to fabricate a dosage structure with complex forms, geometry and spatial distribution of medicines in a single machine [24]. The lowest dose of a medication can be generated using 3D printing, and there is an improved probability of generating different dosage types correctly. The API in any dosage form may be placed strategically by monitoring its availability and, as a result, the manufacturing of complex, staggered, or continuous-release dosage forms can be rendered less difficult [3]. FDM 3D printing is one method that is used to manufacture tablets, along with special geometrical forms [25].

1.5.4 Integration with Healthcare Network

Almost all these developments in AM technologies have led to a transformative improvement in health and medical research, that is being increasingly implemented in many hospitals worldwide. Costs of hospital-tailored implants must meet both the patients' and the hospital's requirements. Unit costs have to be affordable despite the need for individualisation. Small amounts can be manufactured at affordable prices through AM. This production process also offers a high degree of flexibility because a 3D CAD-based implant can be optimised and modified quickly. Ottawa Hospital has been the first hospital to open a robust 3D printing network for education, organising and medical research in Canada. In Madrid, a separate workshop named 'FabLab,' which improves the production of 3D printer innovation at the Hospital General Universitario Gregorio Marañón, has been developed in the medical facility [26,27].

1.5.5 Complex Drug-release Profiles

The manufacture of medicines with complicated drug-release profiles is one of the most commonly studied AM application areas. Additive processing increases the value of rendering multiple medicines consistent with several polymers in one formulation, meaning that various medicines are specifically distributed to different parts of the body and at specified time intervals. The polypill encourages the taking of the pill and promotes the independence of each treatment in patients with various illnesses, including elevated blood pressure, diabetes and chronic kidney disease [28].

1.5.6 Implants and Prostheses

Standard medical replacements and prosthetic limbs can be produced in under 24 hours, whereas the manufacturing procedures are lengthy for spinal, dental and hip replacements. Previously, surgeons had to make metal and plastic sections and graft bone or use cutting equipment to alter implants to accomplish the desired shapes and sizes that match perfectly. The abnormal form of the skull, the standardisation of which is a complicated process, is also the appropriate condition in neurosurgical cases. There are examples of popular 3D printers and prostheses, both commercially and clinically, at BIOMED Research Institute in Belgium where the first 3D-printed mandibular titanium prosthesis was successfully implanted [29]. Permanent surgical implants, which are generally used in dentistry and orthopaedics, involve biomaterials that cannot be broken down. Compared to manufacturing implants using conventional technology, AM can accomplish customised real-time manufacturing of any complicated implant with high dimensional precision and accuracy [30].

A custom cranial titanium implant was developed by Winder et al. using stereolithographic resin implants, which simplifies the procedure greatly. Secondly, state-of-the-art technologies create implants with excellent mechanical characteristics that complement bone. In Germany, Solutions developed a titanium hip implant by selective laser melting (SLM) [31]. Body Labs has developed a device that allows patients to prototype their prosthetics on their own limbs by screening in order to produce a more realistic look and appearance. Furthermore, researchers at the Massachusetts Institute of Technology have attempted to formulate a more compatible prosthetic socket [32].

1.5.7 BIOPRINTING OF TISSUES AND ORGANS

The current solution for the problem is organ transplantation from a deceased or living donor for a patient suffering from loss of organ or tissue due to injuries or birth defects; this is one of the current medical challenges. Only a few individuals receive organs and the majority of them suffer from donor shortfall. Treatment for organ transplantation is costly and beyond the control of normal citizens. Donors with tissue compatibility are difficult to locate, so this is another difficulty with transplantation surgery [33]. The alternative to this major issue is to use individual patients' body cells to develop the proper tissue or organ which minimises the risk of rejection by using AM technology (see Figure 1.3); thereby, the need for immunosuppressants would be substantially reduced. Based on the measurements obtained from computed tomography (CT) and MRI scans, 3D-printed synthetic versions of an adult kidney and a baby's stomach, along with the liver, bones and blood vessels, were made to enable the surgical team to plan and conduct a complicated operation [34,35]. The models helped the team to visualise and play with the position of a kidney and to assess the likelihood of specific abdominal closure [35], according to the transplant staff member Nizam Mamode, a hospital transplant surgeon consultant. By using 3D printers, scientists developed an artificial ear, bone and heart valve. Wang et al. created an artificial liver by layering various cells into different hydrogels [36].

1.5.8 MICRONEEDLES

Transdermal system microneedles have micron clusters of needles on the matrix surface to improve penetration of the drug molecule into the skin. A microneedle is efficient in delivering macromolecules rather than conventional microstructured

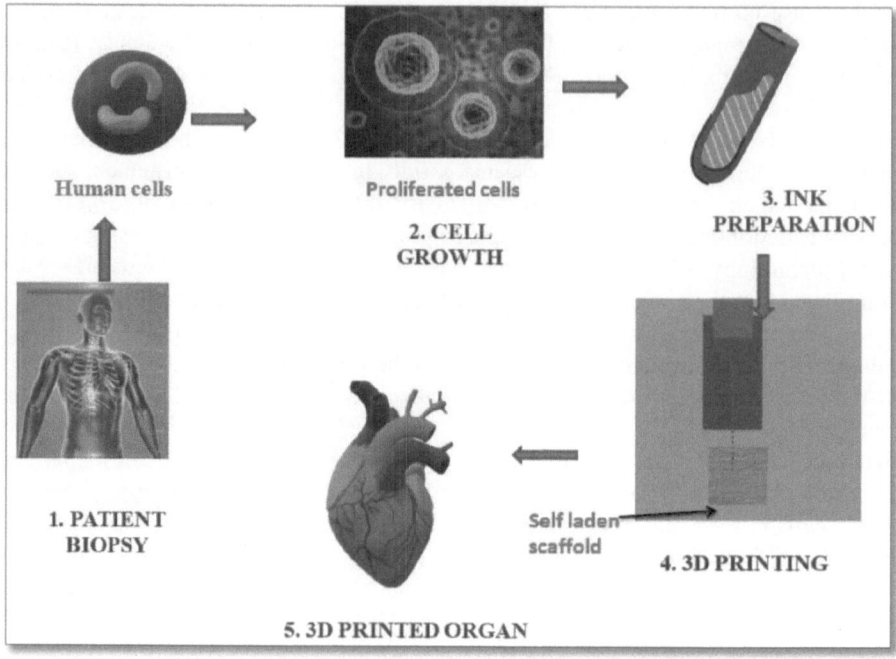

FIGURE 1.3   Bioprinting of organ by additive manufacturing.

molecules [37]. Although conventional micromanufacturing methods are restricted to microneedles with basic geometry, the latest 3D printing technology makes it possible to manufacture microneedles with more complicated and complex geometry. Biodegradable microneedles have been developed. A new micromanufacturing technique with improved resolution has been created. Without a primary guide, an FDM 3D printer with printing parameters was tuned to create microneedles of various sizes, lengths, and concentrations of the series [25]. The study also found that polylactic acid (a reusable, biodegradable, and thermoplastic polymer) degrades in the skin, enabling the medication to be released.

1.5.9 IMPROVING MEDICAL EDUCATION

3D-printed patient-specific models have shown that they can significantly improve efficiency and promote effective learning as well as radically improve results. There is a need for awareness, monitoring and trust of trainees, irrespective of the field of expertise, for safe and efficient use of 3D printing. Reproducibility and security of the 3D-printed model during cadaver dissection, the ability to model various physiological and pathological anatomies from a broad dataset of photographs, and the ability to exchange 3D models among different universities, especially those with fewer resources, are all advantages of 3D printing in education. Anatomical specifics can be accentuated by 3D printers capable of printing with various densities and colours.

1.6   CASE STUDY OF FIRST USFDA-APPROVED TABLET

Until today, Spritam is the only 3D-printed medication on the market that is Food and Drug Administration (FDA)-approved. Founded in 2003, Aprecia Pharmaceuticals had an objective of achieving a unique dosage form made exclusively by 3D printing. A high-dose cardiovascular disease medication was tried for early on-scale trials of its patented devices, offering the first value of getting 1,000 mg of drug loading in a ZipDose system that can disintegrate in seconds and also deliver positive accuracy and comparative bioavailability/bioequivalence. ZipDose technology is a weapon in the understanding that a large range of compounds, especially pharmaceuticals and nutraceuticals, are important to the formulation strategy. The first example of a commercial product created with ZipDose technology is Spritam. The medication substance, levetiracetam, was very important in supporting the development of Spritam, which is currently marketed as immediate capsules, tablets and oral solutions in both branded and generic products. Therefore, it was important to identify an effective regulatory mechanism, backed by the extensive clinical and regulatory background of levetiracetam [38–40].

1.7   REGULATORY PERSPECTIVE

Researchers believe that 3D printing will also be a part of the future of the pharmacy. A personalised 'polypill', which would possibly contain all the medicines a patient needs in a single pill, could be created if common medications were available for chronic diseases on a pharmacist's 3D printer. But this trend is resistant, since controlling and maintaining protection in local pharmacies will be more difficult than in manufacturing sites. The practice also poses questions about 3D printing and intellectual property, software engineering standardisation, business models and the potential for counterfeit drugs.

In the manufacture of traditional or 3D-printed medical equipment, the FDA usually may not approve specialised materials for general use. Regulation in AM is required, but FDA guidelines emphasise that, due to the variety in printing processes, there is no way to include a standardised collection of guidelines. Instead, the FDA recognises finished surgical equipment and devices, etc. For example, the FDA has approved spinal implants made of titanium alloy, but the FDA does not review or authorise the use of titanium in medical devices. The FDA tests the products used in the manufacturing of medical equipment for the protection and usefulness of the product for its intended use. The content is assessed in depth as part of the final product and its planned usage, and the FDA analyses the device as being sufficiently safe and productive for its intended use or approximately comparable to the advantages and risks of the legally sold system. If these requirements are satisfied, the FDA shall approve or refuse (respectively) the approval of particular devices for the stated intended purpose. At the end of the day, this does not give approval or licence for the same material to be included in other devices.

Since the format is so recent, navigating the uncontrolled processes for producing 3D pharmaceuticals is expensive, which poses a challenge for certain players. Since 3D printing techniques vary considerably, even inside solid dose medications, it is premature to identify best practices. The pharmaceutical industry is particularly interested in inkjet 3D printing methods because they have many similarities with current production processes and can provide a more effective, long-term printing solution. However, 3D printing would not fully replace conventional manufacturing processes for some time. Additionally, further study is necessary to develop more effective binding polymers that account for structural differences and patient protection. When businesses send 3D-printed goods to the FDA for approval, the company can gain a greater understanding of industry best practices and regulations [41].

1.8 CHALLENGES AND OPPORTUNITIES

3D bioprinting poses additional problems associated with tissue engineering and regenerative medicine. For instance, consider the issues surrounding internal vascularisation in bioprinted constructs. Numerous experiments have established the viability of developing vascular networks inside organs. Compatibility of materials and cells with the printer and printing methods is one of the problems of printing vascular networks. Additionally, vascular networks can take longer to grow and mature in the tissue structure than cells do. In post-processing, a bioreactor may assist in maintaining the operation of tissue builders and buy time for tissue fusion, remodelling and maturation. Additionally, the normal vascular network is a non-uniform network in terms of scale, steadily decreasing in size from wide to minimal. One potential future approach is to use self-sacrificing materials to 3D print a network of interconnected large-diameter blood vessels. Following implantation, medium- and small-diameter blood vessels will be formed naturally by the host vascular network surrounding the implants, while capillaries will be formed by inducing stem cell differentiation in the printed implants.

Despite the reality that 3D printing has grown very rapidly in the medical industry for several years, there are many other major barriers, particularly technological and regulatory, that need to be overcome in the coming days. The technical difficulties include type and configuration optimisation; pre-and post-processing specifications; error control for all production steps; information supply and multi-material printing difficulties; usability, accuracy and speed for bioprinter tools; changes in resolution specifications; and compatibility concerns for bioprinting. The material to be used in the medicinal product should be chemically stable and customisable, with controlled release kinetics capable of producing non-toxic degradation by-products [41].

1.9 CONCLUSION

Since 2015–16, because of its customisation, reproducibility and durability, AM printing technology has emerged as a genuinely revolutionary medium in multidisciplinary areas, including medicine. The vast spectrum of technology currently available offers a flexible framework for the translation of a concept into a consumer product. The opportunity to create patient-tailored therapeutic devices and customised medication is elucidated by the integration of AM printing with medical techniques. In particular, it facilitates the development of complex patient-specific medical and physiological structures, using the data collected from various imaging techniques such as MRI and CT scans. AM continues to benefit from an additive technique of development in a golden age for the production and process engineering of products through sectors. AM printing is not far from being commonly used almost everywhere in our everyday lives. AM printing has to date been mainly used in manufacturing to build engineering applications. AM printing, however, has the potential to impact large-scale mass customisation of healthcare items and equipment. Several cases have documented the use of AM in a variety of medical applications, including the manufacturing of contact lenses and dental implants. In contrast with mouldings or paste implants, the key benefits of AM printers include the precise anatomy of patients and controlled spatial patterning of materials and polymers in a complex texture. A sufficient collection of regulations to ensure the widespread implementation of different AM printing technologies for manufacturing medical products is required.

REFERENCES

1. Schwab, K. (2020). The Fourth Industrial Revolution: What it means and how to respond. *World Economic Forum*. Retrieved 3 December 2020, from https://www.weforum.org/agenda/2016/01/the-fourth-industrial-revolution-what-it-means-and-how-to-respond/
2. Provaggi, E., & Kalaskar, D. (2017). 3D Printing Families. *3D Printing in Medicine*, 21–42. doi:10.1016/b978-0-08-100717-4.00003-x
3. Ventola, C.L. (2014). Medical Applications for 3D Printing: Current and Projected Uses. *Pharmacy and Therapeutics*, 39(10), 704.
4. Roopavath, U., & Kalaskar, D. (2017). Introduction to 3D Printing in Medicine. *3D Printing in Medicine*, 1–20. doi:10.1016/b978-0-08-100717-4.00001-6
5. Banga, H.K., Kumar, P., & Kumar, H. (2021). 'Utilization of Additive Manufacturing in Orthotics and Prosthetic Devices Development' *IOP Conf. Ser.: Mater. Sci. Eng.* doi:10.1088/1757-899X/1033/1/012083
6. Banga, H.K., Kalra, P., Belokar, R.M., & Kumar, R. (2020). Customized Design and Additive Manufacturing of Kids' Ankle Foot Orthosis. *Rapid Prototyping Journal*, 26(10). doi:10.1108/RPJ-07-2019-0194
7. Banga, H.K., Kalra, P., Belokar, R.M., & Kumar, R. (2020). Design and Fabrication of Prosthetic and Orthotic Product by 3D Printing [Online] First. *IntechOpen*. doi:10.5772/intechopen.94846. Retrieved from https://www.intechopen.com/online-first/design-and-fabrication-of-prosthetic-and-orthotic-product-by-3d-printing
8. Banga, H.K., Kalra, P., Belokar, R.M., & Kumar, R. (2020). 'Effect of 3D-Printed Ankle Foot Orthosis During Walking of Foot Deformities Patients'. In: Kumar H., Jain P. (eds) *Recent Advances in Mechanical Engineering*. Lecture Notes in Mechanical Engineering. Springer, Singapore, pp 275–288.
9. Banga, H.K., Kalra, P., Belokar, R.M., & Kumar, R. (2020). Role of Finite Element Analysis in Customized Design of Kid's Orthotic Product'. In: Singh S., Prakash C., Singh R. (eds) *Characterization, Testing, Measurement, and Metrology*, pp. 139–159 CRC Press, Taylor & Francis Group, USA.
10. Banga, H.K., Kalra, P., Belokar, R.M., & Kumar, R. (2020). Improvement of Human Gait in Foot Deformities Patients by 3D Printed Ankle–Foot Orthosis. In: Singh S., Prakash C., & Singh R. (eds) *3D Printing in Biomedical Engineering*. Materials Horizons: From Nature to Nanomaterials. Springer, Singapore.

11. Banga, H.K., Kalra, P., Belokar, R.M., & Kumar, R. (2018). Fabrication and Stress Analysis of Ankle Foot Orthosis with Additive Manufacturing. *Rapid Prototyping Journal Emerald Publishing*, 24(2), 300–312.

12. Banga, H.K., Belokar, R.M., Madan, R., & Dhole, S. (2017). Three Dimensional Gait Assessments During Walking of healthy people and drop foot patients. *Defence Life Science Journal*, 2, 14–20.

13. Banga, H.K., Belokar, R.M., & Kumar, R. (2017). 'A Novel Approach For Ankle Foot Orthosis Developed By Three Dimensional Technologies', *3rd International Conference on Mechanical Engineering and Automation Science (ICMEAS 2017)*, University of Birmingham, UK Vol. 8 No. 10, pp. 141–145.

14. Banga, H.K., Parveen, K., Belokar, R.M., & Kumar, R. (2014). Rapid Prototyping Applications in Medical Sciences. *International Journal of Emerging Technologies in Computational and Applied Sciences (IJETCAS)*, 5(8), 416–420.

15. LaSelle, R. (2020). The Future of 3D Printing: Five Trends|Jabil. Jabil.com. Retrieved 3 December 2020, from https://www.jabil.com/blog/future-of-3d-printing-additive-manufacturing-looks-bright.html

16. Pravin, S., & Sudhir, A. (2018). Integration of 3D Printing with Dosage Forms: A New Perspective for Modern Healthcare. *Biomedicine & Pharmacotherapy*, 107, 146–154. doi:10.1016/j.biopha.2018.07.167

17. Ali, A., Ahmad, U., & Akhtar, J. (2020). 3D Printing in Pharmaceutical Sector: An Overview. *Pharmaceutical Formulation Design-Recent Practices*. doi:10.5772/intechopen.90738

18. Matthews, K. (2020). How AI and IoT are Changing Daily Operations in Hospitals. Healthcare. *Innovation*. Retrieved 3 December 2020, from https://www.hcinnovationgroup.com/analytics-ai/article/21132663/how-ai-and-iot-are-changing-daily-operations-in-

19. Sarkar, T. (2020). AI and Machine Learning for Healthcare-KDnuggets. KDnuggets. Retrieved 3 December 2020, from https://www.kdnuggets.com/2020/05/ai-machine-learning-healthcare.html

20. Afsana, J.V., Haider, N., & Jain, K. (2019). 3D Printing in Personalized Drug Delivery. *Current Pharmaceutical Design*, 24(42), 5062–5071. doi:10.2174/1381612825666190215122208

21. Yan, Q., Dong, H., Su, J., Han, J., Song, B., Wei, Q., & Shi, Y. (2018). A Review of 3D Printing Technology for Medical Applications. *Engineering*, 4(5), 729–742. doi:10.1016/j.eng.2018.07.021

22. Abdullah, K.A., & Reed, W. (2018). 3D Printing in Medical Imaging and Healthcare Services. *Journal of Medical Radiation Sciences*, 65(3), 237–239. doi:10.1002/jmrs.292

23. Zhu, X., Li, H., Huang, L., Zhang, M., Fan, W., & Cui, L. (2020). 3D Printing Promotes the Development of Drugs. *Biomedicine & Pharmacotherapy*, 131, 110644. doi:10.1016/j.biopha.2020.110644

24. Jiménez, M., Romero, L. Domínguez, I.A., del Mar Espinosa, M., & Domínguez, M. (2019). Additive Manufacturing Technologies: An Overview about 3D Printing Methods and Future Prospects. *Complexity*. Article ID: 9656938. doi: 10.1155/2019/9656938

25. Moussi, K., Bukhamsin, A., Hidalgo, T., & Kosel, J. (2020). Biocompatible 3D Printed Microneedles for Transdermal, Intradermal, and Percutaneous Applications. Retrieved 4 December 2020, from. https://onlinelibrary.wiley.com/doi/full/10.1002/adem.201901358

26. (2017) The Ottawa Hospital launches Canada's first Medical 3D Printing Program. https://www.ottawahospital.on.ca/en/the-ottawa-hospital-launches-canadas-first-medical-3d-printing-program/

27. Perez-Mañanes, R., José, S., Desco-Menéndez, M., Sánchez-Arcilla, I., González-Fernández, E., Vaquero-Martín, J., González-Garzón, J. P., Mediavilla-Santos, L., Trapero-Moreno, D., & Calvo-Haro, J. A. (2021). Application of 3D printing and

distributed manufacturing during the first-wave of COVID-19 pandemic. Our experience at a third-level university hospital. *3D Printing in Medicine*, 7(1), 7. doi: 10.1186/s41205-021-00097-6

28. Aimar, A., Palermo, A., & Innocenti, B. (2019). The Role of 3D Printing in Medical Applications: A State of the Art. *Journal of Healthcare Engineering*, 2019, 1–10. doi:10.1155/2019/5340616

29. Garcia, J., Yang, Z., Mongrain, R., Leask, R. L., & Lachapelle, K. 3D Printing Materials and Their Use in Medical Education: A Review of Current Technology and Trends for the Future. *BMJ Simulation and Technology Enhanced Learning*, 4(1), 27–40, 2017. https://stel.bmj.com/content/4/1/27

30. Fredieu, J., Kerbo, J., Herron, M., Klatte, R., & Cooke, M. (2015). Anatomical Models: A Digital Revolution. *Medical Science Educator*, 25(2), 183–194. doi:10.1007/s40670-015-0115-9

31. Winder, J., R.S. Cooke, J. Gray, T. Fannin & T. Fegan. (1999). Medical Rapid Prototyping and 3D CT in the Manufacture of Custom Made Cranial Titanium Plates. *Journal of Medical Engineering & Technology*, 23, 1, 26–28, doi: 10.1080/030919099294401

32. Nawrat, A. (2018). 3D printing in the medical field: four major applications revolutionising the industry. https://www.medicaldevice-network.com Retrieved 4 December 2020, from https://www.medicaldevice-network.com/analysis/3d-printing-in-the-medical-field-applications/

33. Ali, A., Ahmad, U., & Akhtar, J. (2020). 3D Printing in Pharmaceutical Sector: An Overview. In U. Ahmad, & J. Akhtar (Eds.), *Pharmaceutical Formulation Design – Recent Practices*. IntechOpen. doi: 10.5772/intechopen.90738

34. Hoang, D., Perrault, D., Stevanovic, M., & Ghiassi, A. (2016). Surgical Applications of Three-Dimensional Printing: A Review of the Current Literature & How to Get Started. *Annals of Translational Medicine*, 4(23), 456. doi: 10.21037/atm.2016.12.18

35. Wang, P., Que, W., Zhang, M., Dai, X., Yu, K., Wang, C., Peng, Z., & Zhong, L. (2019). Application of 3-Dimensional Printing in Pediatric Living Donor Liver Transplantation: A Single-Center Experience. *Liver Transplantation*, 25(6), 831–840. doi:10.1002/lt.25435

36. Wang, X. (2019). Bioartificial Organ Manufacturing Technologies. *Cell Transplantation*, 28(1), 5–17. doi:10.1177/0963689718809918

37. Donnelly, R.F., Raj Singh, T.R., & Woolfson, A.D. (2010). Microneedle-based Drug Delivery Systems: Microfabrication, Drug Delivery, and Safety. *Drug Delivery*, 17(4), 187–207. doi:10.3109/10717541003667798

38. Martin, J. (2018). 3D Printing in the Pharmaceutical Industry – Where does it currently stand?. Retrieved 25 December 2020, from https://www.pharmaceuticalonline.com/doc/3d-printing-in-the-pharmaceutical-industry-where-does-it-currently-stand-0002

39. Clinical Trials Arena (2016). Retrieved 21 November 2020, from https://www.clinical-trialsarena.com/projects/spritam-levetiracetam-epilepsy/

40. Retrieved 10 December 2020, from https://www.aprecia.com/news/first-fda-approved-medicine-manufactured-using-3d-printing-technology-now-available

41. Khamkar, P., & Kadam, A. (2021). Regulatory Challenges and Myths about Pharmaceutical 3D Printing, *Manufacturing, Packaging and Logistics, European Pharmaceutical Review* February; 26(1), 26–28.

2 Insights of 3D Printing Technology with Its Types
A Review

Ranbir Singh Rooprai and Jaswinder Singh
Chitkara University Institute of Engineering and Technology,
Chitkara University, Punjab, India

CONTENTS

2.1   INTRODUCTION

3D printing is a revolutionary technique that promises to change the way we design products. This technique is used to build materials in a computer-controlled system

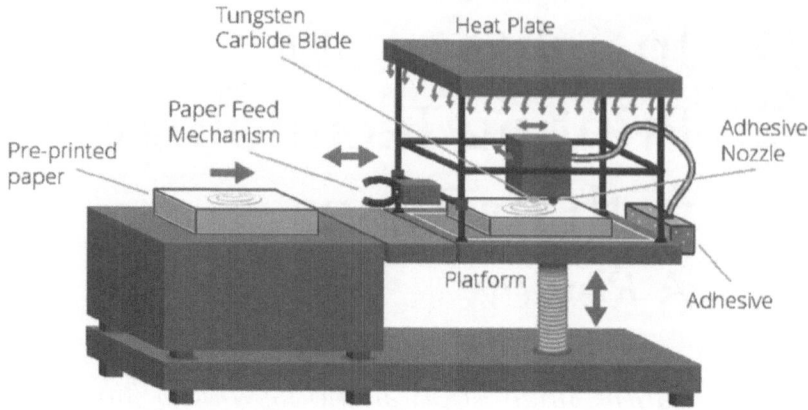

FIGURE 2.1   3D printer.

to create a physical object. The root 3D files are generally divided into several layers and a number of computer-controlled instructions are generated by every layer. Some also call this the third industrial revolution 3D printer and eventual digitisation of manufacturing [1]. The first and second industrial revolutions (textile mechanisation) changed the world irrevocably by destroying old lifestyles and producing new ones with the advent of the automotive assembly line. We must be prepared for 3D printing and industrial digitisation to change the world economically and politically and our lifestyle as radically as possible. The adoption of a wider range of additive manufacturing (AM) approaches was achieved using 3D printing [2]. 3D polymer printing materials are now being manufactured with a wider range of properties. The way goods are made, processed and used by customers constantly changes this creativity. For different types of materials like construction, vehicles, robots, aeronautics and sanitary applications, the use of 3D printing can be credibly used. In designing complex goods, it plays a vital part [3]. It leads to reducing the cost of production and cycles. It is an important tool for the creation of goods in different ways. 3D models are first developed using computer-assisted design (CAD) software in rapid prototyping. 3D printing uses rapid prototyping to create a physical object automatically from a computer model. This includes the STL format to generate the component from the CAD model [4,5]. This software then divides this model by the layer construction in thin cross-sections for part-layers. Rapid prototyping production is one of the first additive applications. This resulted in prototyping being produced much more quickly, enabling concept validation and testing before the development of a finished product [6]. Figure 2.1 gives a view of a 3D printer.

2.2   HISTORY OF 3D PRINTING

The idea of 3D printing was proposed in the 1970s, but the first tests were performed in 1981. Dr Kodama is credited with the first 3D printing attempts to establish a quick technique for prototyping. He was the first to define the concept of manufacturing layer by layer. That defined an ancestor for SLA (or stereolithography). Sadly, just before the deadline, he did not apply the patent criteria. Some years later, Alain Le Mehaute, Oliver de Witte and Jean Claude Andre, a French engineering team, were involved in SLA but were discarded in the absence of a market perspective. This attempt at 3D printing was also done by the stereolithography process. In 1984, Charles "Chuck" Hull was disappointed with his job as a tabletop and furniture producer when he had to create small and custom pieces for several years. Hull, a Bachelor of Engineered Physics undergraduate, worked for Ultra Violet Products in California to make plastics items from photopolymers. In 1986 Hull started his own company named 3D Systems in Valencia, California. In 1988, this company launched the first widely viable 3D printer, the SLA 250.6. Since then, several other companies, such as DTM Corporation, Z Corporation, Solid Scope and Object Geometries, have developed 3D printers for industrial applications. Hull's work, as well as that of other researchers, has revolutionised manufacturing and has been prepared to do the same in many other fields. In 1992, Stratasys obtained the patent for fused deposition modelling (FDM), in which many 3D printers were created. The major actors in the 3D-printing industry evolved from 1993 to 1999 through various methods: Z Corp and binder jetting which created the Z402 – these manufactured models use starch, plaster-centred pulver, a hydraulic liquid binder; Arcam MCP technology and selective laser melting (SLM) using inkjet printing technology used by MIT [6–8]. This technology also helped to revolutionise the production of prosthetics in the late 2000s. The Gartner Hype Cycle for new technologies in 2012 revealed that 3D printing was at the height of inflated expectations. In addition, Gartner indicated that 3D printing had a delay of five to ten years before its efficiency level would be achieved. But the cycle for 2013 has finalised its evaluation by splitting 3D printing into two categories: 3D corporate and 3D consumers [9]. When 3D printing has launched in full, it seems likely that the corporate world, as well as the manufacturing and domestic sectors, will, in other words, undergo a massive shake-up.

2.3   GENERAL PRINCIPLES

2.3.1   MODELLING

3D-printable models can be rendered by means of a CAD modelling kit or 3D scanner. The 3D-modelling approach is used to evaluate and collect information about the structure and appearance of an object. Based on these data, 3D versions of the scanned object can be produced.

2.3.2   PRINTING

A slicer program converts a 3D model into several thin layers. It creates an STL G file that transmits printer commands that involves processing before you print the STL 3D models. A variety of slicer open source programs are available, including Slic3r, KISSlicer and Cura. The G code is followed by the 3D printer, which produces varieties of model instructions by putting the liquid, powder or sheet material in successive layers [10].

2.3.3 Finishing

Although the resolution provided by the printer is enough, the print is a slightly over-dimensional version of many applications. This ordinary object resolution and material removal with more accuracy can be obtained by a higher resolution method.

2.4 TYPES OF 3D PRINTING

2.4.1 Digital Light Processing (DLP)

Digital light processing (DLP), also called a digital micromirror device (DMD), uses aluminium-based mirrors for reflecting the light to make pictures. It refers to the DLP chip. DLP is a 3D-printing procedure in which photopolymer resin is fixed using a projector. DLP technology is similar to the stereolithography (SLA) technique since it interacts through a 3D-printing system with photopolymers. The only difference in DLP is that a protected light is used instead of an ultraviolet laser for the cure of photopolymers. The items are formed in the same manner as SLA. It is taken out from the object so the resin creates space for the untreated part. Then layer-by-layer forming from the base of the container into the tank with a fix on top of the next layer happens. DLP was invented by Larry Hornbeck in 1987 [11]. DLP accepts analogue or digital signals and converts the picture into video, mostly used in cell phones and projectors. It uses a more conventional lamp, which is much simpler and more powerful than SLA and has a crystal show shape. It offers better surface finishing and is better than other methods [12,13]. Figures 2.2 and 2.3 represent a view of the working of DLP. Liquid plastic resin is used as we know in DLP printers. It is hardened and easier to operate than other forms of resin. Due to the high hardness, strength and chemical stability, ceramic materials are used in various industries. At a jerk speed, DLP prints highly compatible products [14,15]. The harder content is rendered easily and quickly by this sort of printer sheet. When one layer is done, it is moved and the next layer begins.

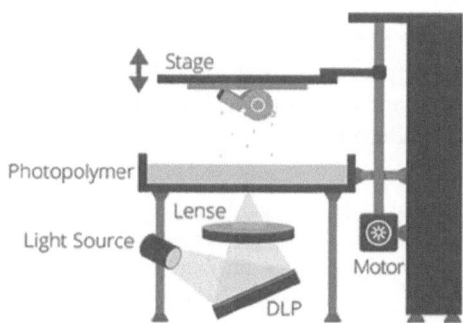

FIGURE 2.2   Digital light processing (DLP).

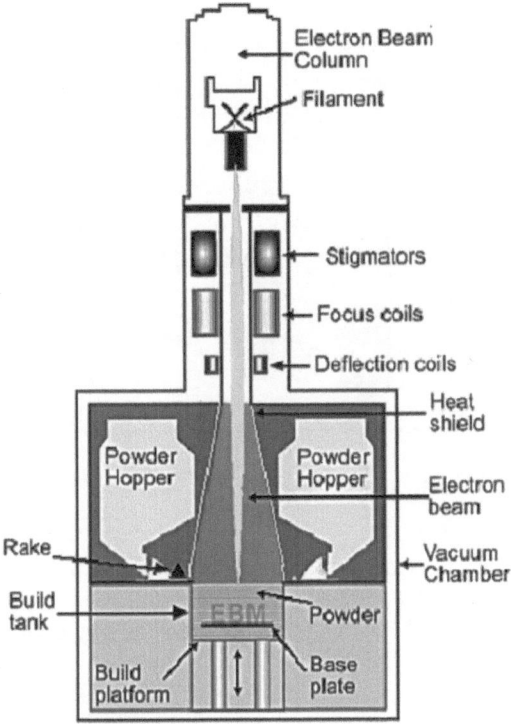

FIGURE 2.3 Electron beam melting (EBM).

2.4.2 ELECTRON BEAM MELTING (EBM)

Electron beam melting (EBM) is a 3D-printing technology that uses an electron beam to melt powder into pieces, using an electron beam to melt metal powder layers, and is an additive layer manufacturing process (ALM). Arcam AB Inc. invented it in 1997. It typically produces a number of alloys with high-density toughness and light weight, making the product economically robust [16]. CAD software is used in this process for the development of 3D models. The CAD.stl file format can be quickly trimmed to be used in an EBM printer. Figure 2.4 shows a schematic representation of the EBM process. This process is carried out using computer-controlled hoppers to disperse metal powder layer by layer. Due to the rising interest in this technology, the industry is making great efforts to make the EBM process more effective [17]. Due to its complicated parts, the EBM process replaces traditional processes such as casting and other processes with greater precision in a short time. Motorsports and medical prostheses are particularly important in the aerospace and defence fields. In this process, the most common materials are used, such as stainless steel, Ti-6Al-4V and Al-Si in powder form. Ti-6Al-4V has the form of a grid that provides greater strength and rigidity. It can render denser components than other traditional processes [18–20]. In comparison, the materials steel and Al-Si can bear

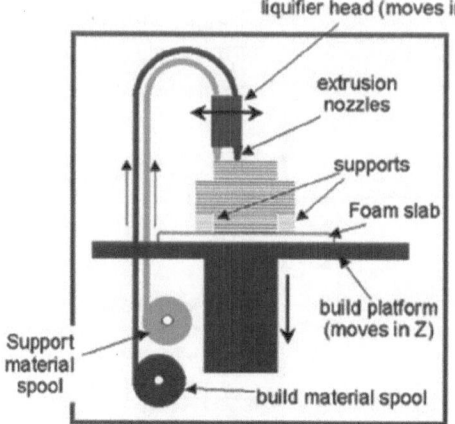

FIGURE 2.4   Fused deposition modelling (FDM).

high temperatures and provide an enhanced surface finish. The substance is highly ductile in this material shape. However, the mechanism is much more sluggish than selective laser melting (SLM). This is the key reason why companies are switching to other processes [21,22].

2.4.3   FUSED DEPOSITION MODELLING (FDM)

Fused deposition modelling (FDM), also called fused filament fabrication (FFF), is a material extrusion 3D printing technology. FDM 3D printers use thermoplastic as the material for components by layer technology. The FDM technique is widely used in the modern world. In 1989, Scott Crump and the Stratasys firm patented the FDM technology. It is a manufacturing process designed to produce high-quality products in a low processing time. In recent years several studies have demonstrated the progress made in this process [23–25]. For the production of end products directly free of the use of machinery instead of any other traditional manufacturing process, the FDM method is used. Figure 2.5 gives a representation of the FDM process. In industry, this technique has become popular for its high accuracy, ease of use and low processing time [26,27]. Parts of FDM modelling are done by CAD software where the file is saved to CAD software in STL file format. Then the file is converted into several slices, so the process works correctly. FDM works with a range of plastics, such as butadiene acrylonitrile (ABS), polylactic acid and polymers [28]. A printhead similar to an inkjet printer is used for an FDM printer. However, heated plastic beads are released as it moves from the printhead into layers rather than into ink. This process is repeated again and again so that the quantity of each deposit can be precisely controlled and shaped by each layer [29]. As the material is heated while extruded, it fuses or binds to the underlying layers. It can have enhanced features such as numerous printheads based on the scope and cost of an FDM printer.

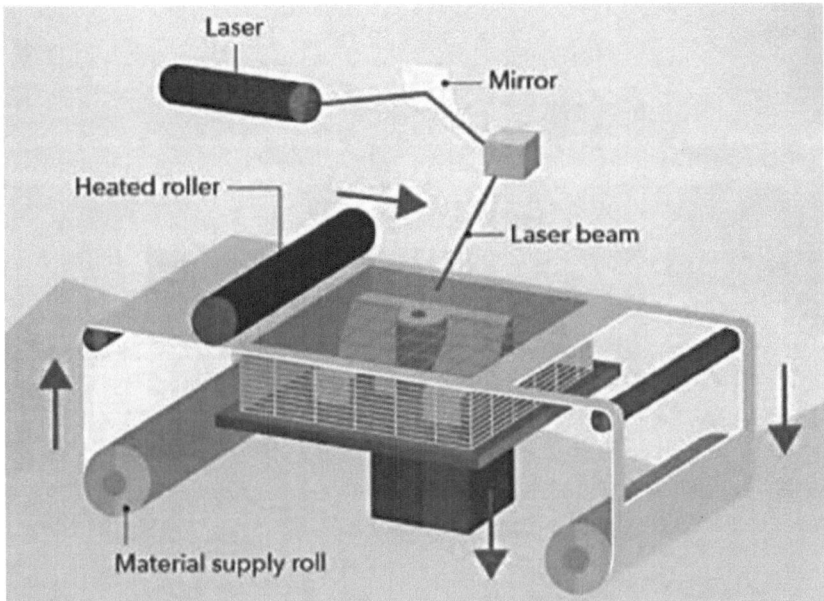

Laser

Mirror

Heated roller

Laser beam

Material supply roll

FIGURE 2.5 Selecting a process by materials.

2.4.4 Laminated Object Manufacturing (LOM)

Laminated object manufacturing (LOM) is a 3D-printing process, which produces products with heat and plastic or paper as a material by using the layering technique. Helisys of Torrance, CA, developed it in 1991. The method offers a large variety of design options for efficient rapid prototyping technology. This is a very efficient method of fast tooling and product design with high precision and low cost of processing [30–32]. It contains various steps. First, translate the CAD file into STL. LOM printers use a continuous adhesive-coated layer placed over a roller-heated substratum. It melts its adhesive on a heated roller that passes through the surface of the material. Then the laser traces the part size you want. The laser often crosses hatches in order to quickly remove any excess material following printing. The platform arrives at its origin when the layering process is completed [33]. A heat roller is used for easy and efficient production of the product. Like a chain loop layer by layer, the operation is repeated again and again. Excessive materials that can be chosen and used after cooling are quickly cut off [34]. These materials are highly resistant and can withstand high temperatures to achieve high surface finish and precision. Figure 2.6 shows a view of LOM.

2.4.5 Selective Laser Melting (SLM)

Selective laser melting (SLM) is a selective laser sintering (SLS) technology that involves high-density powdered material to manufacture products. The material can be totally melted into a solid 3D component. It was invented at the Fraunhofer

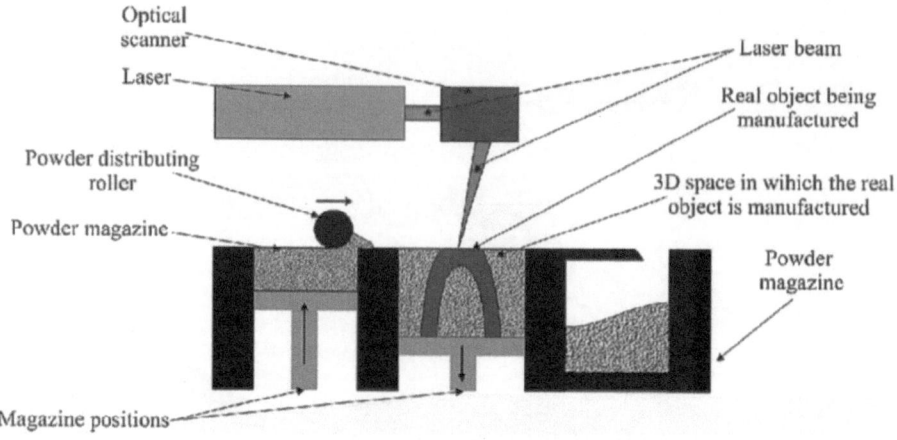

FIGURE 2.6 Laminated object manufacturing (LOM).

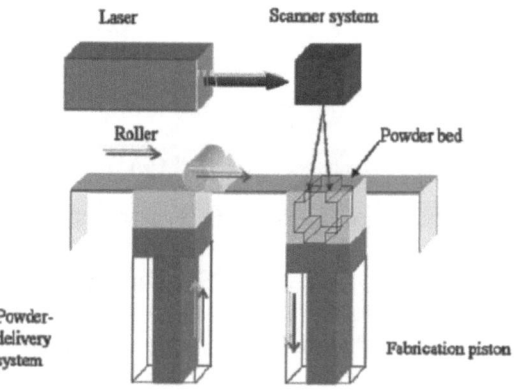

FIGURE 2.7 Selective laser melting (SLM).

Institute in 1995. It is powdered 3D printing, which works by using layer-by-layer technology via CAD file or computer-based software [35,36]. It can also produce the products in order to improve high precision and low processing time surface finish. It is close to other techniques of 3D printing since it also uses CAD tools to cut processes [37,38]. It uses STL file format for fast and accurate processing and replication of pieces. Figure 2.7 gives a view of the SLM process. The powdered metal is mounted on the workplace, where the laser is used to render the process solid by intensive light. Thermal expansion, stress generation and metal changes resulting from the high heating and cooling effects of materials such as Ti-6Al-4V, TA 15 alloy and copper alloy are associated with SLM [39]. These types of defects influence the mechanical and microstructural properties of the components. For their complexity and high precision, these parts can be used in the biomedical, aerospace, automotive and other industries.

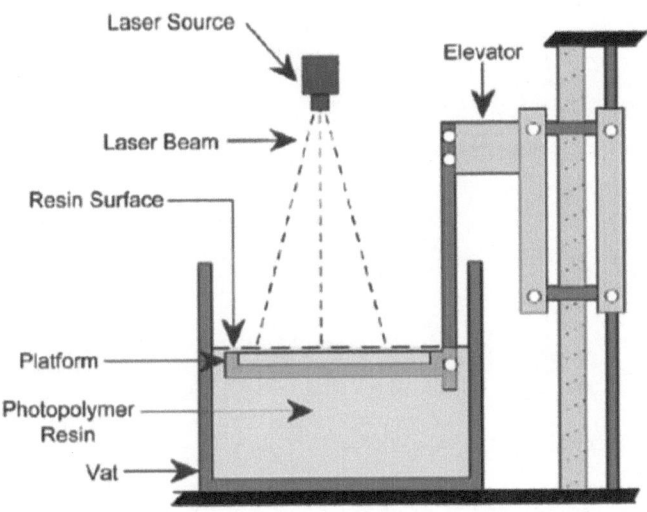

FIGURE 2.8   Selective laser sintering (SLS).

2.4.6   SELECTIVE LASER SINTERING (SLS)

For solid 3D models, SLS printing uses a laser. Carl Deckard and Joe Beaman coined this term in the 1980s. They later participated in the establishment of the Desktop Manufacturing Corporation (DTM). It was acquired by 3D Systems in 2001. This method is used to manufacture solid objects using metal powder with a high surface finish by layer-by-layer technique [40,41]. An SLS printer is used to print different products with powdered content. In the powder, a laser draws the object's outline and fuses them. The process is then set up with a new powder sheet, constructing each layer one by one to form the object. It is then repeated. Laser sintering for metal, plastic and ceramic objects may be used. The level of detail is restricted only by laser precision and powder fineness so that it is possible with this type of printer to construct extremely delicate and complex structures [42]. Figure 2.8 shows a view of the SLS technique. SLS technology uses many materials such as composites, stainless steel, thermoplastics and polymers. Because of its high mechanical working capacity, nylon is the best choice for SLS printing [43,44].

2.4.7   STEREOLITHOGRAPHY (SLA)

SLA is a methodology that renders projects as simple as possible. This is a very ancient procedure that has been used until now. Via rapid prototyping, SLA can transform models into a true 3D object. Charles Hull, the co-founder of 3D Systems Inc. in the 1980s, initially invented this technique. Figure 2.9 represents a view of the SLA technique [45,46]. SLA printed parts with excellent surface finish but depending on the consistency of the printer. It is used to manufacture complex parts with low processing time and cost. In the majority of printers, the object must be processed by

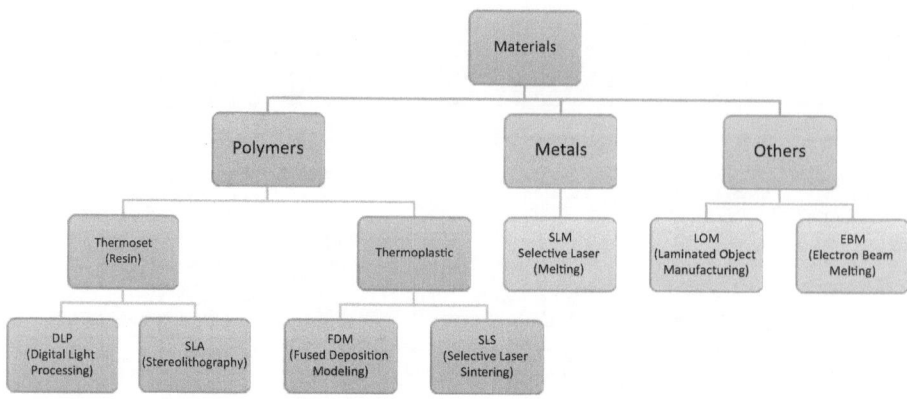

FIGURE 2.9   Stereolithography (SLA).

a CAD register [47,48]. This includes data on an entity's dimension. The CAD file includes a special format for further processing to be transferred to a printer. PPF, thermoset polymers and polylactide materials are used in SLA [49].

2.5   MATERIALS

A complete description of the most core material is designed to prove the tremendous potential of 3D printing, beginning with powdered, sintered metals used in traditional manufacturing, such as casting, injection moulding and carbon fibre. 3D-printing materials include steel, bronze, copper, gold, nickel alloy, aluminium and titanium. These metals are particularly suitable for the production of prototypes, gemstones and other products. 3D-printing materials are typically available in the form of filaments, powders or resins (according to the 3D methods used). Polymers and metals are the two primary classes while others also exist (for example, ceramics or mixtures). Further separating thermoplastics and thermosets into polymers can be accomplished. The 3D-printing method is very simple, as only a few technologies make parts out of some materials. Acrylonitrile butadiene styrene (ABS) has been the most widely used thermoplastic polymer since the start of 3D printing. Figure 2.2 shows the selection process by materials [50]. The material is very durable, very flexible and easy to extrude and is suitable for 3D printing. It requires less extruder force than using another 3D filament, polylactic acid (PLA).

2.6   APPLICATIONS IN DIFFERENT FIELDS

1. **Field of Education:** Nowadays, schools and their curricula use 3D printing a lot. Benefits of 3D printing for education are that they help students to create prototypes without the need for expensive materials in a short time. Students design and build models they can bring with them. In colleges, it is used to create assignments or work projects for students. Students can easily make low-cost complex models with a specific strength.

2. **Mechanical Field:** 3D printing was the first invention for rapid prototyping and processing. It takes hundreds of thousands of dollars to inject a traditional prototype, and it takes several weeks to produce a single mould. AM is a key asset in mechanical design. It offers enhanced power, long service life and a strong mechanical surface finish. Mechanical 3D printing makes it possible to create a batch of traditionally designed components.

3. **Field of Architecture:** All construction methods (such as cement wax, cement plastic and polymers) are also printed. Sintered powder can also be used to obtain a strong surface finish and high-strength models are used in industry and elsewhere [51]. The benefits of such systems include increased complexity and detailed design, lower labour costs, better functional performance and less waste.

4. **Medical Field:** In recent years there have been various 3D printing innovations available in the medical sector. These include bioprinting of tissue-like biomaterials and structures that replicate their natural counterparts with medical devices such as prosthetics. 3D-printing technology allows complex and highly flexible parts to be used in orthopaedic implants easily [52]. 3D printing may be grouped into many broad categories of current medical use: tissue and organ manufacture; prosthetic development, implants and anatomical models; and pharmaceutical investigation into the discovery, distribution and dosing of pharmaceuticals [53]. An analysis of these medical applications is offered as follows. One of the most important ways in which 3D printing affects health is the manufacturing of medical equipment. 3D methods of printing have a wide range of options for manufacturers of medical devices that have been rapidly adopted in this industry [54]. The US Food and Drug Administration (FDA) hosted a workshop in 2014 seeking input on the use of AM in the medical field.

2.6.1 BIOPRINTING TISSUES AND ORGANS

Present organ insufficiency treatment mostly relies on bone marrow transplants from living or dead donors. Age, condition, injury and birth defects caused by tissue or organ failure are severe medical concerns. But there is a persistent lack availability of human organs for transplantation, while inkjet, laser-based or extrusion-based 3D-bioprinting technology is most popular. Several print heads can be used for depositing the various cells (organs, blood cells, muscle cells) [55].

2.6.2 CUSTOMISED IMPLANTS AND PROSTHESES

The conversion of X-rays, MRI or CT scans into digital STL 3D print files will render implants or prostheses in virtually all conceivable geometries. Thus, in the medical industry, 3D printing has been successfully used, often within 24 hours, to manufacture regular and complex, personalised prostheses, arms and surgical implants. Dental, spinal and hip implants have been manufactured using this method [56]. In the 3D printing of prostheses and implants, there have been several other industrial and clinical achievements.

2.6.3 ANATOMICAL MODELS FOR SURGICAL PREPARATION

The variability and complexity of the human body are very suitable for surgical planning using 3D-printed models. It is better to rely solely on MRI or CT scans, which are unlearnable because they are visualising in 2D on a flat screen, if the patient's model of anatomy is tangible to the doctor in order to investigate or simulate a procedure [57]. Using 3D-printed models trained in surgery is also more difficult than training on cadavers, because cadavers are difficult to provide and expensive. Cadavers also lack the required pathology, so that they provide less of a lesson in anatomy than a surgical patient illustration.

2.6.4 IMPROVING MEDICAL EDUCATION

3D models are created in that way as they can increase the efficiency for rapid learning. This learning can be encouraged by improving the understanding, management and trust of the trainees significantly, irrespective of their area of expertise. The benefits of 3D printing in the education sector are reproducibility and safety of its printed model. The rapid prototyping products produced by 3D printing make this technique very popular these days. It can print with different techniques having various densities that can be used for defining anatomical details.

2.6.5 CUSTOMISED 3D-PRINTED DOSAGE

3D-printing technology is already used and promises to be transformative in pharmaceutical research and manufacturing. 3D-printing benefits include accurate droplet size and dose monitoring, re-productiveness and ability to manufacture dosage forms with complex pharmaceutical releasing profiles. The use of 3D printing to make it easier and more feasible could also standardise the complex drug manufacturing processes. In the advancement of personalised medicine, 3D-printing technology may also be very significant.

2.7 CONCLUSION

3D-printing technology has become ever more universal in recent decades. The development of usable structures of multi-materials was happening from time to time. 3D printing is becoming more useful in a variety of fields like medicine, education, construction and many others. The dependency of the manufacturers on 3D-printing techniques is more than other conventional methods. In this study, we have described the history and general principles in the introductory section. In the following part we defined the materials, types and various applications of 3D printing with the help of a literature review. Thus, we have been able to write this review paper of 3D printing.

REFERENCES

1. Pryor, S. (2014). Implementing a 3D printing service in an academic library. *Journal of Library Administration*, 54(1), 1–10.

2. Yang, F., Zhang, M., & Bhandari, B. (2017). Recent development in 3D food printing. *Critical Reviews in Food Science and Nutrition*, 57(14), 3145–3153.

3. Javaid, M., & Haleem, A. (2018). Additive manufacturing applications in medical cases: A literature-based review. *Alexandria Journal of Medicine*, 54(4), 411–422.

4. McCausland, T. (2020). 3D printing's time to shine. *Research-Technology Management*, 63(5), 62–65.

5. Tay, Y. W. D., Panda, B., Paul, S. C., Noor Mohamed, N. A., Tan, M. J., & Leong, K. F. (2017). 3D printing trends in building and construction industry: a review. *Virtual and Physical Prototyping*, 12(3), 261–276.

6. Garmulewicz, A., Holweg, M., Veldhuis, H., & Yang, A. (2018). Disruptive technology as an enabler of the circular economy: What potential does 3D printing hold? *California Management Review*, 60(3), 112–132.

7. Attaran, M. (2017). The rise of 3-D printing: The advantages of additive manufacturing over traditional manufacturing. *Business Horizons*, 60(5), 677–688.

8. Gross, B. C., Erkal, J. L., Lockwood, S. Y., Chen, C., & Spence, D. M. (2014). Evaluation of 3D printing and its potential impact on biotechnology and the chemical sciences. *Analytical Chemistry*, 86(7), 3240–3253.

9. Prince, J. D. (2014). 3D printing: an industrial revolution. *Journal of Electronic Resources in Medical Libraries*, 11(1), 39–45.

10. Gokhare, V. G., Raut, D. N., & Shinde, D. K. (2017). A review paper on 3D-Printing aspects and various processes used in the 3D-Printing. *International Journal of Engineering Research & Technology*, 6, 953–958.

11. Hong, H., Seo, Y. B., Lee, J. S., Lee, Y. J., Lee, H., Ajiteru, O., ... & Park, C. H. (2020). Digital light processing 3D printed silk fibroin hydrogel for cartilage tissue engineering. *Biomaterials*, 232, 119679.

12. Dean, D., Wallace, J., Siblani, A., Wang, M. O., Kim, K., Mikos, A. G., & Fisher, J. P. (2012). Continuous digital light processing (cDLP): Highly accurate additive manufacturing of tissue engineered bone scaffolds: This paper highlights the main issues regarding the application of Continuous Digital Light Processing (cDLP) for the production of highly accurate PPF scaffolds with layers as thin as 60 µm for bone tissue engineering. *Virtual and Physical Prototyping*, 7(1), 13–24.

13. He, R., Liu, W., Wu, Z., An, D., Huang, M., Wu, H., ... & Xie, Z. (2018). Fabrication of complex-shaped zirconia ceramic parts via a DLP-stereolithography-based 3D printing method. *Ceramics International*, 44(3), 3412–3416.

14. Liu, Z., Liang, H., Shi, T., Xie, D., Chen, R., Han, X., ... & Tian, Z. (2019). Additive manufacturing of hydroxyapatite bone scaffolds via digital light processing and in vitro compatibility. *Ceramics International*, 45(8), 11079–11086.

15. Zeng, Y., Yan, Y., Yan, H., Liu, C., Li, P., Dong, P., ... & Chen, J. (2018). 3D printing of hydroxyapatite scaffolds with good mechanical and biocompatible properties by digital light processing. *Journal of Materials Science*, 53(9), 6291–6301.

16. Zäh, M. F., & Lutzmann, S. (2010). Modelling and simulation of electron beam melting. *Production Engineering*, 4(1), 15–23.

17. Galati, M., & Iuliano, L. (2018). A literature review of powder-based electron beam melting focusing on numerical simulations. *Additive Manufacturing*, 19, 1–20.

18. Lunetto, V., Galati, M., Settineri, L., & Iuliano, L. (2020). Unit process energy consumption analysis and models for Electron Beam Melting (EBM): Effects of process and part designs. *Additive Manufacturing*, 33, 101115.

19. Wong, H., Neary, D., Jones, E., Fox, P., & Sutcliffe, C. (2019). Benchmarking spatial resolution in electronic imaging for potential in-situ Electron Beam Melting monitoring. *Additive Manufacturing*, 29, 100829.

20. Del Guercio, G., Galati, M., Saboori, A., Fino, P., & Iuliano, L. (2020). Microstructure and mechanical performance of Ti–6Al–4V lattice structures manufactured via Electron beam melting (EBM): A review. *Acta Metallurgica Sinica (English Letters)*, 33(2), 183–203.
21. Karlsson, J., Snis, A., Engqvist, H., & Lausmaa, J. (2013). Characterization and comparison of materials produced by Electron Beam Melting (EBM) of two different Ti–6Al–4V powder fractions. *Journal of Materials Processing Technology*, 213(12), 2109–2118.
22. Parthasarathy, J., Starly, B., Raman, S., & Christensen, A. (2010). Mechanical evaluation of porous titanium (Ti6Al4V) structures with electron beam melting (EBM). *Journal of the Mechanical Behavior of Biomedical Materials*, 3(3), 249–259.
23. Tyberg, J., & Bøhn, J. H. (1999). FDM systems and local adaptive slicing. *Materials & Design*, 20(2–3), 77–82.
24. Dhinakaran, V., Kumar, K. M., Ram, P. B., Ravichandran, M., & Vinayagamoorthy, M. (2020). A review on recent advancements in fused deposition modeling. *Materials Today: Proceedings*, 27, 752–756.
25. Boparai, K. S., & Singh, R. (2017). Advances in fused deposition modeling. *Reference Module in Materials Science and Materials Engineering*. doi: 10.1016/B978-0-12-803581-8.04166-7
26. Vyavahare, S., Teraiya, S., Panghal, D., & Kumar, S. (2020). Fused deposition modelling: A review. *Rapid Prototyping Journal*, 26, 176–201.
27. Jain, P., & Kuthe, A. M. (2013). Feasibility study of manufacturing using rapid prototyping: FDM approach. *Procedia Engineering*, 63, 4–11.
28. Pramanik, D., Mandal, A., & Kuar, A. S. (2020). An experimental investigation on improvement of surface roughness of ABS on fused deposition modelling process. *Materials Today: Proceedings*, 26, 860–863.
29. Croccolo, D., De Agostinis, M., & Olmi, G. (2013). Experimental characterization and analytical modelling of the mechanical behaviour of fused deposition processed parts made of ABS-M30. *Computational Materials Science*, 79, 506–518.
30. Mueller, B., & Kochan, D. (1999). Laminated object manufacturing for rapid tooling and patternmaking in foundry industry. *Computers in Industry*, 39(1), 47–53.
31. Yi, S., Liu, F., Zhang, J., & Xiong, S. (2004). Study of the key technologies of LOM for functional metal parts. *Journal of Materials Processing Technology*, 150(1–2), 175–181.
32. Wang, W., Conley, J. G., & Stoll, H. W. (1999). Rapid tooling for sand casting using laminated object manufacturing process. *Rapid Prototyping Journal*, 5(3), 134–140.
33. Pang, A., Joneja, A., Lam, D. C., & Yuen, M. (2001). A CAD/CAM system for process planning and optimization in LOM (Laminated Object Manufacturing). *IIE Transactions*, 33(4), 345–355.
34. Liao, Y. S., Li, H. C., & Chiu, Y. Y. (2006). Study of laminated object manufacturing with separately applied heating and pressing. *The International Journal of Advanced Manufacturing Technology*, 27(7–8), 703–707.
35. Kempen, K., Thijs, L., Van Humbeeck, J., & Kruth, J. P. (2012). Mechanical properties of AlSi10Mg produced by selective laser melting. *Physics Procedia*, 39, 439–446.
36. Prashanth, K. G., Scudino, S., Klauss, H. J., Surreddi, K. B., Löber, L., Wang, Z., ... & Eckert, J. (2014). Microstructure and mechanical properties of Al–12Si produced by selective laser melting: Effect of heat treatment. *Materials Science and Engineering: A*, 590, 153–160.
37. Song, B., Zhao, X., Li, S., Han, C., Wei, Q., Wen, S., ... & Shi, Y. (2015). Differences in microstructure and properties between selective laser melting and traditional manufacturing for fabrication of metal parts: A review. *Frontiers of Mechanical Engineering*, 10(2), 111–125.

38. Zhang, B., Li, Y., & Bai, Q. (2017). Defect formation mechanisms in selective laser melting: A review. *Chinese Journal of Mechanical Engineering*, 30(3), 515–527.
39. Yakout, M., Elbestawi, M. A., & Veldhuis, S. C. (2020). A study of the relationship between thermal expansion and residual stresses in selective laser melting of Ti-6Al-4V. *Journal of Manufacturing Processes*, 52, 181–192.
40. Ganeriwala, R., & Zohdi, T. I. (2014). Multiphysics modeling and simulation of selective laser sintering manufacturing processes. *Procedia Cirp*, 14, 299–304.
41. Mercelis, P., & Kruth, J. P. (2006). Residual stresses in selective laser sintering and selective laser melting. *Rapid Prototyping Journal*, 12(5), 254–265.
42. Hoy, M. B. (2013). 3D printing: Making things at the library. *Medical Reference Services Quarterly*, 32(1), 93–99.
43. Paul, R., & Anand, S. (2012). Process energy analysis and optimization in selective laser sintering. *Journal of Manufacturing Systems*, 31(4), 429–437.
44. Yuan, S., Strobbe, D., Li, X., Kruth, J. P., Van Puyvelde, P., & Van der Bruggen, B. (2020). 3D printed chemically and mechanically robust membrane by selective laser sintering for separation of oil/water and immiscible organic mixtures. *Chemical Engineering Journal*, 385, 123816.
45. Manapat, J. Z., Chen, Q., Ye, P., & Advincula, R. C. (2017). 3D printing of polymer nanocomposites via stereolithography. *Macromolecular Materials and Engineering*, 302(9), 1600553.
46. Phillips, B. T., Allder, J., Bolan, G., Nagle, R. S., Redington, A., Hellebrekers, T., ... & Licht, S. (2020). Additive manufacturing aboard a moving vessel at sea using passively stabilized stereolithography (SLA) 3D printing. *Additive Manufacturing*, 31, 100969.
47. Bugeda, G., Cervera, M., Lombera, G., & Onate, E. (1995). Numerical analysis of stereolithography processes using the finite element method. *Rapid Prototyping Journal*, 1(2), 13–23.
48. Kim, K., Yeatts, A., Dean, D., & Fisher, J. P. (2010). Stereolithographic bone scaffold design parameters: osteogenic differentiation and signal expression. *Tissue Engineering Part B: Reviews*, 16(5), 523–539.
49. Kim, K., Dean, D., Wallace, J., Breithaupt, R., Mikos, A. G., & Fisher, J. P. (2011). The influence of stereolithographic scaffold architecture and composition on osteogenic signal expression with rat bone marrow stromal cells. *Biomaterials*, 32(15), 3750–3763.
50. Berman, B. (2012). 3-D printing: The new industrial revolution. *Business Horizons*, 55(2), 155–162.
51. Xia, M., & Sanjayan, J. (2016). Method of formulating geopolymer for 3D printing for construction applications. *Materials & Design*, 110, 382–390.
52. Martelli, N., Serrano, C., van den Brink, H., Pineau, J., Prognon, P., Borget, I., & El Batti, S. (2016). Advantages and disadvantages of 3-dimensional printing in surgery: A systematic review. *Surgery*, 159(6), 1485–1500.
53. Cox, S. C., Thornby, J. A., Gibbons, G. J., Williams, M. A., & Mallick, K. K. (2015). 3D printing of porous hydroxyapatite scaffolds intended for use in bone tissue engineering applications. *Materials Science and Engineering: C*, 47, 237–247.
54. Hurst, E. J. (2016). 3D printing in healthcare: Emerging applications. *Journal of Hospital Librarianship*, 16(3), 255–267.
55. Cui, X., Boland, T., D'Lima, D. D., & Lotz, M. K. (2012). Thermal inkjet printing in tissue engineering and regenerative medicine. *Recent Patents on Drug Delivery & Formulation*, 6(2), 149–155.
56. Ozbolat, I. T., & Yu, Y. (2013). Bioprinting toward organ fabrication: Challenges and future trends. *IEEE Transactions on Biomedical Engineering*, 60(3), 691–699.
57. Banks, J. (2013). Adding value in additive manufacturing: researchers in the United Kingdom and Europe look to 3D printing for customization. *IEEE Pulse*, 4(6), 22–26.

3 3D Printing Technology
An Overview

Raman Kumar
Guru Nanak Dev Engineering College, Ludhiana, India

Harpreet Kaur Channi
Chandigarh University, Gharuan, India

CONTENTS

3.1 INTRODUCTION

3D printing is a way of constructing three-dimensional tangible structures from a digital file and is the main part of 'additive manufacturing' (AM). Additive methods play a significant role in the generation of 3D-printed items. Additive refers to the consecutive addition of thin layers to produce an entity between 16 and 180 microns or more. 3D-printing methods make a layer-by-layer object and create complex shapes. An item is generated in an additive process by identifying successive layers of a matter before the object is constructed. Each layer can be interpreted as a smooth cross-section of the material. 3D printing, for example using a milling machine, is the reverse of subtractive production that cuts out/hollows out a piece of metal or plastic (Shahrubudin, Lee, & Ramlan, 2019). 3D printing makes it possible to create complicated forms with less material than conventional processing methods (Diegel, Singamneni, Huang, & Gibson, 2010a; Diegel, Singh, Singamneni, & Withell, 2010b).

A 3D computer model that can be generated from a series of 3D software applications is a starting point for any 3D printing technique. The CAD 3D region can be opened or scanned using a 3D printer for faster cost-effective programs for designers and customers. The layout is 'sliced' into layers, and the template is transformed into a file for 3D printer scanning. Based on the setup and the technique, the content handling of the 3D printer is then laid down. As noted, a range of 3D technology styles processes diverse materials to create the finished product in several ways. Usable plastics, metals, ceramics and sand are commonly used in industrial prototyping and automotive applications. Analysis of biomaterials for 3D printing and various kinds of food is also being performed (Macy, 2015; Pârvu & Gilbert, 2014). In general, fabrics at the entry point of the market are, therefore, even more stringent. The most popular material used is plastic, usually ABS or PLA, although various alternatives, including nylon, are increasing. There are also a growing variety of accessories, such as sugar and chocolate, adapted for cooking.

Each of the many types of 3D printers uses a different technology that deals with various materials. It is necessary to be mindful that one of the most fundamental drawbacks of 3D printing is the lack of a single approach to materials and applications. Some 3D printers use a specified lightening/thermal supply to convert powdered materials into sine/fuse/powder layers (nylon, plastics, ceramics, metal). Some goods use a light laser to stabilise the resin again in ultra-thin layers. An alternative method of 3D printing is to cast fine droplets in a reminder of 2D inkjet printing but with enhanced tinting and a binder for repairing layers. The proposal is probably the most extensive scale to see the type, and this is the form in many 3D input stage printers. This device extrudes plastics, usually PLA or ABS, into layers through a heated extruder and generates a pre-established filament form. Since parts can be printed directly, substantial and complex objects can be made, even with built-in features that refuse assembly needs (Chaidas, Kitsakis, Kechagias, & Maropoulos, 2016; Tyler, Gullotti, Mangraviti, Utsuki, & Brem, 2016).

But another key point is that no 3D-printing approaches are yet available as plug-and-play applications. Some steps and others are often missed as the part is taken off the printer before clicking. In addition to the fact that the 3D design realities can be overwhelming, especially for components that require complex support through the build process; file preparation and conversion can also be time-consuming and complicated. But there are constant corrections and technological updates for these tasks, and the condition varies. Moreover, these parts must be completed before the printer has been removed. Help removal is apparent for processes that need assistance. Others include sanding, lacquering, or other conventional finishing touches, typically done by hand, requiring expertise and/or time and stamina (Banga, Belokar, Kalra, & Kumar, 2018).

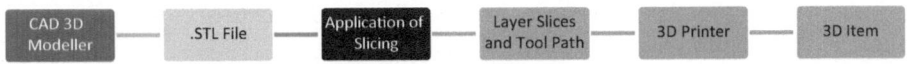

FIGURE 3.1   3D printing steps (Hager, Golonka, & Putanowicz, 2016; Sakin & Kiroglu, 2017).

The steps usually followed for 3D printing are shown in Figure 3.1. There are three main steps in 3D printing. The first step is to schedule the item you want to print when you plan a 3D format, right before printing. It is also possible to build this 3D file using a 3D scanner using CAD software or it can be easily imported from an online shop. You can move to the second level after your 3D file has been reviewed for printing. The actual printing process is the second step. First, pick which material satisfies the specific characteristics necessary for your product. The variety of materials used in 3D printing is wide. All related products include plastics, ceramics, resins, crystals, rocks, cloth, biomaterials and fruit bottles. Some of these products also have several finishing methods that allow you to create the exact outcome you have in mind. Some, including glazing, are still manufactured and not readily available in 3D-printing materials. Phase three is the completion process. Specialised skills and materials are needed for this level. It can also not be used or shipped immediately after the item is first printed before it has been sanded, lacquered or decorated to be completed as expected. The device's selected content will determine the most appropriate printing methods (Liu, Fan, Lu, & Yang, 2014; Van Herpen, 2014).

3.2   3D-PRINTING MATERIALS

Since the production of 3D printers has been going on for a long time, many compounds are also offered, such as powder, ink, pellets, granules, resin, etc. Individual products are also typically built with material properties more specifically adaptable to speciality platforms' applications to conduct dedicated applications, such as dentistry. Instead, this essay will look at the more common forms of material in a more general way (Banga et al., 2018). And some of the textiles are also distinct.

3.2.1   PLASTICS

The synthetic technique typically utilises nylon or polyamide in polish or the fused deposition modelling (FDM) process in the filament form. It is a practical, versatile and enduring, solid plastic material for 3D printing. By default, it is white so that it can be coloured before or after printing. This material can also be combined with powdered aluminium to create another popular 3D-sintering material: aluminide (in powder format) (Sandhu et al., 2020). ABS is also a popular 3D-printing plastic and is commonly used on filament format input stage FDM 3D printers. It is a very versatile plastic with some colours. ABS is sold from a range of non-proprietary sources in filament form, which is another factor in its success (Singh et al., 2020).

For this reason, PLA is a biologically degradable, 3D-printing plastic filament. It is also suitable for DLP/SL resin and FDM filament format applications. It is sold in various colours and as transparent, and is suitable for a wide range of 3D printers. It is not as durable or flexible as ABS. Lay wood, however, is a specially made 3D printing medium for 3D input stage printers. The wood/polymer composite filament shape is also referred to as WPC (Busch et al., 2014).

3.2.2 METALS

For industrial 3D printing, there is a more excellent range of metals and metal composites. In a type of powder, stainless steel for sinter/melt/EBM processes is one of the best and most commonly used metals for 3D printing. The two most popular are aluminium and cobalt-related products. Usually, silver, gold or bronze or other materials may be shielded. A variety of metal materials have been directly 3D-printed with a wide range of gold and silver applications in the jewellery market in the last few years. Titanium is one of the hardest metal materials used for commercial 3D printing. All the products are of extremely solid and powder-like quality. It can be added in powder form to sinter/melt/EBM processes (Gibson et al., 2018).

3.2.3 CERAMICS

Ceramics is a comparatively recent category of products with varying degrees of success that can be used for 3D printing. For these components, the specific thing to remember is that the ceramic parts must experience the same processes after printing as any ceramic component produced using conventional manufacturing methods, including firing and varnishing (Chen et al., 2019).

3.2.4 PAPER

The necessary copying paper A4 is a 3D medium supplied with Mcor Technologies' patented SDL technology. The company has a business model that varies marginally from other 3D printers, whereby the equipment's capital cost is in the middle of the line. Still, the priority is on a cost-efficient, readily available source of local buyable content. 3D paper-printed models are safe, eco-friendly, easy to use and require no post-processing.

3.2.5 BIOMATERIALS

There have been substantial studies on the biomaterial promise of 3D printing for various medical uses and others. Several leading laboratories are researching live tissue to develop applications, including printing human organs for transplants and external tissue for body parts. Additional research in this field concentrates on processing food products with the best beef example (Guvendiren, Molde, Soares, & Kohn, 2016).

3.2.6 FOOD

3D food-printing tests with extruders have significantly improved in recent years. The most popular form is chocolate. There are also sugar printers and tests with pasta and beef. Work is ongoing to render finely balanced whole meals using 3D-printing techniques (Sun, Zhou, Huang, Fuh, & Hong, 2015).

3.2.7 OTHER

Stratasys is only one company with a single offer with its digital materials for Objet Connex 3D-printing applications (proprietary). This allows the mix of traditional Objet 3D printing materials in different and complex print processes to form new materials with the requisite characteristics. By integrating current primary materials in various ways up to 140 other digital materials can be achieved.

Below are listed the most common techniques used for each material category.

3.3 TECHNOLOGY FOR PLASTIC OR ALUMIDE

3.3.1 FUSED DEPOSITION MODELLING (FDM) TECHNOLOGY

This is currently the most common printing technique, due to the number of printers on the market. Compared to other 3D-print technology, FDM is an inexpensive 3D-printing procedure. This technique works by the melting and extrusion of materials by printing a cross-section of each object's layer by a 3D nozzle. The sheet is reduced with every new layer and repeats this step until the item is finished. The layer thickness determines the output of the 3D print. Some FDM 3D printers have two or more printer heads for multicolour printing and can accommodate overhangs in dynamic three-dimensional print areas, as shown in Figure 3.2 (Lu et al., 2021; Shi, Chen, Tuo, Gong, & Guo, 2021).

3.3.2 SELECTIVE LASER SINTERING (SLS) TECHNOLOGY

Laser sintering is a 3D printing method involving constructing an object by melting various powder levels to create an item. Most importantly, the technique makes it possible to build dynamic and interlocking shapes. Plastic and alumide are available for this. The working of SLS technology is shown in Figure 3.3. SLS has several comparisons to stereolithography. However, SLS uses powdered material placed in a vat. On top of the previous layer, a sheet of powdered material with a roller for each layer is set. A laser sintering is then performed in conjunction with a specific pattern to shape the object to be manufactured. Interestingly, it is possible to use the

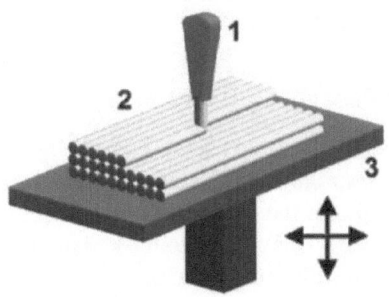

FIGURE 3.2 FDM technology.

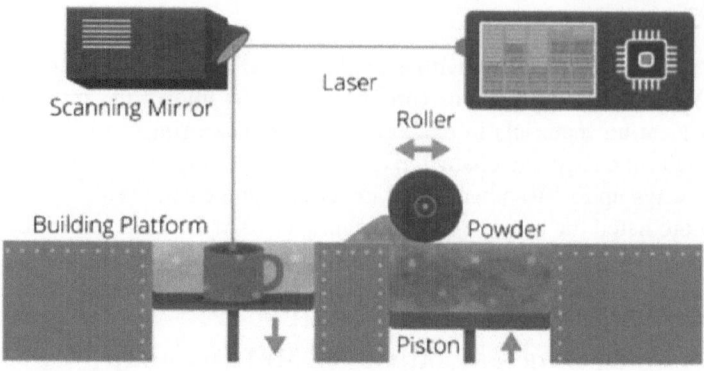

FIGURE 3.3 SLS technology (3D, 2020).

powders' non-sintered component to provide a support structure, and this substance can be recycled until the object is formed for reuse (Yu et al., 2017).

3.4 TECHNOLOGY FOR RESIN OR WAX

The technology needed is photopolymerisation, a technique for solidifying UV-light-sensitive resin. It is used in various 3D-printing systems.

3.4.1 STEREOLITHOGRAPHY (SLA)

Stereolithography (SLA) is used in a resin bowl. The plate is reduced, and the liquid polymer is illuminated, where the UV laser draws the cross-section layer by layer. Until a model is produced, this process is replicated. This film is printed in 3D using the material removed from the resin (underneath), making room for the unformed resin at the bottom of the container to shape the next board. Another way is to print the object in 3D by adding it to the next layer of the tank. The stereolithography uses fluid plastic and layer one as the base medium and turns this fluid into a 3D layer. Fluid resin with a clear rim is mounted on a vat. A UV laser traces a fluid resin pattern from the tube's base to heal and consolidate a resin coating. A lifting platform continually draws up the solidified building, as the laser creates a new prototype for each sheet to create the ideal 3D object shape (Kim et al., 2016). A representation of stereolithography is shown in Figure 3.4.

3.4.2 DIGITAL LIGHT PROCESSING (DLP)

DLP 3D is more like a stereo print that uses a separate light source and a stereo monitor. This technology utilises regular light sources and controls the light micro pieces to monitor the emitted light on the surface of the subject that is being printed. The fluid glass display panel works like a photomask. This method causes an immense amount of light to shine onto the cured surface, quickly hardening the resin. It is a projector used for the treatment of resin in photopolymers. The same is true of the SLA technique except that the photopolymer resin is shielded by a light bulb rather

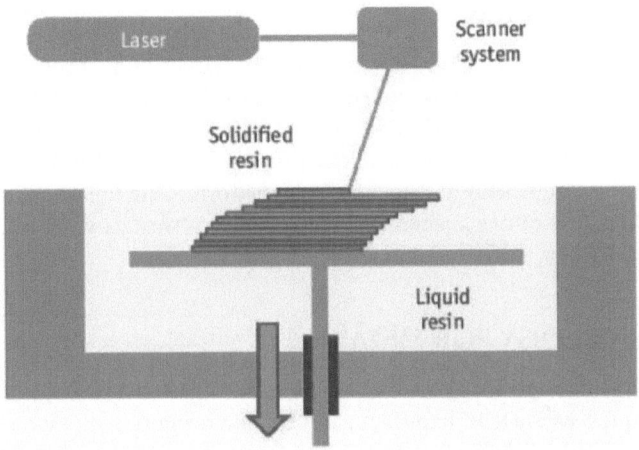

FIGURE 3.4   Representation of stereolithography (Kim et al., 2016).

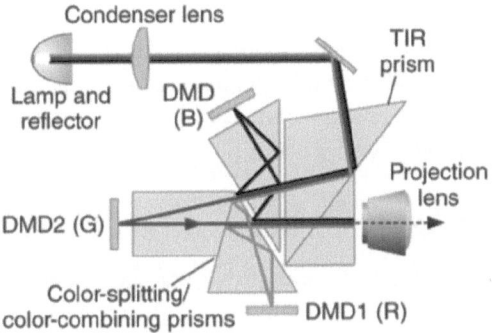

FIGURE 3.5   Digital light processing (Clouds, 2020).

than by a UV laser. Similar to SLA, the substance is created by separating the resin's material, allowing a way for uncured resin on the lower side, making the next layer or returning it to the tank by treating the next layer on the top. In silver and brass 3D printing, Sculpteo uses DLP technology. First, print the wax model in 3D and then use the lost-wax casting method: around the wax, the mould is formed, and the object is molten and filled with silver (Li et al., 2021; Vivero-Lopez et al., 2021). The working of DLP is shown in Figure 3.5.

3.4.3   CONTINUOUS LIQUID INTERFACE PRODUCTION (CLIP)

This operates by projecting a continuous UV image series onto an oxygen-permeable UV transparent window under a fluid resin bath provided by a digital light projection system. A dead-zone region overlying the window preserves the liquid interface under the component. The resin tank is pulled out of the area of care over the dead area (Taki, 2020).

3.4.4   MULTIJET PRINTERS

UV light for high-quality PolyJet and MultiJet 3D-printing processes is used to crossline a photopolymer. It is considered equivalent to stereolithography. A jet printer sprays mini-droplets of photopolymers instead of lasers to cure layers as the first sheet (similar to ink in an inkjet printer). Using UV light, the polymer is attached to the printer head and locks the layer form. The construction foundation cuts with a thickness of one sheet and directly deposits the last layer with fresh material (Brunton, Arikan, & Urban, 2015).

3.5   TECHNOLOGY FOR METAL

In conjunction with the lost-wax casting method, DLP enables the 3D printing of objects. Sculpteo uses DLP manufacturing for 3D printers with silver and brass. A 3D wax print can also be impressed. The technique is known as lost-wax casting which then emerges from it. A paced plate forms around the wax when silver. Direct metal laser sintering (DMLS) uses a laser as a source of power to track a cross-section of material by layer to synthesise metal powder with a laser. Laser sintering direct metal is the same as partial laser sintering. The electron beam is used as a power source employing electron beam melting (EBM) instead of laser in 3D printing. A powder beam of metal in a high vacuum is molten layer by layer and will fully melt the metal powder. This process creates high-density metal components while maintaining material properties.

3.6   MULTICOLOUR

In the making of the detailed 3D prints with colour, binder jetting is common. To disperse a coat of powder onto the building platform, an automatic roller is used. Excess powder must be placed on the sides so that the bed is covered with a compressed powder sheet. The print heads apply a liquid binder to the quick axis to paint the object on the power simultaneously. The lamination of selective deposition is a paper-based 3D press. This method is close to the rapid prototyping procedure for laminated objects (LOM). This technique requires layers of plastic glue (or plastic or metal foil) to be continuously glued onto a heated rolling position, layer by layer of paint into a laser cutter. Each sheet of fresh material is pushed onto a roller, and the process proceeds to the end of the piece. The most sophisticated PolyJet 3D printing method is triple-jetting technology (PolyJet) used in the Stratasys Objet 500 Connex3. With three materials, this technique conducts precise printing and hence makes three-colour mixing possible. It would help if you referred to PolyJet & Multijet to know more about this technology.

3.7   CONCLUDING REMARKS

As 3D printing changes, the number of innovations and processes is increasing slowly. 3D printing continues to develop its hardware, fabrics and methods for artefacts and components. The required 3D-printing process and the right material should be chosen based on various variables such as budget, design or function. Various articles which were historically created only by mass manufacturing may be produced using 3D printing. Because of the cost, time and expertise involved with the printing and finishing processes, Sculpteo is useful as an online 3D-printing business. This challenge may discourage people from using this remarkable technology, but at Sculpteo we use our expertise to help people who can print 3D and simplify additive technology.

REFERENCES

3D (2020). *Selective Laser Sintering (SLS)*. https://formlabs.com/asia/blog/what-is-selective-laser-sintering

Banga, H. K., Belokar, R. M., Kalra, P., & Kumar, R. (2018). Fabrication and stress analysis of ankle foot orthosis with additive manufacturing. *Rapid Prototyping Journal, 24*(2), 301–312. doi:10.1108/RPJ-08-2016-0125

Brunton, A., Arikan, C. A., & Urban, P. (2015). Pushing the limits of 3D color printing: Error diffusion with translucent materials. *ACM Transactions on Graphics, 35*(1). doi:10.1145/2832905

Busch, S., Weidenbach, M., Fey, M., Schäfer, F., Probst, T., & Koch, M. (2014). Optical properties of 3D printable plastics in the THz regime and their application for 3D printed THz optics. *Journal of Infrared, Millimeter, Terahertz Waves, 35*(12), 993–997.

Chaidas, D., Kitsakis, K., Kechagias, J., & Maropoulos, S. (2016). *The impact of temperature changing on surface roughness of FFF process*. Paper presented at the *20th Innovative Manufacturing Engineering and Energy Conference, IManEE*.

Chen, Z., Li, Z., Li, J., Liu, C., Lao, C., Fu, Y., ... He, Y. (2019). 3D printing of ceramics: A review. *Journal of the European Ceramic Society, 39*(4), 661–687.

Diegel, O., Singamneni, S., Huang, B., & Gibson, I. (2010a). *The future of electronic products: Conductive 3D printing?* Paper presented at the *4th International Conference on Advanced Research in Virtual and Physical Prototyping, VRAP*, Leiria.

Diegel, O., Singh, D. P. K., Singamneni, S., & Withell, A. (2010b). *'3D faxing': Rapid prototyping of new product and process systems to help manage multi-national development teams*. Paper presented at the *4th International Conference on Advanced Research in Virtual and Physical Prototyping, VRAP*, Leiria.

Gibson, M. A., Mykulowycz, N. M., Shim, J., Fontana, R., Schmitt, P., Roberts, A., ... Bordeenithikasem, P. (2018). 3D printing metals like thermoplastics: Fused filament fabrication of metallic glasses. *Materials Today, 21*(7), 697–702.

Guvendiren, M., Molde, J., Soares, R. M., & Kohn, J. (2016). Designing biomaterials for 3D printing. *ACS Biomaterials Science Engineering, 2*(10), 1679–1693.

Hager, I., Golonka, A., & Putanowicz, R. (2016). 3D printing of buildings and building components as the future of sustainable construction? *Procedia Engineering, 151*, 292–299.

Kadry, H., Wadnap, S., Xu, C., & Ahsan, F., (2019). Digital light processing (DLP) 3D-printing technology and photoreactive polymers in fabrication of modified-release tablets. *European Journal of Pharmaceutical Sciences, 135*, 60–67.

Kim, G. B., Lee, S., Kim, H., Yang, D. H., Kim, Y.-H., Kyung, Y. S., ... Ha, H. (2016). Three-dimensional printing: Basic principles and applications in medicine and radiology. *Korean Journal of Radiology, 17*(2), 182–197.

Li, L., Zheng, Y., Yang, K., Su, X., Wang, Y., Chen, X., ... Li, B. (2021). Modified three-wavelength phase unwrapping algorithm for dynamic three-dimensional shape measurement. *Optics Communications, 480*. doi:10.1016/j.optcom.2020.126409

Liu, J., Fan, Y., Lu, Q., & Yang, Y. (2014). Design of extendable Tool Path Generation software for 3D printing. Paper presented at the *4th International Conference on Manipulation, Manufacturing and Measurement on the Nanoscale, 3M-NANO 2014*, Taipei, Taiwan.

Lu, D. Z., Mei, Z., Li, X. L., Wang, C. P., Sun, X., Wang, X. W., & Wang, J. W. (2021). Digital design and effect evaluation of three-dimensional printing scoliosis orthosis. *Chinese Journal of Tissue Engineering Research*, *25*(9), 1329–1334. doi:10.3969/j. issn.2095-4344.3758

Macy, B. (2015). Reverse engineering for additive manufacturing. In A. Nee (ed.), *Handbook of Manufacturing Engineering and Technology* (pp. 2485–2504): Springer, London. doi:10.1007/978-1-4471-4670-4_41

Pârvu, O., & Gilbert, D. (2014). Automatic validation of computational models using pseudo-3D spatio-temporal model checking. *BMC Systems Biology*, 1–24. doi:10.1186/s12918-014-0124-0

Sakin, M., & Kiroglu, Y. C. (2017). 3D printing of buildings: Construction of the sustainable houses of the future by BIM. *Energy Procedia*, *134*, 702–711. doi:10.1016/j.egypro.2017.09.562

Sandhu, K., Singh, G., Singh, S., Kumar, R., Prakash, C., Ramakrishna, S., ... Pruncu, C. I. (2020). Surface characteristics of machined polystyrene with 3D printed thermoplastic tool. *Materials*, *13*(12), 2729.

Shahrubudin, N., Lee, T. C., & Ramlan, R. (2019). An overview on 3D printing technology: technological, materials, and applications. *Procedia Manufacturing*, *35*, 1286–1296.

Shi, X., Chen, B., Tuo, X., Gong, Y., & Guo, J. (2021). Study on performance characteristics of fused deposition modeling 3D-printed composites by blending and lamination. *Journal of Applied Polymer Science*, *138*(9). doi:10.1002/app.49926

Singh, G., Singh, S., Prakash, C., Kumar, R., Kumar, R., & Ramakrishna, S. J. P. C. (2020). Characterization of three-dimensional printed thermal-stimulus polylactic acid-hydroxyapatite-based shape memory scaffolds. *Polymer Composites*, *41*(9), 3871–3891. doi:10.1002/pc.25683

Sun, J., Zhou, W., Huang, D., Fuh, J. Y., & Hong, G. S. (2015). An overview of 3D printing technologies for food fabrication. *Food Bioprocess Technology*, *8*(8), 1605–1615.

Taki, K. (2020). A simplified 2D numerical simulation of photopolymerization kinetics and oxygen diffusion-reaction for the continuous liquid interface production (CLIP) system. *Polymers*, *12*(4). doi:10.3390/POLYM12040875

Tyler, B., Gullotti, D., Mangraviti, A., Utsuki, T., & Brem, H. (2016). Polylactic acid (PLA) controlled delivery carriers for biomedical applications. *Advanced Drug Delivery Reviews*, *107*, 163–175. doi:10.1016/j.addr.2016.06.018

Van Herpen, I. (2014). Fabrics: The next step in 3D printing? *WSA*, *20*(7), 10–13.

Vivero-Lopez, M., Xu, X., Muras, A., Otero, A., Concheiro, A., Gaisford, S., ... Goyanes, A. (2021). Anti-biofilm multi drug-loaded 3D printed hearing aids. *Materials Science and Engineering C*, *119*. doi:10.1016/j.msec.2020.111606

Yu, Y., Guo, Y., Jiang, T., Li, J., Jiang, K., & Zhang, H. (2017). Study on the ingredient proportions and after-treatment of laser sintering walnut shell composites. *Materials*, *10*(12). doi:10.3390/ma10121381

4 Use of Additive Manufacturing in Surgical Tools/Guides for Dental Implants

Himanshu Deswal
Dental Officer, ECHS, Polyclinic Sonipat, Haryana, India

Anoop Kapoor
Sri Sukhmani Dental College and Hospital, Dera Bassi (Punjab), India

Komal Sehgal and Vishakha Grover
Dr. H.S.J. Institute of dental sciences, Panjab University Chandigarh, Chandigarh, India

CONTENTS

4.1   ADDITIVE MANUFACTURING (AM)

Additive manufacturing is an emanate field of science that comprises three-dimensional (3D) printing and related technologies for the fabrication of the product via digital images and layer-wise addition of the material. Brown (2015) of the American Society for Testing and Materials (ASTM) defines 'Additive manufacturing is the process of

DOI: 10.1201/9781003301066-4

41

joining materials to make objects from 3D model data, usually layer upon layer, as opposed to subtractive manufacturing methodologies' (Noort 2012). The technique is a consequence of the blending of three diverse areas i.e. materials, creativity and technology together to transform into a new era for the manufacturing process (Brown 2015). The cardinal position of this innovation is that the digitally obtained 3D image is practically composed of individual sections or slices and in the same sequence, these geometrical images are collected from different layers and printed via an attached printed device for the production of the desired outcome. The technique is uniquely versatile in terms of producing objects of diverse design geometry, complexity and shape (Jain et al. 2016, Dawood et al. 2015, Liu et al. 2006).

4.1.1 General Aspects

It emerged as a technique to create models or prototype parts in the field of engineering as rapid prototyping. It is aimed at reducing the labour intensiveness of the process for product development and lowering the cost and time taken. The probability of creating highly complex 3D shapes and designs enabled the use of AM in many fields for application (Ashley 1991, Noorani 2006, Flowers and Moniz 2002, Chua et al. 1998).

Three technologies, i.e. computer numerical control (CNC), computer-aided design (CAD), and computer-aided manufacturing (CAM) working in close coordination have brought in the concept of rapid manufacturing (Noorani 2006, Cooper 2001, Kruth 1991, Wong and Herndez (2012). Charles Hull, an engineer is known as the pioneer in contemporary 3D printing technologies, developed the concept that surface hardening of layers of liquid material to form a 3D shape by using a source of energy such as ultraviolet (UV) light. He came up with this idea while he was working on UV lamps to cure resins. The technology was patented first by Hull in 1986 under the name stereolithography (SL) (See and Meindorfer 2016). This was possibly the first technique that appeared for 3D printing and has been most widely implemented, so much so that in today's world this word is used interchangeably for rapid prototyping. The initial process in which a standard tessellation language (STL) file is created from the CAD software model data, for evaluation of information carried out in each layer as a piece. The basic process is the creation of an STL file for AM process which was evolved by 3D Systems Inc. in 1987.

AM process equipment determines the thickness of the layer and the design features such as the resolution of the product and photo-polymerisation mediates the polymerisation reaction for constructing a polymer from monomeric units (Liu et al. 2006, Cooper 2001, Kruth 1991). Microstereolithography is competent for evolving a higher resolution product, with the thickness of a layer being less than 10 μm and is the better version of the basic technique (Halloran et al. 2011). The process of usage of diverse forms of materials for printing a single product has been termed multiple material stereolithography (Wong and Herndez 2012).

The Society of Manufacturing Engineers in 2004 classified various technologies like stereolithography (SL), laminated object manufacturing (LOM), fused deposition modelling (FDM), selective laser sintering (SLS), 3D printing (3DP) on the basis of criteria identifying processes into solid, liquid and powder-based (Kruth 1991). But the incessant search for better equipment and material, four additional technologies, i.e. prometal, laminated engineered net shaping (LENS), electron beam melting (EBM), and PolyJet were considered in 2012 (Wong and Herndez 2012, Bhushan and Grover 2019).

Nowadays, many treatment options in medicine and dentistry, particularly involving restorative solutions for missing or damaged body parts depend on 3 D planning of the treatment (Bhushan and Grover 2019, Banga et al. 2014, 2017a, 2017b, 2018, 2020a, 2020b, 2020c, 2020d, 2020e, 2021).

A timeline of significant events in the history of additive manufacturing leading to contemporary times, adapted from Wohlers and Gornet (2014) has been given Figure 4.1.

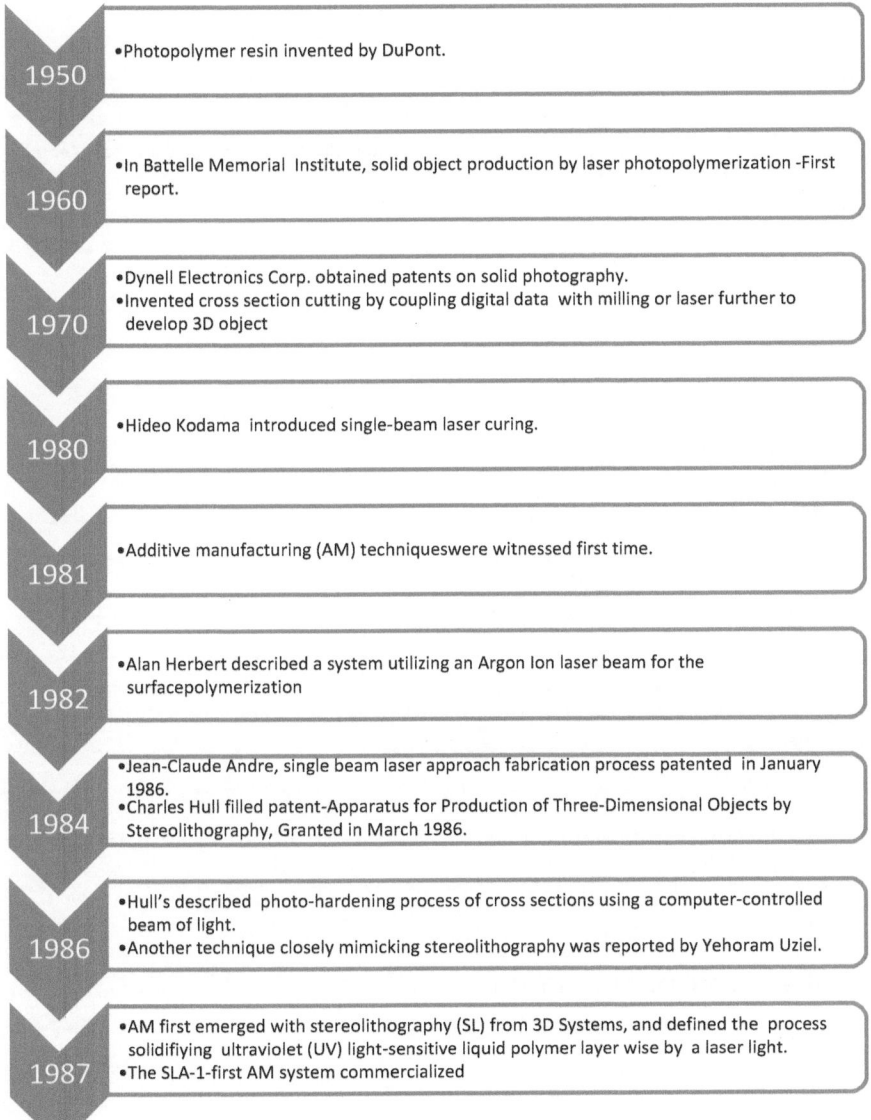

FIGURE 4.1   Timeline

(Continued)

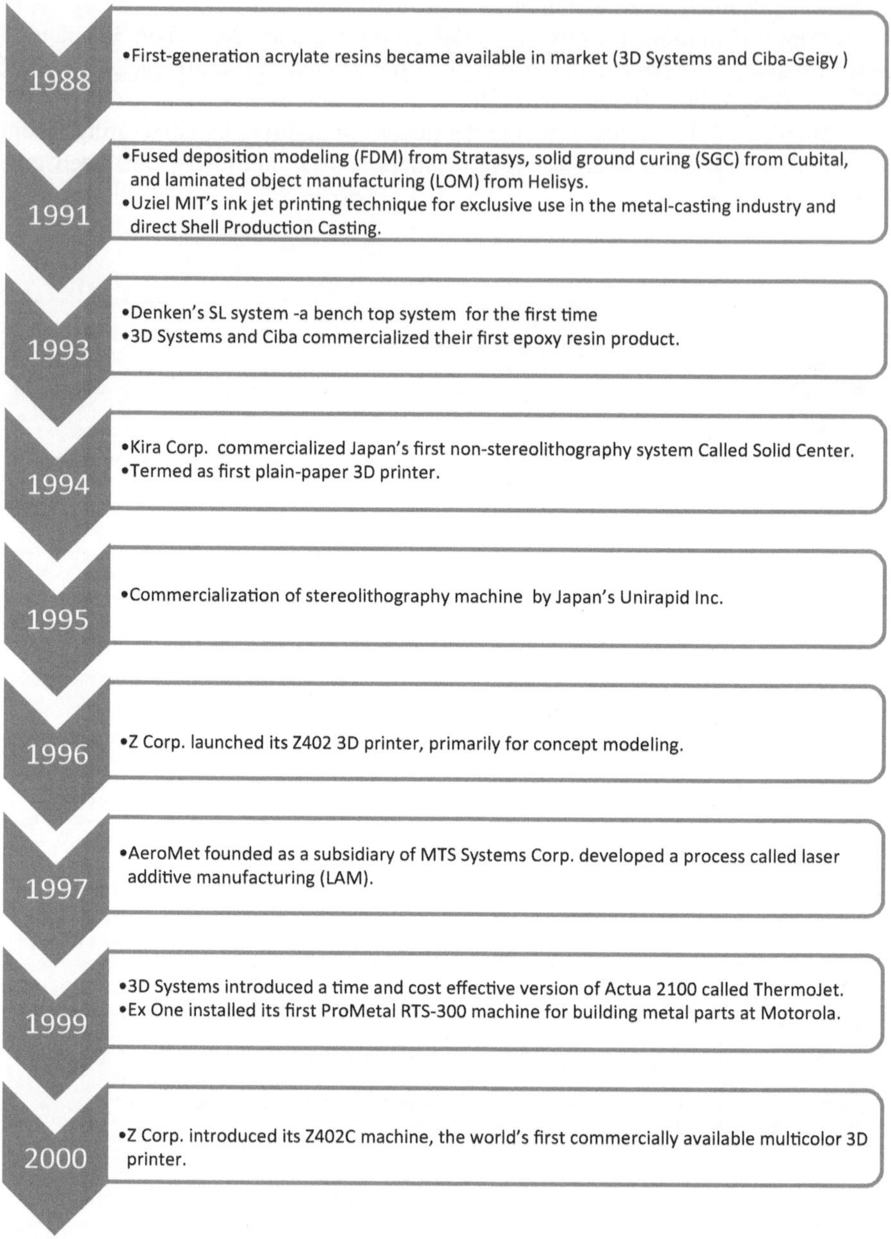

1988
- First-generation acrylate resins became available in market (3D Systems and Ciba-Geigy)

1991
- Fused deposition modeling (FDM) from Stratasys, solid ground curing (SGC) from Cubital, and laminated object manufacturing (LOM) from Helisys.
- Uziel MIT's ink jet printing technique for exclusive use in the metal-casting industry and direct Shell Production Casting.

1993
- Denken's SL system -a bench top system for the first time
- 3D Systems and Ciba commercialized their first epoxy resin product.

1994
- Kira Corp. commercialized Japan's first non-stereolithography system Called Solid Center.
- Termed as first plain-paper 3D printer.

1995
- Commercialization of stereolithography machine by Japan's Unirapid Inc.

1996
- Z Corp. launched its Z402 3D printer, primarily for concept modeling.

1997
- AeroMet founded as a subsidiary of MTS Systems Corp. developed a process called laser additive manufacturing (LAM).

1999
- 3D Systems introduced a time and cost effective version of Actua 2100 called ThermoJet.
- Ex One installed its first ProMetal RTS-300 machine for building metal parts at Motorola.

2000
- Z Corp. introduced its Z402C machine, the world's first commercially available multicolor 3D printer.

FIGURE 4.1 (CONTINUED)   Timeline

(*Continued*)

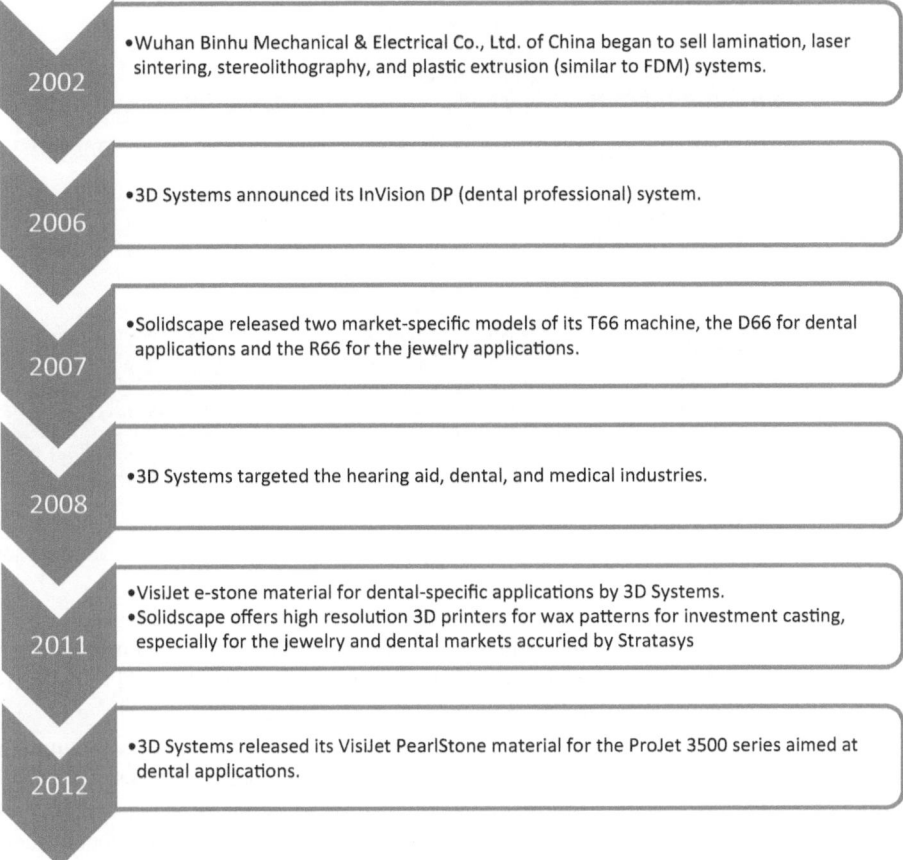

2002 • Wuhan Binhu Mechanical & Electrical Co., Ltd. of China began to sell lamination, laser sintering, stereolithography, and plastic extrusion (similar to FDM) systems.

2006 • 3D Systems announced its InVision DP (dental professional) system.

2007 • Solidscape released two market-specific models of its T66 machine, the D66 for dental applications and the R66 for the jewelry applications.

2008 • 3D Systems targeted the hearing aid, dental, and medical industries.

2011 • VisiJet e-stone material for dental-specific applications by 3D Systems.
• Solidscape offers high resolution 3D printers for wax patterns for investment casting, especially for the jewelry and dental markets accuried by Stratasys

2012 • 3D Systems released its VisiJet PearlStone material for the ProJet 3500 series aimed at dental applications.

FIGURE 4.1 (CONTINUED)   Timeline.

4.2 CLINICAL APPLICATIONS IN ORAL HEALTHCARE

3D printing and digital technology have remarkably enhanced the accuracy and quality of dental prosthesis, restorations and predictability in implantology while using customised surgical templates, etc. In oral surgery, pre-treatment planning by fabricating surgical templates has significantly increased the probability of unintentional damage to the adjoining vital structures.

The technique helped provide educational models of oral tissues and structures such as bone and jaw, so as to physically demonstrate any specific clinical therapeutic procedures as needed to the students for learning purposes (Lal et al. 2006). 3D printing can print biological tissues like bone which can act as a lattice-like structure for the entry of bone-forming cells i.e. osteoblasts for regeneration of bone. 3D alginate peptide hybrid scaffolds can be used for the same purpose. These types of scaffolds are documented to bestow appropriate and a consistent conducive local milieu for the growth and differentiation of the stem cells (Zhou et al. 2014). Calcium sulphate ($CaSO_4$) and calcium phosphate (CaP) based composite scaffolds are printed

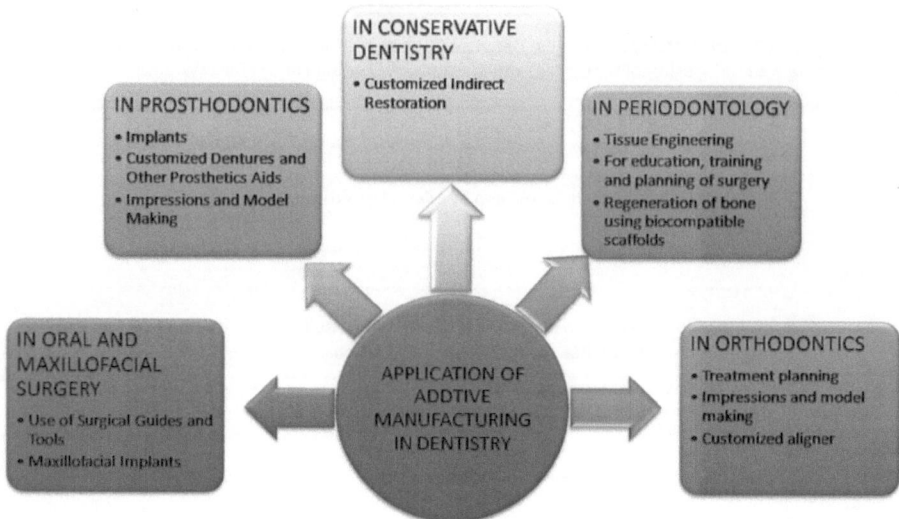

FIGURE 4.2   Applications of AM in the several fields of dentistry.

with AM and used for bone augmentation (Sykes et al. 2004). Such scaffolds have shown promising results by improving the treatment outcomes when used to regenerate the disease destroyed periodontal tissues (Figure 4.2).

Maximum dental lab work is also now digitalised by amalgamating oral scanning, CAD/CAM designing, and 3Dprinting. Contemporary restorative works from endodontics as well as prosthodontics, like bridges, crowns, stone models, and several appliances of orthodontic, are being prepared by these innovative techniques. Furthermore, these AM techniques have enabled the fabrication of the maxillofacial prosthesis with or without functional integration, which depends on the clinical situation of the patient for replacing the damaged, missing or lost part from the face and oral cavity. With the help of 3D printers, maxillofacial reconstruction is done with ease like obturators are being prepared for the reconstruction of the cleft palates and the replacement of lost part of the orbital floor, maxilla, zygoma, mandible due to trauma may surely reduce morbidity and disability associated for such patients and enhance their life quality. Figure 4.1 shows the several fields of dentistry in which AM has been used (Bhushan and Grover 2019).

4.3   EVOLUTION OF GUIDED DENTAL IMPLANT SURGERY

Dental implants have become a standard of care therapy in the field of oral rehabilitation of patients who have partial or complete loss of teeth. It is an alloplastic material or device that is surgically placed into the oral tissues beneath the mucosal or periosteal layer or within the bone for restoration of functional, therapeutic, or aesthetic purposes (Thakral et al. 2014). Implants as a restorative technique have evolved immensely in terms of continuous improvements and innovations in implant materials, surface modifications, surgical techniques and approaches. The very first evidence of implant placement has been reported, a long time back in AD 600 in the

Mayan population where implanted fragments of mandible to replace three lower incisors were found. Pierre Fauchard and John Hunter (eighteenth century) were the pioneer surgeons credited with the transplantation of the teeth of one human to another. The era of modern implant dentistry was ushered in with the introduction of 'titanium implants' in the 1950s, when Per-Ingvar Brånemark, a Swedish professor of anatomy, happen to discover the basic concept of osseointegration while studying bone vascularity in rabbit bone. The direct bone titanium contact allowed the load transfer on the bone tissue and later proved as the foundation of the science of contemporary implantology. Per-Ingvar Brånemark was recognised as the 'father of modern dental implantology'. He identified and reported that titanium is a very strong and non-corrosive metal which resulted in an irreversible attachment to the bone tissue when it was implanted into it. In 1965, he used the first titanium dental implant in a human volunteer, a Swedish individual named Gosta Larsson (Abraham 2014).

In the 1980s and around, in the early years of modern implantology, the concept of implant placement was introduced based on the residual bone available in the area to be restored. Over a period of time, various studies reported that implants placed with this approach usually appeared malpositioned in a lingual or facial location, and refuted the long term successful functioning of restored dentition either compromising the aesthetic concerns or the functional status owing to overload of occlusal forces (Kopp et al. 2003). Such implants which were not appropriately planned and positioned keeping in view, the biomechanical and aesthetic factors ended up with major discrepancies in implant survival and success. This led to the development of the novel concept of contemporary implant science as 'prosthesis-driven implantology', wherein the final functional prosthesis is central for the planning and placement of implant (Kalra et al. 2013).

Even with the new concept, freehand implant surgeries very frequently lead to improper position or angulations in the implant surgical procedures, particularly in the case of young and inexperienced implant surgeons. There arose the need for a method, tool or technique for being precise in implant placements, which was realised by the introduction of implant surgical guides. Initially, surgical guides were prepared on the master cast of the patient made by gypsum (Becker and Kaiser 2000, Almog et al. 2001). These kinds of surgical templates could help to some extent regarding the prosthetic guidance, but could not assess the anatomy of the underlying bone (Amet and Ganz 1997). It was also found that the hard surface of the gypsum master cast may not precisely duplicate the soft tissue morphology also, so this method was not graded as a quality method as considered essential for implant treatment planning purposes (Kalra et al. 2013).

Further, modified guides were developed in which a metal sphere was incorporated along with the positioned guide tubes at model wax-up time and conventional radiographs were taken for the patient. Magnification factor could be calculated with ease and these guides enabled the estimated measurement of the dimension and depth of implant, when the dimension of the metal sphere was known. With the help of such templates, it was feasible to know the direction and the position of the implant at the outset, but the precision of placement was confined to the first drill only. The issue of precise direction, orientation and position of implant within the bone housing was yet not resolved.

4.4 CLASSIFICATION AND TYPES OF IMPLANT SURGICAL GUIDES

Surgical templates used to help obtain the proper surgical placement and angulations of dental implants to ensure precise positioning are known as implant surgical guides (GPT 2005). The main objective of a surgical template is to ensure the precise placement of the implant by positioning the implant drill according to the planned treatment and help guide the surgical removal of bone to place the implant in the best possible position. Conventional radiographic or computer image-guided surgical templates based on preoperatively collected individual patient records are widely used in clinical practice to place the implants into planned positions precisely (Ramasamy et al. 2013).

The proper implant placement is very important to prevent the vital structure from damage, provide a favourable prosthesis and also ensure the long-term success of the result (Le and Nielsen 2015). Consequently, several surgical template techniques have been evolved for the placement of dental implants into the desired position (Le and Nielsen 2015, D'Souza and Aras 2012, Greenberg 2015, Kola et al. 2015). A complete limiting surgical template is the most precise technique (D'Souza and Aras 2012, Greenberg 2015, Kola et al. 2015).

Balshi and Garver (1987) illustrated various types of surgical templates. Three basic surgical templates were used for the placement of implants:

1. The fully edentulous.
2. The partially edentulous.
3. Partially edentulous tooth-supported design.

This classification makes use of the status of the dentition of the patient as the prime parameter. A fully edentulous surgical stent is further divided into a general guide and a specific guide. The general guide is provided to the area of placement of the dental implant while specific guide is provided to the location and angulations of each dental implant requiring placement. A general guide stent is a replica of the transitional denture.

Stumpel in 2008 described a different classification. He used a conceptual approach to illustrate three different types of surgical templates.

1. Non-limiting surgical template – is the one that demonstrates to the dentist where the prosthesis will go in regard to the implant site. It will rely on the surgeon to determine the parameter in relation to the angulations and precise positioning of the implant.
2. Partially limiting design – is the one where some sort of guidance is available that directs only the first drill which is to be used for implant site preparation, whereas the rest of the preparation will be done by the surgeon.
3. Completely limiting design – is the one that will limit instrumentation freehand by the surgeon. Drilling for implant site preparation is guided in mesiodistal and buccolingual planes, and depth is also guided in accordance with the final position of the implant along with the prosthetic components.

(Salem 2019)

As the surgical guides were evolved to be more and more restrictive and precise in terms of guidance, the decision-making and surgical execution of the procedure became more controlled, safe and subject to less error at the operator's end. The two most popular designs used in this context are: cast-based guided surgical template and computer-assisted design and manufacturing (CAD/CAM) based surgical guide (D'Souza and Aras 2012, Vercruyssen et al. 2014).

4.5   CAST-BASED IMPLANT SURGICAL GUIDE

This technique uses clinical examination including transgingival probing and the use of periapical radiograph to assess the underlying bone topography mostly in cases of implant surgeries without reflecting flap along with using an analogue for implant position (Stumpel 2008). Basically, the data regarding the root structures and underlying bone is obtained from the digital conversion of a periapical radiograph and the recorded bone sounding measurements dictate the orientation of the implant drill. A cast-based osteotomy is performed, further, a laboratory analogue along with the guide sleeve based on the implant diameter to be used is placed and an implant surgical guide template is created on the patient's cast (D'Souza and Aras 2012).

4.6   CAD/CAM-BASED IMPLANT SURGICAL GUIDE

In this technique, computerised tomographic scan-based data is used to construct surgical guide. First of all, computed tomography (CT) images are converted into information amenable to be analysed by CT software, which transfers the treatment plan to the surgical site (Marchack 2007, Nikzad and Azari 2008). The virtual views of the volume of bone, morphology, and density are visualised on the computer screen. This helps in the presurgical assessment of any impending risk factors such as reduced bone support compromise bone structure or any vital structures in the vicinity. Keeping in view, all these factors the prosthetic planning using the scanner graphic template is done (Holst et al. 2007); and further, these data can be imported to the laboratories for milling or AM process as may be applied for the construction of the implant surgical guide (Spector 2008).

4.7   DESIGN AND DEVELOPMENT OF CONTEMPORARY IMPLANT SURGICAL GUIDES

Radiographic imaging of the selected implant site was vital for planning the surgical placement of the implant. In fact, it has a pivotal role in the progress of the development of diagnostic implant surgical guides. The success and survival of implants are routinely assessed by the radiographic examination of the peri-implant tissues. In intraoral periapical radiography, the radiographic technique of choice is the paralleling cone technique with projections at right angles to the tangent of the arcuate alignment of the teeth in the areas of interest. Information concerning the mesiodistal dimensions of the region in which implants are considered is evaluated to estimate the potentially available bone so that decisions regarding bone augmentation procedures that are to be performed are taken. But this view is limited to providing details of only two or three teeth, not more than that. However, for treatment planning for implant especially in areas adjacent to the inferior alveolar nerve and maxillary sinus, a wider view is necessary. Panoramic radiography which provides a holistic picture of the maxillofacial structures is preferred to obtain a complete overview of both jaws together on an X-ray. Still, there were some drawbacks of panoramic radiography like unpredictable distortion, low level of reproducibility, and magnification in both vertical and horizontal directions (1.1–1.7 times). It misses out the information about the third dimension i.e. buccolingual or cross-sectional and the alveolar ridge inclines. There can be high chances of errors in angular dimensions and mesiodistal distance due to improper seating of the patient and/or varied jaw curvatures in different individuals. Thick focal trough, blurred images owing to an intensifying screen, etc. are the common concerns associated with the use of this technique. Generally speaking, panoramic radiographs provide inferior images, but still are considered as useful as may be combined with other tools for the assessment to shell out better information. However, they have not been advocated for primary imaging tests for implant planning (Siu et al. 2010).

To overcome these drawbacks of 2D imaging, a novel technique called computed tomography came into being in 1972. It was discovered by Charles Hounsfield and, by the mid-1980s, the use of CT scanners became common in medical settings to effectively replace the earlier techniques used, which were quite cumbersome and laborious. Originally devised for the soft tissue analysis specifically for the human brain, the technique was not really meant for high contrast calcified skeletal structures. However, over a period of time, it was adapted to many diverse applications including skeletal imaging analysis. CT uses X rays to produce high-resolution images in an axial plane ranging from 22 to 30 and from 32 to 35 slices for maxilla and mandible respectively, with a setting of 1.5 mm thickness and 1 mm apart with 0.5 mm overlapping. Further with the settings of thin sections, the scan could be made more contiguous and non-overlapping. To reduce the radiation dose and the time taken for diagnosis, the use of spiral or helical CT was introduced by Heiken et al, in which the thickness of the slice varied between 0.4 to 1 mm without an overlap and spiral CT did not use the conventional films.

This imaging technique has been extensively utilised in treatment planning and surgical procedures pertaining to dental implant surgery. The salient merits in this regard are a high-density resolution and the ability to cast some information regarding adjacent soft tissues, which is essential for dental implant surgical planning. The reformatted CT images provide co-referenced axial, panoramic and cross-sectional images, thus reducing the time for fast correlation of the different views. CT provides a technique with more precise estimates than conventional periapical and panoramic radiography. Anatomical landmarks such as mandibular canal, anterior mandibular buccal depression, etc. are better visualised and analysed. The reformatted images from the CT scan provide a fairly accurate evaluation of the bone characteristics apical to the maxillary sinuses. Very rarely, nephrotoxicity may appear as an adverse drug reaction to the colour dye used for contrast in the image. Few demerits such as hazardous radiation specifically for pregnant women and children, uncomfortable body posture and claustrophobia in susceptible individuals are associated with CT imaging, yet the technique is highly recommended for its potential for the most precise presurgical assessment of bone volume and to plan the most appropriate design and position of the implants, for a specific case by case scenario.

The CT dentascan came up with the intention to obtain true cross-sections of the jawbones via specially developed algorithms. Dentascan imaging provides a very clinician-friendly, simple and programmed display of the imaging details of the patient including reformation and organisation. It works on the in-system referenced panoramic images of the bone housing along with the three-dimensional display of bone, including the curvature of the jaw. Image spacing is approximately 1 mm apart in the digital output to allow accurate prosthetic treatment planning. Some inherent limitations such as false size, magnification, and limited range of the diagnostic information, are critical. On the whole, it provides a reasonable diagnostic date that is accurate, detailed and specific. Usually, a diagnostic template transfers and tailors the three-dimensional treatment plan of the final prosthesis into the bridging step of imaging analysis (Lingam et al. 2013).

Cone beam computed tomography (CBCT) is an imaging method that enables a precise three-dimensional portrayal of mineralised hard tissue structures. This novel imaging modality permits a fine resolution (2 line pair/mm), enhanced diagnostic quality and reduced shorter scanning times. There is a huge difference in the radiation exposure dose from conventional CT scans for maxillofacial imaging, approximately to the amount of 10 times (68 µSv compared with 600 µSv of conventional CT) (Loubele et al. 2009). Further, the technique offers great dimensional accuracy with only about 2 per cent magnification permissible (Kumar et al. 2015). CBCT was preferred for the majority of dental and maxillofacial purposes both diagnostic and therapeutic as this high-resolution imaging facility, was much smaller in size as well as cost-effective as opposed to conventional CT scanning. In two-dimensional imaging, of each slice, every two-dimensional pixel represents a three-dimensional cube or vowels of the area imaged. This two-dimensional limitation was overcome by the use of a cone-shaped incident X-ray beam as compared to the fan-shaped beam of conventional CT. The radiation dose reduction was significant and amounted to approximately equivalent to radiation exposure as occurs in two and eight panoramic radiographs (0.035 to 0.10 mSv). Higher resolution was accomplished due to the smaller voxel size in CBCT scans as opposed to conventional CT. Contemporary commercial CBCT units include NewTom DVT 9000 (Quantitative Radiology, Verona, Italy), i-CAT (Imaging Sciences International, Hatfield, USA), and 3D Accuitomo (J. Morita, Kyoto, Japan) etc. (Siu et al. 2010).

Better imaging results were observed against the multi-slice CT-multidetector-row helical computer tomography (MDCT) unit. Salient merits as described above along with the user flexibility place the CBCT in a distinctly upright position for oral rehabilitation treatment planning with dental implants. Another investigation revealed that the effective dose with the NewTom machine (CBCT) was significantly lower than traditional CT imaging. Radiation dose is an important determinant to analyse the benefit and risks against the applicability of different modalities available for the imaging of the facial skeleton. Radiation exposure levels of cone beam CT systems fitted moderately in between the CT and conventional intraoral radiography. Bennett aptly remarked that cone beam CT scanning is a technique for developing surgical guides for implant dentistry (Siu et al. 2010).

The evolution in hardware has been successively followed by advancements in the planning software which allow three-dimensional reformatted CT based data on a personal computer when developing a treatment plan. A recently developed interactive three-dimensional CT software program (SimPlant; Materialse, Leuven, Belgium) has realised the interactive virtual placement of implant after analysing the recipient bone and adjacent structures in all dimensions. This was the first commercialised software tool that enabled the checking of prosthodontic implications at the same time. But there existed yet lags that the scanning device was to serve as the surgical device, though it was more of a virtual template not a surgical template per se. There is still a missing link that transfers the computer plan into the actual treatment of the patient, which was bridged by the invention of the CAD/CAM technique (Siu et al. 2010).

The physical nature of such models was perceived better as these could function by mimicking the presence of natural tissues and with enhanced direct insights of complex details for the clinician, who were earlier limited from screen images. Though there remained certain issues with existing milling machines such as limited movement, difficulty in programming intricate tissue details, etc. Further, the technique needed skilful human intervention and a learning curve to operate the equipment.

To further simplify the technicality and the development of the implant surgical guide, it was soon realised that the layer-wise digital data format obtained from CT scanned images may be feasible to comply with the digitalised workflow of the rapid prototyping (RP) technology. It was hypothesised that such fusion of technology may obtain fabrication of 3-dimensional products directly from CAD models, irrespective of the complexity of the structure. The physical realisation of CT data was a breakthrough and was popularly termed 'real virtuality' or 'virtual reality'. With this, started the process of, a new therapeutic protocol that included the transfer of the designed and planned data for the construction of custom made stereo lithographic drill guides (Tardieu et al. 2003).

Nowadays, with constant and rapid advancements in all three domains of AM, there are many third-party implant planning software programs commercially available (Mora et al. 2014), which have been listed below in Table 4.1.

TABLE 4.1
Commercially Available Implant Planning Software

Company	Implant Software
Materialise Dental Inc, Glen Burnie, MD, USA	Simplant
Anatomage, San Jose, CA, USA	Invivo5
Nobel Biocare, Goteborg, Sweden	NobelClinician
Cybermed Inc, Seoul, Korea	OnDemand3D
BioHorizons, Inc, Birmingham, AL, USA	Virtual Implant Placement software
Dental Wings Inc, Montreal, CA, USA	coDiagnostiX
BlueSkyBio, LLC, Grayslake, IL, USA	Blue Sky Plan
Sirona Dental Systems, Inc, Charlotte, NC, USA	Galileos system
i-CAT, Imaging Sciences International LLC, Hatfield, PA	TxSTUDIO software
NewTom, Verona, Italy	NewTom implant planning software

4.8   AM IN SURGICAL TOOLS/GUIDES FOR DENTAL IMPLANTS

The term computed tomography (CT) surgical guide is defined as 'a surgical procedure that uses a device (surgical guide) that was additively manufactured from a digital file of the cone beam computed tomography (CBCT)' (GPT 2017, Klein and Abrams 2001, Tyndall et al. 2012). The digital workflow has sequential steps: (1) obtaining the data of patients like CBCT scans and intraoral impressions; (2) digital processing of the information and executing this information by virtual planning of implant via CAD/CAM dental software (Ganz 2015, Tapie et al. 2015); (3) CAD/CAM fabrication of the surgical template (Rosenfeld et al. 2006, Tardieu et al. 2003). Jung and co-workers (Jung et al. 2009) introduced static and dynamic implant guide systems.

Static systems are those that transfer predetermined implant placement sites to identify the location within the patient, s mouth via surgical templates. These are categorised into half-guided preparation and fully guided implant surgery (Kühl et al. 2013).

Instead, the dynamic systems help transfer only the planned prosthesis via visual imaging tools into the computer algorithm rather than intraoral surgical guides physically. Dynamic systems allow the surgeon to intervene in the operative procedure in real time to alter the position of implants (Revilla-León et al. 2020).

4.9   POWER OF DIGITAL PLANNING, DESIGN AND 3D PRINTING

When viewing a CBCT to evaluate potential implant sites, dentists initially use the 3D visualisation software supplied by a CBCT system manufacturer. This native software allows for the visualisation of the patient's alveolar anatomy and possible implant position. In most instances, the CBCT software includes tools for linear measurements that allow for the basic planning of potential implant size and position. Some CBCT manufacturers supply virtual implant libraries that allow for a more specific 3D implant planning and its orientation to the surrounding structures. However, software that is strictly a 'viewer' does not allow for surgical guide design and ordering of a computer guide. Additionally, viewer software does not allow for designing a prosthetic 'blueprint' in the form of a virtual wax-up or incorporation of an actual wax-up. For such task planning, specialised implant treatment planning software caters to the requisites. Common brands include Simplant, Anatomoge, 3Shape and Dental Wings Codiagnostics.

Complex clinical case scenarios are the prime indications for the use of computerised 3 D printed surgical templates such as when surgical spaces are limited, placing angulated implants like in the 'all-on-4' technique, immediate placement and provisionalisation, orthodontic anchorage, multiple adjacent implants and for achieving precision (Valente et al. 2009, Ozan et al. 2009, Arisan et al. 2010, Van Assche et al. 2007, 2012, Van Steenberghe et al. 2002, Stumpel 2008). If anyone plans to order a template than making chairside in one's clinic, then it is mandatory to use a third-party implant planning software. CBCT data are imported in standard format digital imaging and communications in medicine (DICOM) file format into the specialised software in order to plan implant surgery and design and order surgical template.

Software for treatment planning of implant has tools that can easily visualise the final restoration while planning the placement of implant fixture with respect to the recipient area. When making a CBCT scan for patients with few missing teeth, the proposed future teeth may be placed virtually using the software tooth library. If multiple teeth are missing, however, a radiographic guide may be worn by the patient while taking the scan. Alternatively, matching optical scan images of the patient's dentition into CBCT can be used instead of a scan appliance in many cases. In edentulous arches, the radiographic guide must be worn if a mucosa-supported guide is desired. The radiographic guide should be well-fitting and properly positioned in order to accurately transfer the relationship of the prosthesis to the bone. One must avoid the use of a poor-fitting radiographic guide or an unstable guide that can easily be displaced if improperly worn during the scan. If a poor-fitting guide is used, a risk of the implants not being in the planned position exists and this has serious consequences. By using implant treatment planning software, clinicians can create the initial design of the planned restoration. The software can be used to position implants virtually in the proper restorative position. This allows the user to visualise the implant and bone position with the final restoration in mind. Occasionally, deficient bone requires clinicians to change the trajectory of the implant and make a decision in regard to a screw-retained versus cement-retained restoration. Alternatively, decisions can be made to augment the deficient site and allow for a screw-access restoration and a more favourable prosthetic implant trajectory (Guichet 2015).

Various factors affect the fidelity or precision of the surgical guide like intensity, laser speed, building direction and angle, number of layers, interlayer dimensional changes, software, post-curing procedures (Allen and Dutta 1994, Puebla et al. 2012, Alharbi et al. 2016, Brain et al. 2016, Ide et al. 2017, Plooij et al. 2011). A few studies were published regarding the precision of manufacturing of the surgical guide (Schneider et al. 2002, Matta et al. 2017, Neumeister et al. 2017, Sommacal et al. 2018, Schneider et al. 2015, Bell et al. 2018). Slight deviation has been noticed, i.e. less than 0.25 mm due to inaccuracy in the fabrication of the surgical guide by SL (Schneider et al. 2002).

A step-by-step workflow for the construction of a 3D-printed implant surgical guide has been described by Whitley III et al. 2017, as given below:

a. An accurate intraoral scan or impression was taken.
b. Pre-operative CBCT scans were examined using software.
c. A virtual tooth replacing the missing tooth was created.
d. First, a virtual implant to mimic the original implant was created.
e. The surgical guide was planned using parameters that coincided with the guided kits for implant drills.
f. A half or full-arch guide was designed to achieve optimal stability by using the teeth mesial and distal to the edentulous area or from the alveolar ridge in the case of a full-arch guide.
g. The stereolithography (STL) file was exported from the planning software and imported into the 3D printing software to set up and complete the print.
h. The guide was oriented to minimise cross-sectional peeling forces during printing and to allow for the drainage of excess resin, and support points were added in areas that did not interfere with an accurate fit of the guide.
i. The appropriate resin volume used and the settings for the print were 50-mm layers in the z-axis with a print time of 3 hours.

j. The guide was removed from the build platform, rinsed twice with 91% isopropanol for 20 minutes and allowed to air dry. Complete polymerisation was accomplished with a polymerisation chamber by exposure for 10 minutes to 108 watts each of Blue UV-A (315-400 nm) and UV-Blue (400-550 nm) light in a heated environment at 60C.

k. Supports were removed, and a stainless steel guide tube that coincided with the guided surgery size key was inserted. The guide was then autoclave sterilised.

l. The surgical guide was evaluated intraorally, and the guided surgery was performed using a flapless approach.

4.10   MATERIALS USED FOR IMPLANT SURGICAL GUIDES

Desirable properties of implant surgical guide construct material:

- Resistant to chemicals
- Dimensional stability
- Time and cost-efficient to be produced in the laboratory
- Standards of quality marked
- Biocompatibility
- Rigid and strong enough to bear the load intraoperatively
- Transparent to see through during the surgical procedure
- Non-corrosive
- Non-allergic and nontoxic
- Easily manipulable
- Withstand a wide range of temperatures (room, oral and the processing).

Furthermore, various polymer materials are available for the manufacturing of the surgical templates via several AM technologies and 3D printers like 3D systems manufacture VisiJet M3 StonePlast, BEGO manufacture VarseoWax SG, DentalMed manufacture 3Delta guide, Detax manufacture Freeprint splint, Dreve manufacture FotoDent guide and have been summarised in Table 4.2. These materials show different mechanical properties; however, there is no criterion for the confirmation of the sufficient quality and accuracy of 3D printed surgical templates. The precision of AM surgical guide depends on the AM technology and 3D printer which is being used for the manufacturing of surgical guides (Matta et al. 2017, Sommacal et al. 2018).

Sommacal et al. (2018) analysed the precision of two 3D printers with different AM technologies, i.e. digital light processing (DLP) and material extrusion while fabricating the surgical template for eight patients. As material extrusion 3D printer could not be able to place on the working casts, demonstrate inaccuracy. However, this technology is scarcely used for manufacturing surgical templates. When new technologies emerge, it is quite necessary to determine the scope to which the technologies are advantageous as compared to the conventional ones. In vivo and in vitro studies should be conducted to evaluate the new technologies and techniques. It is usually exemplified in the following three different aspects of the final implant placement position viz Coronal, apex and angular deviation of the planned implant and that of the placed implant position (Mora et al. 2014). Table 4.3 summarising contemporary evidence regarding 3D printed implant surgical guides has been provided as supplementary information to the chapter for interested readers.

TABLE 4.2

Various Polymer Materials Available for Manufacturing Surgical Templates via Several AM Technologies

Manufacturer	Material	Polymerisation Wavelength (nm)	Modulus Elasticity (MPa)	Colour	Biocompatibility
3d systems	VisiJet M3 StonePlast	405	1.850	Natural	CE certified USP** plastic class VI
BEGO	VarseoWax SG	405	≥1.500	Transparent blue	Class I
Dentax	Freeprint splint	405378–388 (UV)	NA	Clear transparent	Class I,IIa
DentalMed	3Delta guide	385	NA	Transparent	Class I
Dreve	FotoDent guide	385	≥1.900	Clear transparent	NA
		405	≥1.700	Clear transparent	NA
EnvisionTec	E-Guide tint	365–405	2.000	Translucent orange	Class I
	Clear guide	365–405	1.920	Clear transparent	USP** plastic class VI
FormLabs	Dental SG Resin	(315–400 nm) + UV-blue (400–550 nm)	1.500	Transparent orange	Class I
NexDent	NexDent-SG	Blue UV-A + UV-Blue 315–400 + 400–550	≥ 2.000	Translucent orange	Class I, CE certified
Shera	SHERAprint ortho plus	405	1.900–2.100	Clear transparent	Class IIa
	SHERAprint ortho plus UV	385		Clear transparent	
Stratasys	MED610(Clear-Bio)	200–300	2.000–3.000	Clear	Up to 24 h certified for mucosal membrane contact USP** plastic class VI

NA not available.

** USP: United States Pharmacopoeia Plastic Designations Classification.

TABLE 4.3
Literature Review

Van Assche VN et al. (2007): In this pilot study on human cadavers the authors evaluated that whether a CBCT reformatted image can be accurately used for 3D implant planning in partially edentulous jaws. For this four formalin fixed cadaveric jaws were used. A setup was established to simulate in vivo scanning condition by constructing a radiographic guide for the cadaveric jaws and to export the data for 3D planning. A postoperative scan was taken using the same settings. A fusion analysis was done. The mean linear deviation was 1.1 mm at the hex and 2mm at tip. The average angular deviation was 2°. The study concluded that flat panel CBCT images may be useful for computer aided rapid prototyping of surgical guide for partial edentulous conditions.

Arisan V et al. (2010): The purpose of this study was to compare and assess surgical and postoperative outcomes of guided surgery with that of standard techniques in totally edentulous patients. 52 patients were enrolled for the study. Initially a panoramic radiograph and clinical examination of all patients were done. 3 groups i.e. implants placed with standard technique implants placed with mucosa supported and implants placed with bone supported SLA guides were categorised. For guided surgery group a radiopaque scan prosthesis was fabricated and the patients had undergone CBCT wearing the radiopaque scan prosthesis. 2 parameters assessed were duration of surgery (in min) occurrence of pain or haemorrhage number of analgesic consumed and level of swelling on 3rd and 7th day. The mean surgical duration and number of analgesics consumed were minimum in flapless group than bone supported and standard technique. Variations in pain scores (VAS) between groups post operatively were statistically significant with score for flapless surgery significantly lower. The study concludes that mucosa supported single SLA guides for flapless implant placement may help reduce the duration of surgery pain intensity and other typical complication post-operatively.

Orentlicher G & Abboud M (2011): In the review on guided surgery for implant therapy the authors state that with the introduction of newer imaging technologies like cone beam computed tomography and treatment planning concepts like virtual implant planning there have been an interdisciplinary approach for planning and placement of dental implants. In guided surgery the ideal restorative plan is first created virtually on the software followed by implant placement planning leading to a prosthetically driven implant placement as opposed to the old notion of placing the implant where there is bone and deciding the prosthesis part later. During virtual planning the size of dental implants its proximity to vital anatomic structures relationship to the planned restoration can be assessed beforehand thereby increasing the accuracy and predictability of dental implant placement.

Van Assche VN et al. (2012): The authors conducted a systematic review with the purpose of assessing the accuracy of static guided implant placement along with its indications and limitations. This review included clinical preclinical and in vitro studies with the focus on the following four parameters: deviation of the implant at entry point deviation of the implant at apex deviation of the axis of implant deviation of height/depth. After the electronic search 19 articles were finally segregated for the review. The comparison in all the selected studies were based on fusion of preoperative and post-operative CBCT data. The overall mean deviation of implants was 1.09 mm at entry a mean deviation of 1.28 mm at the apex and 3.9° in angulation. Nevertheless randomised controlled trials for a specific factor were lacking. The review concluded that computer guided implant placement can be accurate but randomised controlled trials are needed to analyse impact of individual parameters for optimising the technique.

Kühl S. et al. (2012): The purpose of this study was to compare the accuracy between a fully guided and a half guided implant surgery. Five formalin fixed human mandibles were used and a preoperative CBCT taken for virtual implant planning. 28 implants divided equally in both the groups were inserted using the template. A postoperative CBCT was obtained and images were manually aligned using the anatomic landmarks. The mean total deviation between virtual and actual implant positions between both the groups were 1.52 mm and 1.56 mm at implant base 1.55 mm and 1.84 mm at the tips 3.6° and 4.3° of axial deviation. These differences were statistically non-significant but data showed that fully guided surgery was of additional benefit in the cases of proximity to vital structures.

(Continued)

TABLE 4.3 (CONTINUED)
Literature Review

Verhamme et al. (2013): Aim of study was to develop a relevant method to compare the virtual planned implant position to the ultimately achieved implant position and to evaluate in case of discrepancy the cause for it. In this study five edentulous patients receive implants in the maxilla. Preoperatively a cone-beam CT (CBCT) scan was acquired followed by virtual implant planning. A surgical template was designed and endosseous implants were inserted using the template as a guide. To assess any differences in position the postoperative CBCT scan was matched to the preoperative scan. The accuracy of implant placement was validated three-dimensionally (3D) and the implant position orthogonal projection (IPOP) validation method was applied. Errors introduced by virtual planning surgical instruments and validation process were evaluated. The results of the study indicate that bucco-lingual deviations were less obvious than mesio-distal deviations and a maximum linear tip deviation of 2.84 mm shoulder deviation of 2.42 mm and angular deviation of 3.41° were calculated in mesio-distal direction. Deviations included errors in planning software (maximum 0.15 mm) for surgical procedure (maximum 2.94°) and validation process (maximum 0.10 mm).

Beretta et al. (2014): The aim of the present study was to evaluate the *in vivo* accuracy of flapless computer-aided implant placement by comparing the three-dimensional (3D) position of planned and placed implants through an analysis of linear and angular deviations. Implant position was virtually planned using 3D planning software based on the functional and aesthetic requirements of the final restorations. Computer-aided design/computer-assisted manufacture technology was used to transfer the virtual plan to the surgical environment. The 3D position of the planned and placed implants in terms of the linear deviations of the implant head and apex and the angular deviations of the implant axis was compared by overlapping the pre- and postoperative computed tomography scans using dedicated software. The study concluded that computer-aided flapless implant surgery seemed to provide several advantages to the clinicians as compared to the standard procedure; however linear and angular deviations are to be expected. Therefore accurate pre surgical planning taking into account anatomical limitations and prosthetic demands is mandatory to ensure a predictable treatment without incurring possible intra- and postoperative complications.

Cassetta M et al. (2014): The authors did a comparative CBCT-CT in vitro study to assess any differences between the bone density values obtained through both the modalities and to assess any differences between them. A radiographic template with lead shots incorporated was used for taking the scan. The obtained images were overlapped using a software. 30 measurements were made and the set of values were divided into six groups: cancellous-cortical bone CBCT grey density values (VV) cancellous-cortical bone CT grey density values (HU) cancellous bone CBCT grey density values (VV) cancellous bone CT grey density values (HU) cortical bone CBCT grey density values (VV) cortical bone CT grey density values (HU). There is a linear correlation between the grey density values. The differences observed in the values in all the six groups were statistically significant. The dimensional accuracy of both CBCT and CT are comparable. The study concludes that CT can be substituted by CBCT during dental implant planning because of low radiation and cost effectiveness of CBCT. The authors also devise an approximate conversion ratio of 0.7 for CBCT (0.7*CBCT values = CT values).

Correa LR et al. (2014): The study compared the variations in implant sizes (Width & Length) when planned using digital panoramic radiograph (D-Pan) CBCT generated panoramic images (CBCT-Pan) and CBCT generated cross sections (CBCT cross). A total of 71 patients with 103 implant sites (maxillary premolars and mandibular molars) were assessed. D-pan CBCT-pan CBCT cross were obtained for each patient and were measured using dedicated software. Three observers performed assessment at the same time. For premolar sites the width differed significantly between D-PAN and CBCT Pan with wider implants in CBCT Pan while there were no significant differences in implant length when all implant sites were considered. The study concluded that on average majority of the implants changed to a smaller size in either width or length while using CBCT cross for planning as compared to D-Pan or CBCT Pan view.

(Continued)

TABLE 4.3 (CONTINUED)
Literature Review

Mora MA et al. (2014): The study reviewed the use of cone beam computed tomography as an essential tool in the diagnosis and planning for implant dentistry using different commercially available virtual implant planning software. This review analyses essential characteristics of the entire implant-guided surgery planning process and points out potential sources of error that could affect clinical accuracy outcomes. Clinical accuracy of surgical guides can be affected by: errors in image acquisition; errors in orientation and cross-sectional principles; errors in surgical guide manufacturing; type of surgical guide support or guide fixation full versus partial guidance during the osteotomy preparation full versus partial guidance during implant placement. The authors have detailed different software tools that facilitate implant planning in clinical practice and has also emphasized the need to develop a strict planning protocol that results in successful outcomes.

Stübinger (2014): The aim of the study was to evaluate deviations between virtually planned and placed implants by the use of skeletally supported stereolithographic templates. In this study 10 consecutive patients were selected for virtual 3D implant planning CBCT images were obtained in the pre- and postoperative phase. No control group or randomization was used in this study. Four deviation parameters (i.e. global angular depth and lateral deviation) were defined and calculated between the planned and the placed implants using the coordinates of their respective apical and coronal points. The study results indicate deviations at the coronal positions appeared to be smaller as compared with apical positions. But only the difference with regard to lateral measurements appeared to be statistically significant. Overall there was a slight tendency for higher values for more distal locations. The study concluded that slight deviations between planned and placed implants may occur even with skeletal-supported templates and the clinician should be aware not to overestimate advocated surgical safety by using static navigation tools.

Vercryssen M et al. (2014): In this article the authors review the accuracy and efficacy of the guided surgery. With the introduction of 3D imaging mainly CBCT in implant dentistry various different concepts of 3D planning like computer-guided static and dynamic surgical techniques had been proposed. Accuracy of the guided surgery defined as matching of the virtually planned positions in the software with actual position of the implant in patients. This accuracy had been mainly defined on the basis of four parameters deviation at the entry point deviation at apex deviation of the long axis and deviation in height and depth. Possible sources of errors can be due to errors in positioning in scan prosthesis. Techniques for surgical guide production positioning and stabilization of the surgical template tolerance of the drills learning curve of operator. Efficacy can be assessed by comparing the implant survival or success rates and prosthesis survival following guided implant placement. Overall deviation during the production of a stereolithographic guide is <0.25 mm which might occur during the CBCT scan of patient image segmentation and data procession and generation of model or during rapid prototyping. The survival rates of the implant placed with guided technique were comparable with those for conventional treatment. There is a certain limit of inaccuracy of the range of ±2.0 mm which is less than non-guided surgery and a reduction of inaccuracy below 0.5 mm seems to be quite difficult.

Geng W et al. (2015): This study was done to evaluate the clinical outcome and accuracy of dental implants placed by using different types of CAD/CAM surgical guides. The study procedure includes fabrication of a radiopaque diagnostic template a preoperative CT scan of the patient virtual implant planning designing of the two different types of guides tooth supported and mucosa supported surgical guides and a postoperative CT scan. Total of 111 implants were placed 52 implants by tooth-guided and 59 by mucosa-guided implant guides. Both the preoperative and postoperative CT scans were overlapped for accessing the accuracy. Mean angular deviation mean deviations in position at neck and apex and mean depth deviation were measured. Significant differences were observed between the values of tooth- and mucosa-supported guides with tooth-supported guides showing greater accuracy and being more stable.

(Continued)

TABLE 4.3 (CONTINUED)
Literature Review

Kühl S et al. (2015): Aim of the study was to determine the accuracy of printing surgical templates using a surface scan of a cast model. For this cast models and virtual planning data of nine patients who had undergone guided implant insertion. The original cast were incorporated with titanium pins. Accuracy measurements were performed between the positions of these titanium pins in the cast Positions of the sleeves in the virtually planned models and the real positions of sleeves in the printed templates. A mean 3D deviation of 0.22 mm in the centre of sleeve top 0.24 mm at sleeve base and angular deviation of 1.5°compared with virtual position. Study concludes that high accuracy can be achieved by using printed templates by accounting all the potential sources of inaccuracies. The factors affecting the accuracy may originates from accuracy of scanning procedures accuracy of the virtual designing software accuracy of the 3D printers accuracy of the template fit on the cast and accuracy of execution on the surgical sites.

Lin Y et al. (2015): In an in vitro simulation of implant surgery based on augmented reality the authors compares the geometric positioning of virtually planned implants to the osteotomy sites prepared with augmented reality guided surgery. For this four fully edentulous mandible models and four partially edentulous maxillary models were prepared by taking the scan of the patients with the same conditions and printing the models through rapid prototyping techniques. Forty osteotomy sites were prepared in these models and immediately after surgical simulations a postoperative CT was undertaken. These preoperative and postoperative images were analyzed using Fusion criteria of multimodality image registration. The mean and SD of the discrepancy between planned and prepared site at the entry point were 0.50 ± 0.33 mm 0.96 ± 0.33 mm at apex. $2.70 \pm 1.55°$ of angular accuracy a lateral deviation of 0.86 ± 0.34 mm and a depth deviation of long axis was 0.3 ± 0.27 mm. They concluded that by using the augmented reality along with stereolithographic printed surgical template the deviation was reduced significantly but the result should be interpreted with certain cautions because the main limitation of the study was that it was an in vitro study done on models not on cadavers or in vivo.

Shen P et al. (2015): The purpose of this study was to assess the accuracy of implant placement using surgical guide templates and to compare the results with implant placement based on computer-aided design (CAD) planning merely. In this study a total of 60 patients with dentition defects were included and were equally divided into group I and group II. Preoperative cone beam computed tomography (CBCT) was performed and preoperative planning was designed with Simplant software for all patients. Implant were placed in group I patients based on the preoperative planning without surgical guide templates. Implant surgical guide templates for group II patients were designed and produced by a rapid prototyping (RP) technique and implant was inserted with the assistance of surgical templates in them. Postoperative CBCT was performed for all patients. Image registration was carried out between postoperative CBCT data and that of preoperative planning data to compare the deviations of the implant between the actual and planned positions. There were no infection or pain in the surgical site both in group I and group II. All the implants had achieved osseointegration. Variation at the implant shoulder in group II was 1.18 ± 0.72 mm apex 1.43 ± 0.74 mm angulation 4.21 ± 1.91 mm and depth 0.54 ± 0.29 mm whereas the variation in group I was 2.07 ± 0.51 mm ($P < 0.01$) 2.89 ± 1.02 mm ($P < 0.01$) 8.84 ± 4.64 mm ($P < 0.05$) and 0.78 ± 0.33 mm ($P > 0.05$). The study concluded that the use of surgical guide templates can achieve higher precision and accuracy in implant shoulder apex and angulation which is much more suitable for complicated procedures and conditions such as the flapless method immediate loading aesthetic restoration and insufficient bone height.

Scherer U et al. (2015): Aim of the study was to assess the influence of template-guided vs non-guided drilling protocols on the diameter of drill holes in an in vitro model using fresh cadaveric porcine mandibles. Four groups were created for this experimentation. Group 1 consists of free-hand drilling with an inexperienced operator Group 2 consists of free-hand drilling by an experienced oral surgeon Group 3 consists of template-guided drilling by an inexperienced operator and Group 4 consists of template-guided drilling by an experienced oral surgeon. A total of 180 drilled holes were analysed. The results state that template-guided drilling procedure enhanced the accuracy significantly irrespective of the clinical experience of the operator. These results should be confirmed in large clinical trials.

(Continued)

TABLE 4.3 (CONTINUED)
Literature Review

Cristache & Silviu C M (2017): The aim of this study was to evaluate by superimposition of 3D digital files the accuracy of computer guided dental implant insertion in partially edentulous patients using a stereolithographic template with sleeve structure incorporated into the design. Avoiding the second CBCT. A pre-operative CBCT and digital impression were taken and a stereolithographic surgical template was designed and printed. Sixty-five implants were placed in twenty-five consecutive patients with the help of the 3D printed surgical template. After surgery digital impression was taken and 3D inaccuracy of implants position at entry point apex and angle deviation was measured using an inspection tool software. Mann–Whitney U test was used to compare accuracy between maxillary and mandibular surgical guides. A p value <.05 was considered significant. Mean (and standard deviation) of 3D error at the entry point was 0.798 mm (±0.52) at the implant apex it was 1.17mm (±0.63) and mean angular deviation was 2.34 (±0.85). A statistically significant reduced 3D error wasobserved at entry point $p = .037$ at implant apex $p = .008$ and also in angular deviation $p = .030$ in mandible when comparing to maxilla. The study concluded that the surgical template use has proved high accuracy for implant insertion.

Deeb G R et al. (2017): The aim of the study was to check the accuracy of implant surgical guides produced with in-office desktop stereolithographic 3D-printers. The study design was planned to mimic a single implant placement in the maxillary anterior region where esthetics is deemed utmost importance and therefore the precision of implant placement is critically crucial. They used 3shape Implant Studio software for treatment plan of #8 using a digital intraoral scan from a Trios scanner and cone-beam computed tomography (CBCT). Stereolithographic guides were printed using a 3D printer and the implant was inserted. Pre- and postimplant insertion digital scans were superimposed to determine distance and angulation differences in mesiodistal and faciolingual position of the implants compared to the planned position. They found that the mean difference in mesiodistal direction at the alveolar crest between planned and placed implants was 0.28 mm (range 0.05–0.62 mm) and the difference in the faciolingual direction was 0.49 mm (range 0.08–0.72mm). The mean mesiodistal angulation deviation was 0.84 degrees (range 0.08–4.48) and the mean faciolingual angulation deviation was 3.37 degrees (range 1.12–6.43). So they concluded that in-office fabricated stereolithographic implant surgical guides demonstrate similar accuracy to laboratory or manufacturer prepared guides. And the technique provided a convenient and cost-effective means of assuring proper implant placement.

Matta R.E (2017): The aim of the study was to evaluate the impact of the fabrication method on the 3D accuracy. Templates designed for 13 patients were investigated in this study same virtual planning based on a scanned plaster model was used to fabricate a conventional thermo-formed and a 3D-printed surgical guide for each of patients (single tooth implants). Both templates were acquired individually on the respective plaster model using an optical white-light scanner and the virtual data obtained were superimposed. Using the 3D geometry of the implant sleeve The coordinate system was adjusted to the sleeve in the following sequence: x plane in the vestibule-oral direction y plane in the mesio-distal direction and z plane in the cranio-caudal direction the deviation between both surgical guides was evaluated. The mean discrepancy of the angle was 3.479. Concerning the three-dimensional position of the implant sleeve the highest deviation was in the Z-axis at 0.594 mm. The study concluded that thermo-formed and three-dimensionally printed surgical templates which were produced using the same planning differed significantly. Nevertheless both methods were able to transfer a predetermined implant position into the clinical situation.

Bemcharit S et al. (2018): The purpose of this retrospective study was to measure and compare the deviations and angulation differences in fully and partially guided implant surgery by using a tooth guided implant surgical guide fabricated using in office 3D printing technology. Treatment plan and designing of the guides were done on 3 shape implant studio v 2016. Guided osteotomy with free handed implant placement was done in a partialy guided while guided osteotomy and guided implant placement was done in fully guided. The deviations for fully guided are 0.17 ± 078 mm in mesial 0.44 ± 0.78 mm in distal 0.23 ± 1.08 mm in buccal −0.22 ± 1.44 in lingual −0.32 ± 2.36° angular. The deviations for partially guided are 0.33 ± 1.38 for mesial −0.03 ± 1.59 for distal 0.62 ± 1.15 for buccal −0.275 ± 1.6 for lingual 0.59 ± 6.83° angulation.

TABLE 4.3 (CONTINUED)
Literature Review

Caitlyn K. Bell (2018): The purpose of this study was to evaluate the accuracy of placed implants using two different guided implant surgery materials: thermoplastic vs 3D-printed surgical guides. Twenty duplicate mandibular models ten thermoplastic and ten 3D-printed surgical guides were used. Twenty implants were placed following the guided surgery protocol. Cone beam computed tomography scans of placed implants and the control implant were superimposed to measure deviations. The thermoplastic group showed average deviations of 3.4 degrees 1.3 mm at the head and 1.6 mm at the apex of the implant compared to 2.36 degrees 0.51 and 0.76 mm for the 3-D printed group; $p = 0.143$ $p < 0.001$ and $p < 0.001$ respectively. The study concluded that there is a significant difference in the accuracy of the location of the implant head and apex between thermoplastic and 3D-printed surgical guides.

Ma B et al. (2018): The purpose of this study was to evaluate the errors in implant placement by using CBCT and plaster cast model scan in posterior teeth by using universal digital surgical guides. 28 posterior implants were included and divided into two groups Group 1: implant planning based on CBCT and Group 2: implant planning based on overlapping the optical scanned cast and CBCT. A digital surgical guide was printed using three dimensional printers. Planned position referred to pre-surgical positions and inserted implant position referred to actual position a postoperative CBCT was undertaken. Inserted model was generated by scanning the cast made by putting the lab analogue in the impression of the placed implants. A planned model generated by scanning the cast made by connecting a lab cylinder screw a lab cylinder body and lab analogue to the printed surgical guide. Preoperative and postoperative data obtained in both the cases were overlapped using a software. The parameter assessed for analysing the accuracy are angle deviations coronal apical depth deviation for both the conditions for virtually planned and actual positions of the implants. A statistically significant difference was found between deviation of CBCT and that of the scanned cast. The model analysis showed lower deviation value compared to CBCT analysis.

Schnutenhaus S (2018): The aim of this study was to investigate differences between the virtually planned and clinically achieved implant positions in completely template-guided implantations as a function of the type of edentulous space the residual natural dentition and the surgical implementation. In this study 56 patient with a total of 122 implants were evaluated retrospectively. Placement of dental implants was completely template guided. Data of the planned implant positions were overlapped with the actual clinical implant positions measurement of the 3D deviations were obtained for: radial deviation height deviation and axial deviation. There are no statistically significant differences regarding the surgical approach for any of the parameters assessed. The study concluded that template-guided implantation offers a high degree of accuracy even in the presence of different configurations of the residual dentition or different surgical approaches. And the clinically achievable accuracy can be described as sufficient for further prosthetic treatment.

Younes F et al. (2018): This randomized controlled trial was done for a comparative evaluation of the effectiveness of free-hand pilot drill-guided and fully guided implant surgery using apical global deviation (AGD) in partially edentulous patient. In addition to this primary outcome an additional comparison was done for financial cost and time spent both preoperative and intra operative. Thirty three partially edentulous patient were enrolled for the study and were randomly allocated to one of the treatment group. Accuracy in implant placement was assessed by comparing the planned implant position to its actual position with apical global deviation as primary outcome variable. Secondary analysis was done on cost incurred and time spent. Efficiency of guided surgery both partially and fully guided was also assessed by an incremental cost effectiveness ratio (ICER) which was defined as an extra cost incurred to decrease the apical global deviation. In terms of surgical accuracy fully guided (FG) surgery (AGD 0.97 mm) was most effective and free-hand (FH) implant placement (AGD 2.11 mm) was least effective. Total time invested preoperative and postoperative did not differ significantly between all the three groups (P = 0.811). A significant additional cost was found in partially guided and fully guided group). The study concludes that fully guided is most efficient surgical approach and the extra operational cost is acceptable to reduce the recurrent apical global deviation.

(Continued)

TABLE 4.3 (CONTINUED)
Literature Review

Frösch L et al. (2019): This in vitro trial was done to compare the heat generation during guided osteotomy preparation to that of conventional one. Four study groups were defined for sequential and single drilling procedures with and without surgical guides. Osteotomies were performed in polyurethane foam blocks and the temperature was measured using infra red camera. Guided osteotomy showed statistically significant higher temperature than single conventional approach for the 2.2, 3.5, and 4.2 mm drills. Higher heat generation and longer duration of latent heat production was observed during sequential drilling. Duration of the heat exposure over the critical temperature was for less than one minute except for 4.2 mm drill guide for which it was 76 seconds. Results of this study suggest that guided surgical drill use generates more heat and special care should be taken to avoid heat development and potential complications.

Omami G & Al Yafi F (2019): The purpose of this review was to assess the usefulness of CBCT in implant dentistry and whether or not it should be routinely used for each and every case of implants planning. Clinical assessment and conventional 2D radiographs often provide inadequate diagnostic data for proper implant placement. Cone beam CT (CBCT) enables 3D visualisation of the alveolar ridge aiding clinicians with identification of vital anatomic structures and pathologies. CBCT provides accurate linear measurements at low radiation dose compared with conventional CT scan which helps in diagnosis and treatment planning particularly in complex implant cases. Even though straightforward implant surgery can be performed with careful clinical and 2D radiographic assessment CBCT should be considered. It provides the unparalleled benefit of computer-aided implant planning leading to improved clinical outcomes and reduced complications. Radiation dose should always be optimized with a field of view limited to area of interest.

Santis DD et al. (2019): The purpose of this pilot trial was to evaluate accuracy of implant placed using two types of surgical guides (fully guided and pilot drill guided) using Noble Bio care and to define factors influencing accuracy. 20 patients were enrolled 10 in each group and an OPG and CT was done for each patient. Radiographic template designed for completely edentulous patients for fully guided group osteotomies and implants were placed with the help of guide while for pilot drill guided only 1st drill osteotomy done by guide and sequential drilling and implant placement done free-hand.

Smitkarn P et al. (2019): This randomized controlled clinical trial compares the accuracy of single tooth in partially edentulous patients. Implants were placed using fully digital guided surgery and free hand implant surgery. A total of 52 patients were enrolled for study digital implant planning was performed for both groups of patient using data from CBCT post-operative CBCT was obtained 2 weeks after surgery using same protocol as pre-operative. The median (IQR) deviation in angles shoulders and apexes were $2.8(2.6)°$ $0.9(0.8)$mm and $1.2(0.9)$mm in guided group and $7.0(7.0)°$ $1.3(0.7)$mm and $2.2(1.2)$mm in free hand group. The study concludes that static guided surgery produces more accuracy in implant positions than free hand implant placement.

Yafi AF et al. (2019): This study reviews the workflow for computer-aided implant surgery and the factors affecting the accuracy and the clinical outcomes of the static guided implant surgical guide. The digital workflow consist of a number of steps for a prosthetically driven 3D virtual plan. The plan is then transferred to the surgical site using a surgical guide. Guided implant surgery tends to increase the accuracy and predictability of the placed implant decrease the operative time compared with the free-hand implant surgery. Deviations in the guided surgery may occurs between virtually planned implant and the original position of the implant due to accumulation of errors throughout the digital workflow and also due to patient-related and surgery-related factors. These deviations can also occur due to the surgical learning curve of the guided surgery.

(Continued)

TABLE 4.3 (CONTINUED)
Literature Review

Varga Jr et al. (2020): The purpose of this randomised parallel group of clinical trial was to access the accuracy of free hand implant placement pilot drill guided partially guided and fully guided implant placement protocols. A total of 207 implants were placed in both maxilla and mandible. All the cases were digitally planned. A post operative CBCT was taken with same specification as pre operative CBCT one to three days after surgery and comparison was performed using medical image analysis using a detected software. Angular deviation was taken as a primary outcome variable. A significant amount of improvement seen in Angular deviation as the guidance was increased from free handed to fully guided it was $(3.04° \pm 1.51)$ for all the secondary outcome variable all the guided protocol were superior to free hand placement significantly. The study concludes that static guided surgery significantly improved the accuracy of dental implant surgery as compared to free hand implant placement. Any levels of guidance is better than free hand and as the guidance increases the accuracy increases. Digital techniques could be used to improve localisation and targeting of implant placement and reduce the inherent invasiveness of surgery.

Sarment et al. (2003) studied related to precision of implant placement by using stereolithographic surgical templates on epoxy mandibles compared with those constructed by CAD/CAM template to those constructed conventionally. When there is comparison between virtual planning of implant placement and actual placement reveals marked deviation in surgical placement of implant using conventional one as compared to CAD/CAM template. Distance between the centre of the head of the virtually planned and actual implant differ by 1.5 ± 0.7 mm for conventional guide and by 0.9 ± 0.5 mm for the CAD/CAM guide. The distance between the center of the apex of the virtually planned and actual implant differ by 2.1 ± 0.97 mm for conventional guide and by 1.0 ± 0.6 mm for the CAD/CAM guide. And regarding angle which is formed between the long axis of virtually planned and actual implant placed differ by 8.0 ± 4.5 degrees for conventional guide and by 4.5 ± 2.0 degrees for the CAD/CAM guide. Studies suggested that CAD/CAM guides improve the precision. Moreover studies reveal that CAD/CAM surgical guides permit ideal placement of multiple implants and facilitate prosthetically driven implant positioning based on anatomic limitations. However further studies were necessary to validate its clinical use.

Tardieu et al. (2003) presented a case of immediate loading of mandibular implants using a five-step procedure. The first step consisted of building a scannographic template the second step consisted of taking a computerised tomographic (CT) scan and the third step consisted of implant planning using SurgiCase software. The final two steps consisted of implant placement using a drill guide created by stereolithography and placement of the prosthesis. Using a CT scan-based planning system the surgeon was able to select the optimal locations for implant placement. By incorporating the prosthetic planning using a scannographic template the treatment was optimized from a prosthetic point of view. Furthermore the use of a stereolithographic drill guide allowed a physical transfer of the implant planning to the patient's mouth. The scannographic template was designed so that it could be transformed into a temporary fixed prosthesis for immediate loading and the definitive restoration was placed 3 months later.

Di Giacomo et al. (2005) used CAD/ CAM for manufacturing tooth-born and multiple bone guides for various twist drills of size 2.2, 3.2, and 4.0 mm. SimPlant (DENTSPLY Implants Waltham Mass.) was then applied according to the SurgiGuide protocol. On the basis of pre and post-operative computed tomography scans variation at the head of the implant was 2.45 ± 1.42 mm with a range of 0.2–4.5 mm while variation at the apex of the implant was 2.99 ± 1.77 mm with a range of 0.8–7.1 mm and while comparing the angulations which was 7.25 ± 2.67 degrees with a range of 3.6–12.2 degrees.

Matta et al. (2017) from the same virtual planning based on a scanned plaster model compared the accuracy of the implant sleeve from the conventional thermo-formed and AM surgical guides. Both manufacturing processes varied significantly with respect to the 3D positioning of the implant sleeve as well as its angle. The average deviation ranged from 0.266 to 0.864 mm and 3.5° for the angle. The largest deviation in all spatial directions was found in the Z-axis (0.594 mm). Both methods were found as appropriate for clinical use.

(Continued)

TABLE 4.3 (CONTINUED)
Literature Review

Van Steenberghe D et al. (2002) evaluated the precision of Nobel Guide surgical guides (Nobel Biocare Zurich) compared the virtually planned versus actual placement of 10 implants in the completely edentulous maxilla of two cadaver jaws. Using fiducially related markers pre and post-surgical computed tomography scans were compared revealing close vicinity between the actual location and planned location of implants placed. On average there was 0.8 mm of deviation between the virtually planned and actual implant placed at the head of the implant while 0.9 mm of deviation can be seen at the apex of the implant and 1.8 degree deviation of implant placement relative to the angle in which the implant was virtually planned to be placed. To increase the precision of placement of implant position Marchack and Moy (2003) showed that use of software for surgical planning and CT scans bears great chances of survival of implants. When CT scans and software for surgical planning were used for creation of the fixed prosthesis for an immediate load treatment the survival rate of implants was 92 percent over a period of 24 months. Despite the capacity of CAD/ CAM guides for accurate implant placement exists there is still divergence in the degree of precision with computer generated guides. There are far fewer clinical studies which use CAD/CAM guides to determine implant placement precisely. Further studies continue to reveal diversion in precision of placement of implant. Another clinical study using CT-based Nobel Guide surgical guides and Nobel Guide protocol looked at the difference in precision of placement of implant. To examine the placement of implant precision patients had undergone post insertion scans using a triple scan technique: guide scan guide and patient pre-placement scan and guide and patient post-placement scan (Marchack and Chew 2015).

4.11 CONCLUSION

Implant surgical guide plays an important link between planning and execution, as it contributes to functionally and cosmetically precise implant-supported prosthetic restoration. Nevertheless, a guide-based system, where the planning is solely based on a wax-up, helps in implant positioning for restorative treatment, whereas the planning based on volume image data can take into account the internal bone anatomy considerations too. In most clinical situations, oral implants can be inserted without a guiding system for the transfer of pre-operative planning, but precision is of utmost importance for the long term durability and successful outcome for the healthful functioning of the restored dentition. Guided surgery can be used with or without elevating a full-thickness flap. The flapless approach is taken into account when patients have adequate keratinised tissue and they also possess adequate bone volume so that no grafting procedure is required. It is the preferred approach and gaining popularity all the more in recent times, as lack of flap elevation and intact blood supply support better healing outcomes owing to fewer chances for postoperative complications or discomfort, surgical time, healing time, and bone loss is also reduced. Further, implants placed with a guided surgical approach not only remain better positioned and healed, rather in addition in complex clinical situations such as inadequate housing of bone and very close vicinity of vital structures such as maxillary sinus (maxilla) and inferior alveolar nerve (mandible) are better planned, treated well with implants and serve with better patient outcomes.

REFERENCES

Abraham, C.M. (2014). A brief historical perspective on dental implants, their surface coatings and treatments. *Open Dentist J*, 8, 50–55. doi:10.2174/1874210601408010050

Alharbi, N., Osman, R., & Wismeijer, D. (2016). Effect of build direction on the mechanical properties of 3D printed complete coverage interim dental restorations. *J Prosthet Dent*, 155, 760–767.

Allen, S., & Dutta, D. (1994). On the computation of part orientation using support structures in layered manufacturing. In: *Proceedings of the Solid Freeform Fabrication Symposium*, Austin, TX, pp. 259–269.

Almog, D.M., & Torrado, E., Meitner, S.W. (2001). Fabrication of imaging and surgical guides for dental implants. *J Prosthet Dent*, 85, 504–508.

Amet, E.M., & Ganz, S.D.(1997). Implant treatment planning using a patient acceptance prosthesis, radiographic record base, and surgical template. Part 1: Presurgical phase. *Implant Dent*, 6, 193.

Arısan, V., Karabuda, C.Z., Özdemir, T. (2010a). Implant surgery using bone-and mucosa-supported stereolithographic guides in totally edentulous jaws: surgical and post-operative outcomes of computer-aided vs. standard techniques. *Clini Oral Implants Res*, 21(9), 980–988.

Arısan, V., Karabuda, Z.C., & Ozdemir, T. (2010b). Accuracy of two stereolithographic guide systems for computer-aided implant placement: a computed tomography-based clinical comparative study. *J Periodontol*, 81(1), 43–51. doi: 10.1902/jop.2009.090348.

Ashley, S. (1991). Rapid prototyping systems. *Mech Eng*, 113(4), 34.

Balshi, T.J., & Garver, D.G. (1987). Surgical Guide stents for placement of implants. *J Oral Maxillofac Surg*, 45, 463–466.

Banga, H.K., Belokar, R.M., & Kumar, R. (2017b). 'A Novel Approach For Ankle Foot Orthosis Developed By Three Dimensional Technologies'. In: *3rd International Conference on Mechanical Engineering and Automation Science (ICMEAS 2017)*, University of Birmingham, UK, Vol. 8 No. 10, pp. 141–145.

Banga, H.K., Belokar, R.M., Madan, R., & Dhole, S. (2017a). Three dimensional Gait assessments during walking of healthy people and drop foot patients. *Defen Life Sci J*, 2, 14–20.

Banga, H.K., Kalra, P., Belokar, R.M., & Kumar, R. (2020a). Customized design and additive manufacturing of kids' ankle foot orthosis. *Rap Prototyping J*, 26(10). doi:10.1108/RPJ-07-2019-0194

Banga, H.K., Kalra, P., Belokar, R.M., & Kumar, R. (2020b). Design and fabrication of prosthetic and orthotic product by 3D printing [Online First]. *IntechOpen*, doi:10.5772/intechopen.94846. Available from: https://www.intechopen.com/online-first/design-and-fabrication-of-prosthetic-and-orthotic-product-by-3d-printing

Banga, H.K., Kalra, P., Belokar, R.M., & Kumar, R. (2020c). Effect of 3D-printed ankle foot orthosis during walking of foot deformities patients. In: Kumar H., Jain P. (eds) *Recent Advances in Mechanical Engineering*. Lecture Notes in Mechanical Engineering. Springer, Singapore, pp. 275–288

Banga, H.K., Kalra, P., Belokar, R.M., & Kumar, R. (2020d). Role of finite element analysis in customized design of kid's orthotic product. In: Singh S., Prakash C., Singh R. (eds) *Characterization, Testing, Measurement, and Metrology*, pp. 139–159 CRC Press Taylor & Francis Group, USA

Banga, H.K., Kumar, P., & Kumar, H. (2021). Utilization of Additive Manufacturing in Orthotics and Prosthetic Devices Development. In: *IOP Conference Series: Materials Science and Engineering*. doi:10.1088/1757-899X/1033/1/012083

Banga, H.K., Parveen, K., Belokar, R.M., & Kumar, R. (2014) Rapid prototyping applications in medical sciences. *Int J Emerg Technol Comput Appl Sci (IJETCAS)*, 5(8), 416–420.

Banga, H.K., Parveen, K., Belokar, R.M., & Kumar, R. (2018). Fabrication and stress analysis of ankle foot orthosis with additive manufacturing. *Rapid Prototyping J Emerald Publ*, 24(2), 300–312.

Banga, H.K., Parveen, K., Belokar, R.M., & Kumar, R. (2020e). Improvement of human gait in foot deformities patients by 3D printed ankle–foot orthosis. In: Singh S., Prakash C., Singh R. (eds) *3D Printing in Biomedical Engineering*. Materials Horizons: From Nature to Nanomaterials. Springer, Singapore

Becker, C.M., & Kaiser, D.A. (2000). Surgical guide for dental implant placement. *J Prosthet Dent*, 83, 248–251.

Bell, C.K., Sahl, E.F., Kim, Y.J., Rice, D.D. (2018). Accuracy of implants placed with surgical guides: thermoplastic versus 3D printed. *Int J Periodontics Restor Dent*, 38, 113–119. doi: 10.11607/prd.3254. PMID: 29240212.

Bhushan, J., & Grover, V. (2019). Additive manufacturing: Current concepts, methods, and applications in oral health care. In: Prakash C. et al. (eds) *Biomanufacturing*. Springer, Cham.

Brain, M., Jimbo, R., & Wennenberg, A. (2016). Production tolerance of additive manufactured polymeric objects for clinical applications. *Dent Mater*, 32, 853–861.

Brown, C. (2015). Additive manufacturing: It's a positive thing. *Inside Dent Technol*, 6(3), 50–51.

Cassetta, M., Stefanelli, L.V., Pacifici, A., Pacifici, L., & Barbato, E. (2014). How accurate is CBCT in measuring bone density? A comparative CBCT-CT in vitro study. *Clin Implant Dent Relat Res*, 16(4), 471–478.

Chua, C.K., Chou, S.M., Lin, S.C., Eu, K.H., & Lew, K.H. (1998). Rapid prototyping assisted surgery planning. *Int J Adv Manuf Technol*, 14(9), 624–630.

Cooper, K. (2001). *Rapid Prototyping Technology*. Marcel Dekker, New York.

Correa, L.R., Spin-Neto, R., Stavropoulos, A., Schropp, L., da Silveira, H.E., & Wenzel, A. (2014). Planning of dental implant size with digital panoramic radiographs, CBCT-generated panoramic images, and CBCT cross-sectional images. *Clin Oral Implants Res*, 25(6), 690–695.

Cristache, C.M., & Silviu, G. (2017). Accuracy evaluation of a stereolithographic surgical template for dental implant insertion using 3D superimposition protocol. *Int J Dent*, 2017, 1–9 doi:10.1155/2017/4292081

D'Souza, K.M., & Aras, M.A. (2012). Types of implant surgical guides in dentistry: A review. *J Oral Implantol*, 38, 643–652.

Dawood, A., Marti, B., Sauret-Jackson, V., & Darwood, A. (2015). 3D printing in dentistry. *BrDent J*, 219(11), 521–525.

Deeb, G.R., Allen, R.K., Hall, V.P., Whitley III, D., Laskin, D.M., & Bencharit, S. (2017). How accurate are implant surgical guides produced with desktop stereolithographic 3-dimentional printers?. *J Oral and Maxillofac Surg*, 75(12), 2559–e1.

Di Giacomo, G.A., Cury, P.R., de Araujo, N.S., Sendyk, W.R., & Sendyk, C.L. (2005). Clinical application of stereolithographic surgical guides for implant placement: Preliminary results. *J Periodontol*, 76(4), 503–507.

Flowers, J., & Moniz, M. (2002). Rapid prototyping in technology education. *Technol Teach*, 62(3),7.

Frösch, L., Mukaddam, K., Filippi, A., Zitzmann, N.U., & Kühl, S. (2019). Comparison of heat generation between guided and conventional implant surgery for single and sequential drilling protocols-An in vitro study. *Clin Oral Implants Res*, 30(2), 121–130. doi:10.1111/clr.13398. Epub 2019 Jan 28. PMID: 30578579.

Ganz, S.D. (2015). Three-dimensional imaging and guided surgery for dental implants. *Dent Clin North Am*, 59, 265–290.

Geng, W., Liu, C., Su, Y., Li, J., & Zhou, Y. (2015). Accuracy of different types of computer-aided design/computer-aided manufacturing surgical guides for dental implant placement. *Int J Clin Exp Med*, 8(6), 8442.

Glossary of Prosthodontic Terms. (2005). *J Prosthet Dent*, 94, 10–92. [PubMed: 16080238].

Glossary of Prosthodontic Terms. (2017). 9th Ed. *J Prosthet Dent*, 117, e24.

Greenberg, A.M. (2015). Digital technologies for dental implant treatment planning and guided surgery. *Oral Maxillofac Surg Clin North Am*, 27, 319–340.

Guichet, D. (2015). Digitally enhanced dentistry: The power of digital design. *J Calif Dent Assoc*, 43(3), 135–141. PMID: 25864301.

Halloran, J.W., Tomeckova, V., Gentry, S., Das, S., Cilino, P., Yuan, D., Guo, R., ..., Long, D. (2011). Photopolymerization of powder suspensions for shaping ceramics. *J Eur Ceram Soc*, 31(14), 2613–2619.

Holst, S., Blatz, M.B., & Eitner, S. (2007). Precision for computer-guided implant placement: Using 3D planning software and fixed intraoral reference points. *J Oral Maxillofac Surg*, 65, 393–399.

Ide, Y., Nayar, S., Logan, H., Gallagher, B., & Wolfaardt, J. (2017). The effect of the angle of acuteness of additive manufactured models and the direction of printing on the dimensional fidelity: Clinical implications. *Odontology*, 105(1), 108–115. doi:10.1007/s10266-016-0239-4. Epub 2016 Mar 19. PMID: 26995273.

Jain, R., Bindra, S., & Gupta, K. (2016). Recent trends of 3-D printing in dentistry: A review. *Ann Prosthodont Restrorat Dent*, 2(4),101–104.

Jung, R.E., Schneider, D., Ganeles, J., Wismeijer, D., Zwahlem, M., Hämmerle, C.H., & Tahmaseb, A. (2009). Computer technology applications in surgical implant dentistry: A systematic review. *Int J Oral Maxillofac Implants*, 24, s92–109.

Kalra, M., Aparna, I.N., & Dhanasekar, B. (2013). Evolution of surgical guidance in implant dentistry. *Dent Update*, 40(7), 577–578, 581–582. doi: 10.12968/denu.2013.40.7.577. PMID: 24147389.

Klein, M., & Abrams, M. (2001). Computer-guided surgery utilizing a computer-milled surgical template. *Pract Periodontics Aesthet Dent*, 13, 165–169.

Kola, M.Z., Shah, A.H., Khalil, H.S., Rabah, A.M., Harby, N.M., Sabra, S.A., & Raghav, D. (2015). Surgical templates for dental implant positioning; current knowledge and clinical perspectives. *Niger J Surg*, 21, 1–5.

Kopp, K.C., Koslow, A.H., & Abdo, O.S. (2003). Predictable implant placement with a diagnostic/surgical template and advanced radiographic imaging. *J Prosthet Dent*, 89, 611–615.

Kruth, P.P. (1991). Material incress manufacturing by rapid prototyping techniques. *CIRP Ann Manuf Technol*, 40(2), 603–614

Kühl, S., Payer, M., Zitzmann, N.U., Lambrecht, J.T., & Filippi, A. (2015). Technical accuracy of printed surgical templates for guided implant surgery with the co diagnostic X TM software. *Clin Implant Dent Relat Res*, 17, e177–e182.

Kühl, S., Zürcher, S., Mahid, T., Müller-Gerbl, M., Filippi, A., & Cattin, P. (2013). Accuracy of full guided vs. half-guided implant surgery. *Clin Oral Implants Res*, 24, 763–769. doi:10.1111/j.1600-0501.2012.02484.x.

Kumar, M., Shanavas, M., Sidappa, A., & Kiran, M. (2015). Cone beam computed tomography – know its secrets. *J Int Oral Health*, 7(2), 64–68.

Lal, K., White, G.S., Morea, D.N., & Wright, R.F. (2006). Use of stereolithographic templates for surgical and prosthodontic implant planning and placement. *Part I. The concept. J Prosthodont*, 15, 51–58.

Le, B., & Nielsen, B. (2015). Esthetic implant site development. *Oral Maxillofac Surg Clin North Am*, 27, 283–311.

Lin, Y.K., Yau, H.T., Wang, I.C., Zheng, C., & Chung, K.H. (2015). A novel dental implant guided surgery based on integration of surgical template and augmented reality. *Clin Implant Dent Relat Res*, 17(3), 543–553.

Lingam, A.S., Reddy, L., Nimma, V., & Pradeep, K. (2013). Dental implant radiology- Emerging concepts in planning implants. *J Orofac Sci*, 5, 88–94.

Liu, Q., Leu, M.C., & Schmitt, S.M. (2006). Rapid prototyping in dentistry: Technology and application. *Int J Adv Manuf Technol*, 29, 317–335.

Loubele, M., Bogaerts, R., Van Dijck, E., Pauwels, R., Vanheusden, S., Suetens, P., ... Jacobs, R. (2009). Comparison between effective radiation dose of CBCT and MSCT scanners for dentomaxillofacial applications. *Eur J Radiol*, 71(3), 461–468.

Ma, B., Park, T., Chun, I., & Yun, K. (2018). The accuracy of a 3D printing surgical guide determined by CBCT and model analysis. *The J Advan Prosthodontics*, 10(4), 279–285. doi:10.4047/jap.2018.10.4.279

Marchack, C., & Moy, P. (2003). The use of a custom template for immediate loading with the definitive prosthesis: A clinical report. *J Calif Dent Assoc*, 31(12), 925–929.

Marchack, C.B. (2007). CAD/CAM-guided implant surgery and fabrication of an immediately loaded prosthesis for a partially edentulous patient. *J Prosthet Dent*, 97, 389–394.

Marchack, C.B., & Chew, L.K. (2015). The 10-year evolution of guided surgery. *J Calif Dent Assoc*, 43(3), 131–134. PMID: 25864300.

Matta, R.E., Bergauer, B., Adler, W., Wichmann, M., & Nickenig, H.J. (2017). The impact of the fabrication method on the three-dimensional accuracy of an implant surgery template. *J Cranio Maxillofac Surg*, 45, 804–808.

Mora, M.A., Chenin, D.L., & Arce, R.M. (2014). Software tools and surgical guides in dental-implant-guided surgery. *Dent Clin North Am*, 58(3), 597–626. doi:10.1016/j.cden.2014.04.001.PMID: 24993925.

Neumeister, A., Schulz, L., & Glodecki, C. (2017). Investigations on the accuracy of 3D printed drill guides for dental implantology. *Int J Comput Dent*, 20, 35–51.

Nikzad, S., & Azari, A. (2008). A novel stereolithographic surgical guide template for planning treatment involving a mandibular dental implant. *J Oral Maxillofac Surg*, 66, 1446–1454.

Noorani, R. (2006). *Rapid Prototyping—Principles and Applications*. Wiley, Hoboken.

Noort, R.V. (2012). The future of dental devices is digital. *Dent Mater*, 28, 3–12.

Omami, G., & Al Yafi, F. (2019). Should cone beam computed tomography be routinely obtained in implant planning? *Dent Clin North Am*, 63(3), 363–379. doi:10.1016/j.cden.2019.02.005. Epub 2019 Apr 12. PMID: 31097132.

Orentlicher, G., & Abboud, M. (2011). Guided surgery for implant therapy. *Oral Maxillofac Surg Clin North Am*, 23, 239–256.

Ozan, O., Turkyilmaz, I., Ersoy, A.E., McGlumphy, E.A., & Rosenstiel, S.F. (2009). Accuracy of three types of CT SLA surgical guides in implant placement. *J Oral Maxillofac Surg*, 67(2), 394–401.

Plooij, J.M., Maal, T.J., Haers, P., Borstlap, W.A., Kuijpers-Jagtman, A.M., & Bergé, S.J. (2011). Digital three-dimensional image fusion processes for planning and evaluating orthodontics and orthognathic surgery: A systematic review. *Int J Oral Maxillofac Surg*, 40(4), 341–352. doi:10.1016/j.ijom.2010.10.013. Epub 2010 Nov 20. PMID: 21095103.

Puebla, K., Arcaute, K., Quintana, R., & Wicker, R.B. (2012). Effects of environmental conditions, aging, and build orientations on the mechanical properties of ASTM type I specimens manufactured via stereolithography. *Rap Prototyp J*, 18 (5), 374–388. doi:10.1108/13552541211250373.

Ramasamy, M., Giri, R.R., Subramonian, K., & Narendrakumar, R. (2013). Implant surgical guides: From the past to the present. *J Pharm Bioallied Sci*, 5(Suppl 1), S98–S102. doi:10.4103/0975-7406.113306. PMID: 23946587; PMCID: PMC3722716.

Revilla-León, M., Sadeghpour, M., & Özcan, M. (2020). An update on applications of 3D printing technologies used for processing polymers used in implant dentistry. *Odontology*, 108(3), 331–338. doi:10.1007/s10266-019-00441-7. Epub 2019 Jul 1. PMID: 31264008.

Rosenfeld, A.L., Mandelaris, G.A., & Tardieu, P.B. (2006). Prosthetically directed implant placement using computer software to ensure precise placement and predictable prosthetic outcomes. Part 1: Diagnostics, imaging, and collaborative accountability. *Int J Periodontics Restor Dent*, 26, 215–221.

Salem, D. (2019). Surgical guides for dental implants; a suggested new classification. *J Dent Oral Health*, 6, 1–8.

Santis, D.D., Malchiodi, L., Cucchi, A., Cybulski, A., Verlato, G., Gelpi, F., & Nocini, P.F. (2019). The accuracy of computer-assisted implant surgery performed using fully guided templates versus pilot-drill guided templates. *BioMed Res Int*, 2019, 1–10. Article ID 9023548, doi:10.1155/2019/9023548

Sarment, D.P., Sukovic, P., & Clinthorne, N. (2003). Accuracy of implant placement with a stereolithographic surgical guide. *Int J Oral Maxillofac Implants*, 18(4), 571–577.

Scherer, U., Stoetzer, M., Ruecker, M., Gellrich, N.C., & von See, C. (2015). Template-guided vs. non-guided drilling in site preparation of dental implants. *Clin Oral Invest*, 19(6), 1339–1346.

Schneider, D., Schober, F., Grohmann, P., Hammerle, C.H., & Jung, R.E. (2015). In-vitro evaluation of the tolerance of surgical instruments in templates for computer-assisted guided implantology produced by 3-D printing. *Clin Oral Implants Res*, 26, 320–325.

Schneider, J., Decker, R., & Kalender, W.A. (2002). Accuracy in medicinal modelling. *Phidias Newsl*, 8, 5–14.

Schnutenhaus, S., Edelmann, C., Rudolph, H., Dreyhaupt, J., & Luthardt, R.G. (2018). 3D accuracy of implant positions in template-guided implant placement as a function of the remaining teeth and the surgical procedure: A retrospective study. *Clin Oral Investig*, 22(6), 2363–2372. doi:10.1007/s00784-018-2339-8. Epub 2018 Jan 22. PMID: 29356920.

See, C.V., & Meindorfer, M. (2016). 3D printing: Additive processes in dentistry. *Laboratory*, May 2016.

Shen, P., Zhao, J., Fan, L., Qiu, H., Xu, W., Wang, Y., Zhang, S., & Kim, Y.J. (2015). Accuracy evaluation of computer-designed surgical guide template in oral implantology. *J Cranio Maxillofac Surg*, 43(10), 2189–2194.

Siu, A.S., Chu, F.C., Li, T.K., Chow, T.W., & Deng, F.L. (2010) Imaging modalities for preoperative assessment in dental implant therapy: An overview. *Hong Kong Dent J*, 7, 23–30.

Smitkarn, P., Subbalekha, K., Mattheos, N., & Pimkhaokham, A. (2019). The accuracy of single-tooth implants placed using fully digital-guided surgery and freehand implant surgery. *J Clin Periodontol*, 46(9), 949–957. doi:10.1111/jcpe.13160. Epub 2019 Jul 19. PMID: 31241782.

Sommacal, B., Savic, M., Filippi, A., Kühl, S., & Thieringer, F.M. (2018). Evaluation of two 3D printers for guided implant surgery. *Int J Oral Maxillofac Implants*, 33, 743–746.

Spector, L. (2008). Computer-aided dental implant planning. *Dent Clin North Am*, 52, 761–775.

Stübinger, S., Buitrago-Tellez, C., & Cantelmi, G. (2014). Deviations between placed and planned implant positions: An accuracy pilot study of skeletally supported stereolithographic surgical templates. *Clin Implant Dent Relat Res*, 16(4), 540–551.

Stumpel, L.J. (2008). Cast-based guided implant placement: A novel technique. *J Prosthet Dent*, 100, 61–69.

Sykes, L.M., Parrott, A.M., Owen, C.P., & Snaddon, D.R. (2004). Applications of rapid prototyping technology in maxillofacial prosthetics. *Int J Prosthodont*, 17, 454–459.

Tapie, L., Lebon, N., Mawussi, B., Fron, H.C., Duret, F., & Attal, J.P. (2015). Understanding dental CAD/CAM for restorations—the digital workflow from a mechanical engineering view-point. *Int J Comput Dent*, 18, 21–44.

Tardieu, P.B., Vrielinck, L., & Escolano, E. (2003). Computer assisted implant placement. A case report: Treatment of the mandible. *Int J Oral Maxillofac Implants*, 18, 599–604.

Thakral, G., Thakral, R., Sharma, N., Seth, J., & Vashisht, P. (2014). Nanosurface – the future of implants. *J Clin Diagnostic Res: JCDR*, 8(5), ZE07–ZE10. doi:10.7860/JCDR/2014/8764.4355

Tyndall, D.A., Price, J.B., Tetradis, S., Ganz, S.D., Hildebolt, C., & Scarfe, W.C. (2012). Position statement of the American Academy of Oral and Maxillofacial Radiology on selection criteria for the use of radiology in dental implantology with emphasis on cone beam computed tomography. *Oral Surg Oral Med Oral Pathol Oral Radiol*, 113, 817–826.

Valente, F., Schiroli, G., & Sbrenna, A. (2009). Accuracy of computeraided oral implant surgery: A clinical and radiographic study. *Int J Oral Maxillofac Implants*, 24(2), 234–242.

Van Assche, N., Van Steenberghe, D., Guerrero, M.E., Hirsch, E., Schutyser, F., Quirynen, M., & Jacobs, R. (2007). Accuracy of implant placement based on pre-surgical planning of three-dimensional cone-beam images: A pilot study. *J Clin Periodontol*, 34(9), 816–821.

Van Assche, N., Vercruyssen, M., Coucke, W., Teughels, W., Jacobs, R., & Quirynen, M. (2012). Accuracy of computer-aided implant placement. *Clin Oral Implants Res*, 23, 112–123.

Van Steenberghe, D., Naert, I., Andersson, M., Brajnovic, I., Van Cleynenbreugel, J., & Suetens, P. (2002). A custom template and definitive prosthesis allowing immediate implant loading in the maxilla: A clinical report. *Int J Oral Maxillofac Implants*, 17(5), 663–670.

Varga, E. Jr, Antal, M., Major, L., Kiscsatári, R., Braunitzer, G., & Piffkó, J. (2020). Guidance means accuracy: A randomized clinical trial on freehand versus guided dental implantation. *Clin Oral Implants Res*, 31(5), 417–430. doi:10.1111/clr.13578. Epub 2020 Jan 31. PMID: 31958166.

Vercruyssen, M., Hultin, M., Van Assche, N., Svensson, K., Naert, I., & Quirynen, M. (2014). Guided surgery: Accuracy and efficacy. *Periodontol*, 2000, 66(1), 228–246.

Verhamme, L.M., Meijer, G.J., Boumans, T., Schutyser, F., Bergé, S.J., & Maal, T.J. (2013). A clinically relevant validation method for implant placement after virtual planning. *Clin Oral Implants Res*, 24 (11), 1265–1272.

Whitley III, D., Eidson, R.S., Rudek, I., & Bencharit, S. (2017). In-office fabrication of dental implant surgical guides using desktop stereolithographic printing and implant treatment planning software: A clinical report. *J Prosthet Dent*, 118(3), 256–263. doi:10.1016/j.prosdent.2016.10.017. Epub 2017 Feb 20. PMID: 28222882.

Wohlers, T., & Gornet, T. (2014) History of additive manufacturing. *Wohlers Rep*. http://wohlersassociates.com/history2014.pdf

Wong, K.V., & Herndez, A. (2012). A review of additive manufacturing. *ISRN Mech Eng*, 2012, 1–10. doi:10.5402/2012/208760 (Article ID 208760).

Yafi, A.F., Camenisch, B., & Al-Sabbagh, M. (2019). Is digital guided implant surgery accurate and reliable?. *Dent Clin North Am*, 63(3), 381–397.

Younes, F., Cosyn, J., De Bruyckere, T., Cleymaet, R., Bouckaert, E., & Eghbali, A. (2018). A randomized controlled study on the accuracy of free-handed, pilot-drill guided and fully guided implant surgery in partially edentulous patients. *J Clin Periodontol*, 45(6), 721–732. doi:10.1111/jcpe.12897. Epub 2018 May 10. PMID: 29608793.

Zhou, Z., Buchanan, F., Mitchell, C., & Dunne, N. (2014). Printability of calcium phosphate: Calcium sulfate powders for the application of tissue engineered bone scaffolds using the 3D printing technique. *Mater Sci Eng C Mater Biol Appl*, 38, 1–10.

5 Materials for 3D Printing in Medicine

Metals, Polymers, Ceramics, Hydrogels

Kamal Kishore, Roopak Varshney, Param Singh, and Manoj Kumar Sinha

National Institute of Technology Hamirpur, Hamirpur, India

CONTENTS

5.1 INTRODUCTION

Nowadays, technological advances have led to the development of a modern technologically driven society where demands are inclined towards personalisation rather than mass customisation. This results in the integration of cyber-physical systems into the conventional manufacturing practices eventually leading to the evolution of

DOI: 10.1201/9781003301066-5

additive manufacturing. Additive manufacturing (AM) is not new in the manufacturing domain; earlier it was popular as rapid prototyping (RP) and 3D printing. The development of new materials, advanced tools and more user-friendly design software has increased the application domain of AM. These developments help in establishing the AM as a complete manufacturing process. As adopted by the American Society for Testing and Materials (ASTM), 'AM is a regenerative process of direct printing physical models from designing software using layer-by-layer fabrication techniques.' AM's flexible and versatile nature has rapidly increased its demands in almost every sector. Specifically, in the medical field, AM has been adopted for organ printing, implant printing and so on (Banga et al., 2021). A wide range of materials including metal powders, polymers, hydrogels, ceramics, nanocomposites and living cells are widely used in AM. Specifically, with the development of biocompatible and printable materials, AM provides tremendous opportunities for its application in the medical industry (Banga et al., 2017a, 2017b). Additionally, AM is also a pioneer in surgical planning, organ printing, the printing of implants and drug delivery systems. The application of AM is also being extended in medical education and research. Figure 5.1 represents a few specific uses of AM in the biomedical field.

5.2 BIOMATERIALS

In the twenty-first century, scientists and researchers' focus is shifted toward the development of biodegradable materials rather than the utilisation of traditional materials such as steel, polymer, etc., for medical applications. It can be achieved either by altering the properties of traditional materials by alloying them or developing a unique multi-material mixture for surface treatment by various coating techniques. Especially for the medical field, biomaterial must have properties such as high biocompatibility with living cells (bioactive glass and hydrogel), ease of manufacturing, high durability and ductility. The biomedical field is patient-specific. Therefore, there is an urgent need to manufacture medical devices, implants, delivery systems, stents, scaffolds, etc., which should be individual-specific (Banga et al., 2014, 2018). AM techniques, at this point, provide an attractive and ultimate solution. The different types of biomaterials with their uses in the biomedical field and corresponding AM techniques used for their fabrication are presented in Table 5.1.

5.3 METALS

In old age, health problems like bone fracture and tissue losses are more common. These problems require metals for fixation, replacement and reconstruction of tissue and bone. These metals provide support to the patient for immediate mobilisation (Niinomi, 2007). Metals and their alloys have better mechanical characteristics such as high strength, high elasticity, better anti-wear and corrosion resistance. Nowadays, around 75 per cent of medically used implants are made of metals like stainless steel, titanium alloys (Banerjee & Williams, 2013), cobalt-chromium alloys (Hsu et al., 2005), niobium, nitinol and tantalum (Black, 1994). But in recent years,

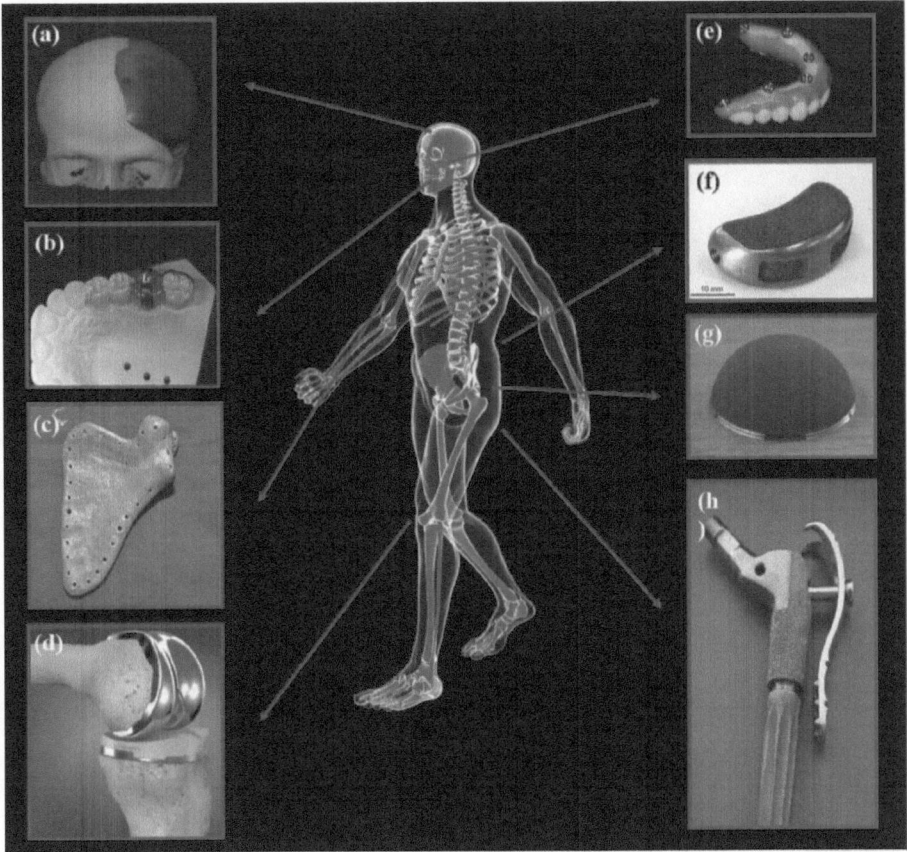

FIGURE 5.1 The biomedical application of 3D printing of bio-metals includes (a) cranial prosthesis (b) surgical guide; (c) scapula prosthesis; (d) knee prosthesis; (e) dental implants; (f) interbody fusion cage; (g) acetabular cup; and (h) hip prosthesis(Ni et al., 2019).

biodegradable metals such as magnesium (N. Li & Zheng, 2013), zinc (Xiang et al., 2014), iron (Vorndran et al., 2011) and calcium are more in use for the manufacturing of implants. Table 5.2 presents a brief of different types of metals used in the biomedical field. For medical applications, AM-based metal and their alloys are classified into three groups as mentioned below:

  i. Conventional metals and their alloys
 ii. Biodegradable metals
iii. Shape-memory alloys

5.3.1 Conventional Metals and Their Alloys

Different metals in the form of high-quality metal powder such as titanium alloys, stainless steel, aluminium, cobalt, etc. are used in AM for biomedical applications.

TABLE 5.1

Different Types of Materials Used in the Biomedical Field with Their Printing AM Techniques (Tappa & Jammalamadaka, 2018)

Type	AM Techniques	Application	Advantages	Limitations
Metals and their alloy e.g. stainless steel, nickel, aluminium, tungsten	SLS, SLM, LDMD, SEBM, LIFT, NPJ	Hip implants, acetabular cups, rod inserts, knee and shoulder implants, orthopaedic tools	High-quality surface, easy to fabricate, good mechanical properties	Corrosive, non-biodegradable
Ceramics e.g. calcium phosphate, glass, oxide of aluminium and titanium	Extrusion printing, DLP, TPP, inkjet printing	Implant coating, scaffolds, dental implants, bone implants	High material strength, corrosion resistance and biocompatibility	Excessive elastic modulus and difficult to mould
Polymers e.g. polycaprolactone, polycarbonates, polyurethanes, PLA	FDM, SLA, inkjet printing, extrusion	Drug delivery systems, prostheses	Easily mouldable and readily available, biodegradable, biocompatible and suitable mechanical strength	Leachable in body fluids and hard to sterilise
Hydrogels e.g. natural, synthetic and composite	SLA, inkjet printing, FDM and laser-based	Drugs delivery system, scaffold, synthetic ECM and biosensors	Biocompatible, biodegradable	Brittle, fragile, poor and mechanical strength

Titanium and its alloys are the most commercially used metals in the biomedical field because of their biocompatibility. In 1970 for the first time, titanium was used for biomedical applications due to its favourable mechanical characteristics. Titanium is mainly used to make artificial hearts, joints, and cardiac valve prostheses (Khorasani et al., 2015). Nowadays, Ti6Al4V and pure titanium (CP-Ti) almost covers 90 per cent of the traditional orthopaedic implants. Hollander et al. (2006) made vertebra with Ti6Al4V alloy through selective laser melting (SLM) techniques. The outcome of the study showed that Ti6Al4V has good biocompatibility and can be used to replace biological parts of the human body. In 2015, for the first time a successfully printed 3D-printed titanium prosthesis was implanted into the palm (Punyaratabandhu et al., 2017).

Tantalum finds its wide application starting in the 1940s in the orthopaedic and dental fields because of its good chemical stability and biocompatibility. However, the use of tantalum is limited because of the difficulty in fabrication and associated high manufacturing costs (Balla et al., 2010). In comparison, porous tantalum is mainly used for bone graft substitute and in surgery of the hip, knee and spinal prostheses. Both solid and porous tantalum parts are fabricated by new AM techniques

TABLE 5.2
Different Types of Metals Used in the Biomedical Field

Name	Properties	AM Techniques	Biomedical Use	References
Titanium and its alloy	Excellent biocompatibility, high ratio strength and good corrosion resistance	SLM, EBM	Bone screws and plates, dental and orthopaedic implants, artificial hearts, artificial joints, cardiac valve prostheses, pacemakers and cornea backplates	Banerjee & Williams (2013)
Tantalum	Good chemical stability and excellent biocompatibility	Spark plasma sintering and SLM	Radiographic bone markers, nerve repair, vascular clips and cranial-defect repair	Black (1994)
Cobalt-chromium alloy	Excellent corrosion resistance, high strength, high-temperature resistance, excellent wear resistance and outstanding biocompatibility	SLM	Dental and oral applications (teeth), artificial joints	Hsu et al. (2005)
Magnesium	Biocompatible with human bone and biodegradable	Laser powder bed fusion, SLM	Bone screws, cardiovascular stents and bone plates	N. Li & Zheng (2013)
Iron	Biodegradable and non-toxic	Direct metal printing (DMP), inkjet printing	Scaffolds and stents implants.	Vorndran et al. (2011)
Zinc	Antiatherogenic, non-toxic, antibacterial and biodegradable	SLM	Cardiovascular stents and dental implants	Xiang et al. (2014)
Liquid metals (mercury, gallium, francium, caesium and rubidium)	High thermal and electrical conductivity, high surface tension, extremely low evaporation and chemical stability	Metal jet printing	Nerve connection and repair, tumour treatment and human skin	Yi & Liu (2017)

such as laser engineered net shaping (LENS) (Balla et al., 2010) and SLM (Wauthle et al., 2015). The first surgery for implementing a 3D-printed tantalum artificial joint to repair a deficient knee joint of an 84-year-old male patient's body was successfully done in the year 2017 (Ni et al., 2019).

Cobalt-chromium alloys are extensively used specifically in oral and dental bio-fields (Sinnett-Jones et al., 2005). The application of these alloys is preferred where a nickel-free component is required. The part fabricated by Co-Cr has excellent mechanical properties like high strength, outstanding wear resistance, high-temperature resistance and excellent biocompatibility (Niinomi et al., 2015).

5.3.2 Biodegradable Metals (BMs)

The metals which are expected to decay gradually in the body after completing their task without having any side effects on the host are termed biodegradable metals. According to ASTM-F3160 standards, 'the term absorbable metallic material is equivalent to biodegradable metals'. The BMs are generally classified into three types. They are (Qin et al., 2019; Zheng et al., 2014):

   i. Mg-based BMs (high biocompatibility)
  ii. Fe-based BMs (high strength and easy to manufacture)
 iii. Zn-based BMs (lower corrosion rates).

5.3.2.1 Mg-based BMs

In 1878, Edward Huse investigated Mg for clinical use. He successfully stopped haemorrhaging blood vessels through the use of pure Mg wire (Witte, 2010). For the first time in 1990, Payr utilised tubular Mg connectors for anastomosis of vessels (Witte, 2010). Its demand increased due to the high biocompatibility, but at the same time, its low strength is a matter of concern. To improve its ductility, strength and biocompatibility, many other materials are alloyed with it. Mg alloys such as Mg-Zn, Mg-Ca, Mg-Si, Mg-Mn, Mg-Ag, and Mg-RE (rare earth metals such as Nd, Y etc.) are now an attractive solution for the biodegradable implants.

5.3.2.2 Zn-based BMs

Zinc is an essential element of the human body because it is involved directly in nucleic acid metabolism, enzyme synthesis, signal transition, gene expression, tissue generation and apoptosis regulation. Demir et al. (2017) proposed a parameter for fabricating biodegradable pure Zn implants using the SLM process. The fabrication of degradable medical implants (cardiovascular stent and dental implant) made by zinc has an ideal degradation rate compared to iron and magnesium-based implants.

5.3.2.3 Fe-based BMs

The root of using Fe as an implant is dated back to 200AD when a human body with an iron dental implant was found in Europe. Many doctors used the Fe wires as sutures and for fracture fixation in the seventeenth century. Iron's mechanical strength is one of the best characteristics of its application in the biomedical field. However, its slow degradation rate and ferromagnetic characteristics sometimes cause infection in the body parts which presents a negative essence on its biocompatibility (Ratner et al., 2004). Hence many pieces of research were carried out to develop Fe-based alloys with modified chemical and microstructure compositions. Fe-Mn, binary Fe-X (X= Mn, Co, Al, W, Sn, B, C, S) Fe-Mn-Pd, Fe-Mn-Si are some examples.

5.3.3   SHAPE-MEMORY ALLOYS (SMA)

Shape-memory alloys are smart materials which may be defined as materials having the ability to change their strength, execute and control movement, generate signals due to changes in geometry or property when exposed to external stimuli such as heat, magnetic field, etc. There are two stable phases for shape-memory alloys; one is at a high temperature called austenite and the other at a low temperature called martensite (Mantovani, 2000). Firstly in 1938, copper-zinc alloy and copper-tin alloy were developed as shape-memory alloys by Greninger and Mooradian. Initially, the pace of research and development related to SMA was slow and therefore it took nearly 30 years to patent the first SMA (Mehl et al., 1938). Further, in 1965, Buehler and his co-worker developed a nitinol (nickel-titanium) based smart alloy in a naval ordnance laboratory and named it (Heilig, 1994). Consequently, some other smart metal alloys were also developed in due time, such as copper-aluminium-nickel, copper-zinc-aluminium and iron-manganese-silicon. Still, NiTi alloy is widely used due to its biocompatibility and high strength. The nickel-titanium alloys can be produced by vacuum melting techniques such as electron-beam melting and vacuum induction melting (Mahan, 2019). However, its processing is very difficult as it is externally compositional sensitive and also the machinability of such SMA is relatively poor. Hence, AM technologies such as SLM are being considered as potential solutions to fabricate parts from NiTi alloys. NiTi is used to make bone clamps, stents, catch baskets for kidney stones, metal guide wires, orthodontics, etc. (Strittmatter et al., 2019).

5.4   CERAMICS

Ceramics have exceptional properties over other materials such as high hardness, high stiffness, wear resistance, corrosion resistance and chemically stability. Most importantly, ceramics have a unique property to withstand high temperatures up to or well above 2000°C. These materials also possess high compressive strength and high hot strength which enable them to be widely used in manufacturing the products to be harsh working conditions. Low tensile strength, high cost, and difficulty in forming are a few equally significant limitations that limit the fabrication of ceramics parts through conventional processes such as ceramics injection moulding. The application of AM technology in ceramics can solve these problems to some extent. As per the literature, For the first time, AM technique was used for ceramics in the 1990s. The 3D printing of ceramics generally required clay-based formulation as ceramics undergoes plastic deformation when mixed with an organic or aqueous medium. Also, sometimes curable monomers resin is added with ceramics to provide sufficient green strength to the manufactured part. Despite the accuracy or flexibility of AM technology, material selection limitation is always a concern as sintering is generally used for post-processing of the 3D-printed ceramics part, which is costly

TABLE 5.3

Different Types of Ceramics Feedstock forms Used for Different AM Techniques (Z. Chen et al., 2019)

Feedstock Form	Ceramic 3D Printing Technology Type
Slurry-based	Stereolithography
	Digital light processing
	Two-photon polymerisation
	Inkjet printing
	Direct ink writing
Powder-based	Three-dimensional printing
	Selective laser sintering
	Selective laser melting
Bulk solid-based	Laminated object manufacturing
	Fused deposition modelling

and time-consuming. Inkjet (suspension), powder bed fusion, stereolithography and paste extrusion are a few commonly used methods for 3D printing of ceramics. 3D-printing technologies used for ceramics with their feedstock form are illustrated in Table 5.3.

5.4.1 BIOCERAMICS

The ceramics used for the repair or replacement of the damaged parts of the body is termed bioceramics. Generally, bioceramics are of two types (Jayaswal et al., 2010):

   i. Bioinert ceramics
   ii. Bioactive glass and glass ceramics.

5.4.1.1 Bioinert Ceramics

The first use of bioinert ceramics as a biomaterial for humans and animals was patented by Rock in 1933 in Germany. This patent mainly consists of the detail about alpha-alumina. These materials are of high strength compared to other forms of bioceramics. This patent remained in shadow until 1965 when CBS's clinical use in the dental implant system was introduced by Sandhaus in 1965 (Jayaswal et al., 2010). Zirconia and alumina are frequently used as bioinert ceramics for prosthetic devices (Koch et al., 2012). Generally, bioinert ceramics are divided into two categories (Corrado, 2017): oxide and non-oxide. Oxide bioinert ceramics are widely used as a biomaterial due to their properties like resistance to corrosion, low wear volume and static nature of wear debris. These are commonly used in hip and knee replacements. Ceramics of carbon and nitrides fall under non-oxide bioinert ceramics. They are generally used as a coating for biometals to improve their surface integrity. The details of different types of bioinert ceramics and their uses are shown in Table 5.4.

TABLE 5.4
Different Types of Bioinert Ceramics with Their Biomedical Uses (Corrado, 2017)

Materials		Biomedical Applications
Oxides	Alumina	Ball heads and inserts for THR bearings
	Zirconia	Dental implants, dental blanks for CAD/CAM
	ZTA/ATZ	The ball head and inserts for THR bearings, knee replacements, components for disc replacement, hip resurfacing
Non-Oxides	Carbon	Heart valves, haemo-compatible coating
	Diamond-like carbon	Coating of bearing component in joint replacement
	Titanium nitride	Coating in joint replacement
	Zirconium nitride	Coating in knee replacement
	Silicon nitride	Spinal cages, ball head and inserts for THR bearings, components for knee replacement, dental implants

5.4.1.2 Bioactive Glass or Glass-ceramics

Glass-ceramics are preferably used for support of other biomaterials. The term bioactive indicates the ability of the material to form bonds with the bones. For specific material, the level of bioactivity indicates the time taken by more than 50 per cent of the interface to form bonds with the bone (Juhasz & Best, 2012). The bioactivity index is denoted as I_B which is calculated as $I_B = 100/t_{0.5bb}$, where $t_{0.5bb}$ = time taken by more than 50 per cent of the interface to form bonds with the bone (Jones, 2007). Table 5.5 indicates the types of bioactive material based on I_B:

In the 1970s, Professor L.L. Hench discovered the particular types of glass that contain SiO_2, CaO, Na_2O, P_2O_5, B_2O_3 and CaF_2 in a specified proportion. These were the first material that forms a bond with both the hard and soft tissue of living beings. Hence, they are termed bioactive glasses (El-Ghannam & Ducheyne, 2017). Two techniques are generally applied to manufacture these bioactive glasses namely: the sol-gel technique and the derived melt technique (X. Chen et al., 2008, Hupa, 2011). Table 5.6 gives details about some bioglass samples manufactured by these two techniques. The bioactive glass particles were first marketed in 1993 under the name of Perioglass. These glasses generally have brittle nature and have poor mechanical strength. Generally, the bioactive glasses were so designed that they contain minerals like calcium and phosphorous in large amounts. They can form hydroxyapatite or

TABLE 5.5
Classification of Bioactive Materials Based on Their I_B Value (Jones, 2007)

I_B Value	Material Class	Examples
$I_B > 8$	Class A (form bond with both hard and soft tissues)	Bioactive glass
$0 < I_B \leq 8$	Class B (form bond with hard tissues)	SHA (sintered hydroxyapatite)

TABLE 5.6
Different Types of Bioglass with Their Composition and Manufacturing Technique (Catteaux & Grattepanche-Lebecq, 2013)

Sr.No.	Sample Bioglass	Method	Composition
Sol-gel synthesis (Low temperature)			
1	Si47C	HCL catalyst	21.5%Na_2O-26.5% CaO-5% P_2O_5-47% SiO_2
2	Si47N	HNO3 catalyst	21.5%Na_2O-26.5% CaO-5% P_2O_5-47% SiO_2
3	Si47PST	Organic	48% CaO-5% P_2O_5-47% SiO_2
4	Si47PSQ	Organic	21.5% Na_2O-26.5% CaO-5% P_2O_5-47% SiO_2
5	Si47M	Melting	21.5% Na_2O-26.5% CaO-5% P_2O_5-47% SiO_2
Melt quench synthesis (high temperature)			
1	45S5	Melting	24.5% Na_2O-24.5% CaO-6% P_2O_5-45% SiO_2
2	52S4.6	Melting	21% Na_2O-21% CaO-6% P_2O_5-52% SiO_2
3	55S4.3	Melting	19.5% Na_2O-19.5% CaO-6% P_2O_5-55% SiO_2

carbonate hydroxyapatite like layers on their surfaces when they are in use. These layers ensure a robust and stable chemical bond between tissues and implants. The bioactive glasses are usually used in addition to biometals, either in composites or coatings.

5.5 POLYMERS

The polymer is a Greek term made by two words 'polus' meaning many and 'meros' meaning part or piece. Hermann Staudinger in his macromolecular hypothesis defines polymers as macromolecules that consist of a large number of structural units connected by many covalent bonds (Jones et al., 2008). But at that time, he was heavily criticised by the scientific community for his hypothesis, but today's human existence cannot be imagined without polymers (Günay et al., 2013). Figure 5.2 represents the percentage contribution of polymers in different AM processes.

According to the International Union of Pure and Applied Chemistry (IUPAC), a polymer can be defined as 'a molecule of high relative molecular mass, the structure of which essentially comprises the multiple repetitions of the unit derived, actually or conceptually, from molecules of low relative molecular mass'(Jones et al., 2008). Major classifications of the polymer are based on the source of their extraction processes which are natural polymers and synthetic polymers. Details of both types of polymers (types, manufacturing method, biomedical use and AM techniques) are shown in Tables 5.7 and 5.8, respectively. The AM technologies used to print 3D products using polymer-based powders, liquid resins, filaments and films are described in Figure 5.3. A few essential characteristics of polymers are listed below as (Puppi & Chiellini, 2020):

i. Polymers can be soluble or insoluble in a solution
ii. Chemically stable and viscoelastic

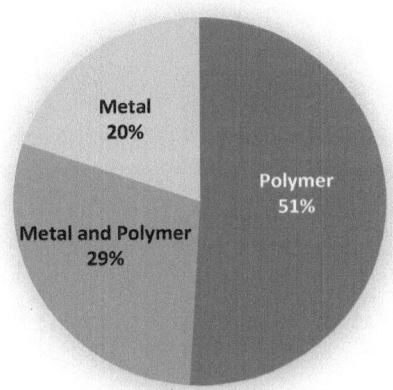

FIGURE 5.2   Parts currently produced by AM systems in the industry (Wohlers, 2013).

   iii.   Due to their cross-link nature, they can be easily formulated into the gel
   iv.   Ability to bind the component and material due to their adhesive nature
   v.   Low density and higher strain at failure.

5.5.1   SHAPE-MEMORY POLYMERS (SMPs)

Shape-memory polymers were initially commercialised in the 1990s and have some ability similar to that of SMAs. The demand for thermally stimuli polymers in industries and research multiplied many folds than any other external stimuli polymers. In thermally induced polymers, temperature plays a vital role in the switching shape-memory effect (Sabahi et al., 2020). Temperature is commonly associated with either melting temperature or transition temperature of the polymers. As compared to smart alloys, whose recoverable strain value is 8 per cent, the recoverable strain value for SMPs is even greater than 200 per cent. The AM techniques such as stereolithography (SLA) based on photo-polymerisation and fused deposition (FDM) are commonly used for manufacturing 3D-printed parts of SMPs. Zarek et al. (2016) made a personalised tracheal stent using synthesised polycaprolactone (PCL) dimethacrylate shape-memory resins using the SLA technique. Senatov et al. (2017) conducted several experiments to study the shape-memory effect and mechanical property of PLA hydroxyapatite and PLA (pure) by pining bone scaffolds using the FDM technique. This polymer responds to changes in temperature, pH, electric field and light intensity promptly. Based on stimuli and functionality, these polymers are classified into three categories (Pattanashetti et al., 2017):

   I. PH sensitive
   II. Thermosensitive
   III. Stimuli-responsive
        a. Light
        b. Electro field
        c. Magnetic.

TABLE 5.7
Polymers Obtained from Nature with Their Biomedical Uses

Type		Source of Extraction	Biomedical Use	AM Techniques	References
Proteins	Collagen	Bovine or porcine skin, Achilles' tendon of bovine or equine	Skin repair, blood vessel, bone and cartilage	Binder jet and SE-AM	Dhand et al. (2016)
	Gelatine	Denaturation of collagen by hydrolysis of the amide group	Biological glues, haemostatic sponges and insulin	SE-AM and SLA	Yamada et al. (1997)
	Fibrin	Blood	Adhesives for skin graft attachment, haemostats in surgery and sealants in colostomy closure	Bioprinting and inkjet printing	Spotnitz (2010)
	Silk Fibroin	Extraction from the protein fibre formed by silkworms and spiders	Wound dressing, sutures, scaffolds and haemostatic devices	SE-AM and SLA	Kundu et al. (2013)
Poly-saccharides	Alginate	Found in marine brown algae (Ascophyllum nodosum, Laminaria hyperborea) and soil bacteria (e.g. Azotobacter vinelandii)	Wound healing, drug delivery and tissue engineering	SE-AM and SLA	Nair & Laurencin (2007)
	Chitosan	Extract from the exoskeleton of crustaceans, insects and some fungi	Chitosan-based scaffolds for various human tissue engineering, including bone, cartilage, skin, liver and nerve	SE-AM and SLA	Croisier & Jérôme (2013)
	Plant and Bacterial Cellulose	Extracted from lignocellulosic material in forests, algae, agricultural residues, bacteria biosynthesis, and chemical synthesis	Wound dressing and bone engineering	SE-AM, ME-AM, FDM and SLA	Sulaeva et al. (2015)
	Hyaluronic Acid	Found in animal tissues or microbial fermentation	Reconstruction surgery, tissue augmentation, ophthalmic surgery and TE and cells encapsulation	SE-AM and SLA	Highley et al. (2016)
Microbial Polyesters or Polyhydroxyalkanoates (PHA)		Formed by gram-negative bacteria and gram-positive	Orthopaedic screws, scaffolds, implantable, injectable systems for drug delivery and skin patches	SLS, ME-AM and SE-AM	Nigmatullin et al. (2015)

TABLE 5.8

Polymer Made by Synthesis Processes with Their Biomedical Uses

Types		Processing Method	Biomedical Use	AM Techniques	References
Poly (ε-caprolactone) (PCL)		Synthesised by ROP of ε-caprolactone monomer in presence of higher alcohol by using tin bis (2-ethyl hexanoate) (stannous octoate) as the catalyst	Polymeric rods, contraceptive implants, fixation devices and tissue repairing patches	ME-AM, SE-AM, SLS and SLA	Manavitehrani et al. (2016)
Poly (α-hydroxy acids)	Poly(lactide) (PLA)	Synthesised by ring-opening polymerisation of dilactide (3,6-dimethyl-p-dioxane-2,5- dione), the cyclic dimer of lactic acid	Long-lasting sutures, suture reinforcements, suture anchors, meniscal darts, tissue regeneration barrier, osteosynthesis, and orthopaedic fixation	ME-AM, SE-AM, SLS, BJ and SLA	Doppalapudi et al. (2014)
	Poly(glycolide) (PGA)	Synthesised by ROP of glycolide, the cyclic dimer of glycolic acid	Internal bone pins and drug delivery systems	FDM	Burns (1995), Banga et al. (2020a, 2020b)
Polypropylene fumarate (PPF)		Two-step reaction of DEF and propylene glycol through a bis(hydroxypropyl) fumarate diester intermediate	Tissue repairing and helps in bone-forming cell	SLA and SE-AM	Yaszemski et al. (1995)
Polyurethanes (PUs)		Obtained by the reaction of an aliphatic or aromatic diisocyanate, a macrodiol and a chain extender such as diol or a diamine.	Manufacturing of elastics and cavity liners for dentistry, cardiovascular catheters and cardiac valves, breast implants, wound dressing membranes, bone adhesives, and condoms	ME-AM and SE-AM	Alves (2012)
Poly (trimethylene carbonate) (PTMC)		Synthesised by ring-opening polymerisation of trimethylene carbonate	Soft tissue engineering, development of copolymer generally with glycolides, flexible suture and orthopaedic screw	SLA and FDM	Brannigan & Dove (2017)
Poly (vinyl alcohol) (PVA)		Free-radical polymerisation of vinyl acetate, followed by alkaline hydrolysis (alcoholysis) of polyvinyl acetate	Water treatment, detergent products and food packaging	BJ, SE-AM and ME-AM	Chong et al. (2013)

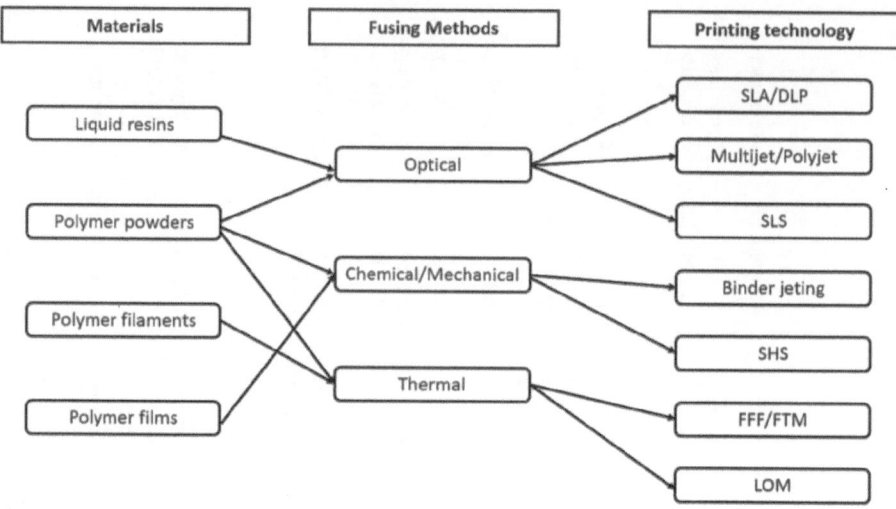

FIGURE 5.3 Overview of type of polymers material, mechanisms and AM methods (Stansbury & Idacavage, 2016).

5.6 HYDROGELS AND THEIR TYPE

The hydrogel is a mixture of polymer, organic compound, or cell with water. It appeared to be a solid jelly-like material due to the 3D-crosslinked network structure present in it (Hoffman, 2012). This network structure helps to retain the liquid part in the form of gel where liquid prevents the network from collapsing. At the gel point condition, the hydrogels abruptly changed into a solid phase and appeared like soft tissue (Gerlach & Arndt, 2009). The hydrogels are widely used in biocompatible applications such as in tissue engineering (Drury & Mooney, 2003; Lee & Mooney, 2001; Banga et al., 2020c, 2020d, 2020e), delivery systems (drug, cell, protein, and gene) (Hamidi et al., 2008; Jabbari et al., 2016), microfluidics (Dong & Jiang, 2007), making of synthetic extracellular matrix (ECM) (Kharkar et al., 2013; Seliktar, 2012), biosensors (Culver et al., 2017; Jung et al., 2017) and regenerative medicines (Annabi et al., 2014). As hydrogels are delicate, the printing techniques used for hydrogels have a slightly mild condition than other printing materials with some modifications in the printing machines. Hydrogels are classified based on their physical properties, sources, cross-linking type, synthetic method and degradation rate. The classification of hydrogels based on the source is shown in Figure 5.4.

As the name suggests, natural polymer hydrogels are obtained from living organisms such as plants, animals and micro-organisms; hence they are also called biopolymers. They have excellent biocompatibility and cell affinity (Francis et al., 2016; Kirchmajer et al., 2015). Synthetic polymer hydrogels are synthesised from their monomers' units and are primarily based on the synthesis method. They are of four types: homopolymer hydrogels; copolymer hydrogels; multipolymer hydrogels; and interpenetrating polymer hydrogels (Kumar & Erothu, 2016). The most commonly used synthetic polymers are poly (ethylene glycol) hydrogels (PEG) in

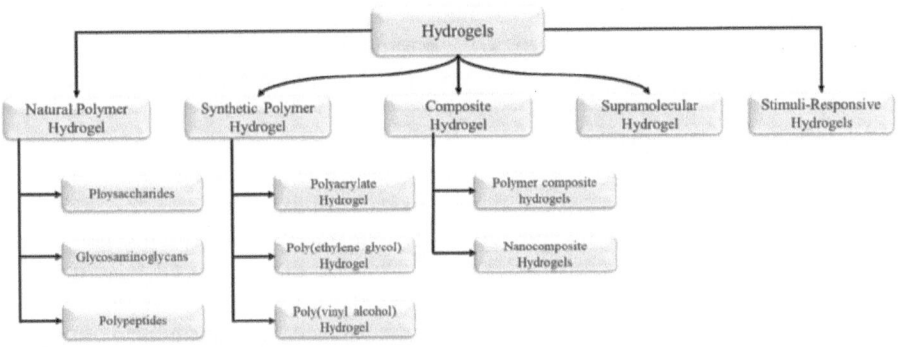

FIGURE 5.4   Different types of hydrogel.

the biomedical domain (see Tables 5.7 and 5.8 for the broad classification of natural and synthetic polymers). The natural and synthetic polymer hydrogels are brittle, fragile and weak in mechanical strength; therefore, to improve hydrogels' mechanical properties, composite hydrogels are introduced. They are prepared by blending two types of hydrogels such as natural-natural polymer hydrogels (Gellan gum-carrageenan, Dextran-hyaluronic acid) (Fernández-Ferreiro et al., 2015), natural-synthetic polymer hydrogels (Alginate-PAAm, Dextran-PEG) (T. Li et al., 2017) and synthetic-synthetic polymer hydrogels (PVA-PAA, PAAm-PVA) (Liu et al., 2018). The inorganic nanomaterial has excellent mechanical strength as compared to organic polymer hydrogels. The organic-inorganic hybrid nanocomposite is found everywhere in nature. These are also quite common in bone, teeth and nacre. To replicate the excellent mechanical properties of these nanocomposites, hydrogels are introduced. Nanocomposite hydrogels are a hybrid mixture of organic and inorganic material that is physically or chemically cross-linked together and have inorganic nanomaterial as a functional group. They are extensively used in bone regeneration, making biosensors and drug delivery systems, etc. (Schexnailder & Schmidt, 2009).

Supramolecular hydrogels and stimuli-responsive hydrogels are dynamic nature hydrogels that are closer to biological function. Supramolecular (cyclodextrin-based host-guest supramolecular hydrogels system) has properties such as self-healing adaptability, molecular recognition and bio-adhesive (Feng et al., 2016). Whereas the hydrogels in which polymer networks respond to the environmental condition such as temperature, light, pH changes, enzymes fall under stimuli-responsive hydrogels some examples are gelatin, agarose, etc. (Crompton et al., 2007; Qu et al., 2017).

5.6.1   Bio-inks and Biomaterials Inks

For 3D printing of functional biological products, the materials that are generally used are termed 'bio-ink'. This term was introduced in 2003 along with the term 'biopaper'. The concept was that the hydrogels in which living cells or tissues were inserted are termed biopaper and living cells or tissues are called bio-ink. But with the development of bioprinting, the adaption of new printing principles and under-standing of the rheological properties of printing materials consequently unified the whole concept of bio-ink (Mironov, 2003). The bio-inks are generally divided into four types: support bio-inks, fugitive bio-inks, structural bio-inks and functional bio-inks (Williams et al., 2018).

The other term, biomaterials inks, can be defined as the biomaterial that can be printed and then planted with the living cell called biomaterial inks, as shown in Figure 5.5. These materials are generally sacrificial and their importance gets dimin-ished when their work is completed without affecting the living cell – for instance, polycaprolactone, polypropylene (Schuurman et al., 2011).

The following are some important factors to be considered during formulating and printing with bio-inks and biomaterials:

I. Properties of bio-inks: The properties of bio-inks mainly depend on the composition, structure, properties and processability of hydrogels mate-rial as well as the type of living cell, their molecular weight, concentration and another component. Rheological properties (such as viscosity, shear-thinning and yield stress) of bio-inks are essential for 3D bioprinting.

II. Parameters of 3D bioprinters: The parameters like nozzle diameter, printing speed, and fabrication time should be optimised for uniform and precise placement of filament of hydrogels.

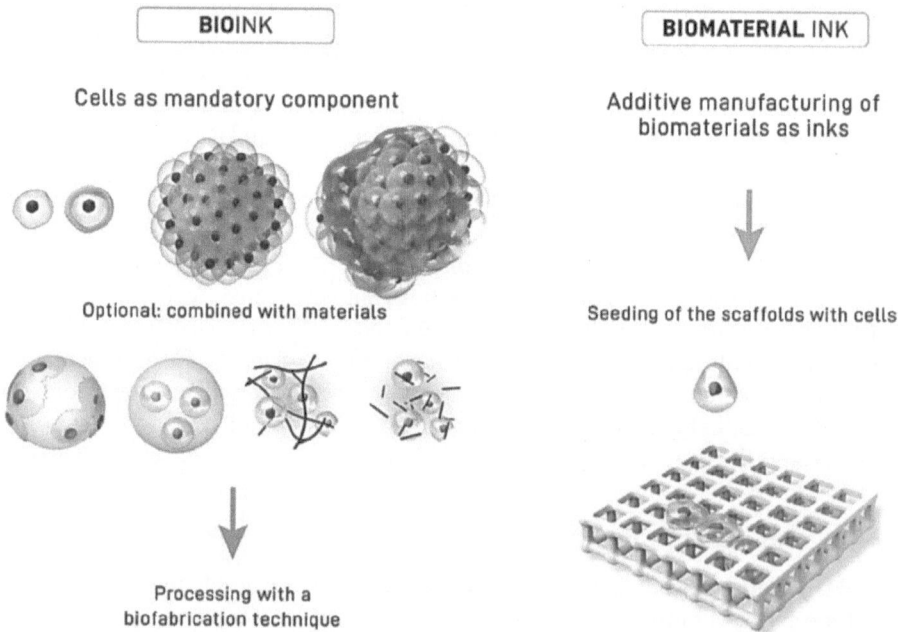

FIGURE 5.5.   Some factors to be considered during formulating and printing with bio-inks and biomaterials inks (J. Li et al., 2020a).

TABLE 5.9

Different Types of Smart Hydrogel with Their Environmental Stimuli and Their 3D-Printed Structure (J. Li et al., 2020b; Wang et al., 2015)

Environmental Factors	3D-printed Structure	Example
Thermoresponsive hydrogels	Porous	Pluronic F127
Magnetic hydrogels	Scaffolds shape in response to the magnetic field	Biopolymer hydrogels with magnetic nanoparticles
PH responsive	Porous	Collagen
Photo cross-linked hydrogels	Desired shape	Gellan gum methacrylate, gelatin
Electro responsive	The shape can be modulated through electric signals	Poly (acrylic acid) sodium salt-modified pluronic

III. Cell viability and biocompatibility: The printed bioproduct is estimated to be non-toxic and hortative in nature for the function of cells embedded in it, such as migration, adhesion, signalling, differentiation and proliferation.

IV. Properties of printed bioproduct: The prepared bio-inks should be reliable so that during and after the printing of the bioproduct should be dimensionally and geometrically stable for a given period.

5.6.2 SMART HYDROGELS

Smart hydrogels have properties of hydrogels along with the ability to stimulate according to environmental factors. In today's scenario, smart hydrogels are very appealing for biomedical applications. Smart hydrogels have some advantages over traditional hydrogels, such as controllable sol-gel transition, self-healing property and so on. A 3D-printing method based on extrusion, inkjet and laser is widely used for fabricating scaffolds, ECMs and drug delivery systems. The smart hydrogels with their shape and structure of the printed part are shown in Table 5.9.

5.7 SUMMARY

Additive manufacturing (AM) is expanding its domain, particularly in the field of medicine and surgery. In the last few decades, there is an exemplary growth of the research describing different medical industry materials' potential exploited by different AM techniques. As the medical field is directly related to human beings' comfort, survival and development, the research on 3D-printable materials and allied industries is gaining unprecedented attention. The global reach and support of the stakeholders are contributing immensely to the development, trial and commercial utilisation of various exotic materials. The present book chapter incorporates sincere effort and a scientific approach to summarise the ongoing research in the realm of multiple materials usages, and their limitations. The chapter also briefly highlights the future possibilities of 3D-printable materials in order to serve humankind in a better way.

ANNEXURE FOR ABBREVIATIONS

AM	Additive manufacturing
ATZ	Alumina toughened zirconia
BJ	Binder jetting
CBS	Crystalline bone screw
DLP	Digital light processing
ECM	Extracellular matrix
FDM	Fused deposition modelling
FFF	Fused filament fabrication
LDMD	Laser direct metal deposition
LENS	Laser engineered net shaping.
LOM	Laminated object manufacturing
ME-AM	Melt extrusion-additive manufacturing
NPJ	Nanoparticle jetting
PAA	Polyacrylic acid
PAAm	Polyacrylamide
PEG	Polyethylene glycol
PLA	Polylactic acid
PCL	Polycaprolactone
PVA	Polyvinyl alcohol
SE-AM	Solution extrusion-additive manufacturing
SEBM	Selective electron-beam melting
SHS	Selective heat sintering
SMA	Shape-memory alloy
SLA	Stereolithography
SLM	Selective laser melting
SLS	Selective laser sintering
TPP	Sodium tripolyphosphate
ZTA	Zirconia toughened alumina

REFERENCES

Alves, P. (2012). *Polyurethane: Properties, Structure and Applications: Biomedical Polyurethane-Based Materials*. NY, US: Nova Science Publishers, Inc. Ardis, A, 2.

Annabi, N., Tamayol, A., Uquillas, J. A., Akbari, M., Bertassoni, L. E., Cha, C., Camci-Unal, G., Dokmeci, M. R., Peppas, N. A., & Khademhosseini, A. (2014). 25th anniversary article: Rational design and applications of hydrogels in regenerative medicine. *Advanced Materials*, 26(1), 85–124.

Balla, V. K., Banerjee, S., Bose, S., & Bandyopadhyay, A. (2010a). Direct laser processing of a tantalum coating on titanium for bone replacement structures. *Acta Biomaterialia*, 6(6), 2329–2334. https://doi.org/10.1016/j.actbio.2009.11.021

Balla, V. K., Bodhak, S., Bose, S., & Bandyopadhyay, A. (2010b). Porous tantalum structures for bone implants: Fabrication, mechanical and in vitro biological properties. *Acta Biomaterialia*, 6(8), 3349–3359. https://doi.org/10.1016/j.actbio.2010.01.046

Banerjee, D., & Williams, J. C. (2013). Perspectives on titanium science and technology. *Acta Materialia*, 61(3), 844–879. https://doi.org/10.1016/j.actamat.2012.10.043

Banga, H. K., Belokar, R. M., & Kumar, R., (2017b). 'A Novel Approach For Ankle Foot Orthosis Developed By Three Dimensional Technologies', *3rd International Conference on Mechanical Engineering and Automation Science (ICMEAS 2017)*, University of Birmingham, UK Vol. *8* No. 10, pp. 141–145.

Banga, H. K., Belokar, R.M., Madan, R., & Dhole, S. (2017a). Three dimensional Gait assessments during walking of healthy people and drop foot patients, *Defence Life Science Journal*, 2, 14–20.

Banga, H. K., Kalra, P., Belokar, R. M., & Kumar, R. (2020a). Customized design and additive manufacturing of kids' ankle foot orthosis, *Rapid Prototyping Journal*, *26*(10). https://doi.org/10.1108/RPJ-07-2019-0194

Banga, H. K., Kalra, P., Belokar, R. M., & Kumar, R. (2020b). Design and fabrication of prosthetic and orthotic product by 3D printing [Online First], *IntechOpen*, doi:10.5772/intechopen.94846. Available from: https://www.intechopen.com/online-first/design-and-fabrication-of-prosthetic-and-orthotic-product-by-3d-printing

Banga, H. K., Kalra, P., Belokar, R. M., & Kumar R. (2020c). Effect of 3D-printed ankle foot orthosis during walking of foot deformities patients'. In: Kumar H., Jain P. (eds) *Recent Advances in Mechanical Engineering*. Lecture Notes in Mechanical Engineering. Springer, Singapore, pp. 275–288

Banga, H. K., Kalra, P., Belokar, R. M., & Kumar R. (2020d). Role of finite element analysis in customized design of kid's orthotic product. In: Singh S., Prakash C., Singh R. (eds) *Characterization, Testing, Measurement, and Metrology*, pp. 139–159 CRC Press Taylor & Francis Group, USA

Banga, H. K., Kalra, P., Belokar, R. M., & Kumar, R. (2020e). Improvement of Human Gait in Foot Deformities Patients by 3D Printed Ankle–Foot Orthosis. In: Singh S., Prakash C., Singh R. (eds) *3D Printing in Biomedical Engineering*. Materials Horizons: From Nature to Nanomaterials. Springer, Singapore.

Banga, H. K., Kumar, P., & Kumar, H. (2021). Utilization of additive manufacturing in orthotics and prosthetic devices development *IOP Conference Series: Materials Science and Engineering*. https://doi.org/10.1088/1757-899X/1033/1/012083

Banga, H. K., Parveen, K., Belokar, R. M., & Kumar, R. (2014). Rapid prototyping applications in medical sciences, *International Journal of Emerging Technologies in Computational and Applied Sciences (IJETCAS)*, *5*(8), 416–420.

Banga, H. K., Parveen, K., Belokar, R. M., Kumar R, (2018). Fabrication and stress analysis of ankle foot orthosis with additive manufacturing. *Rapid Prototyping Journal Emerald Publishing*, *24*(2), 300–312.

Black, J. (1994). Biologic performance of tantalum. *Clinical Materials*, *16*(3), 167–173.

Brannigan, R. P., & Dove, A. P. (2017). Synthesis, properties and biomedical applications of hydrolytically degradable materials based on aliphatic polyesters and polycarbonates. *Biomaterials Science*, *5*(1), 9–21. https://doi.org/10.1039/c6bm00584e

Burns, A. E. (1995). Biofix fixation techniques and results in foot surgery. *Journal of Foot and Ankle Surgery*, *34*(3), 276–282. https://doi.org/10.1016/S1067-2516(09)80060-4

Catteaux, R., & Grattepanche-Lebecq, I. (2013). Synthesis, characterization and bioactivity of bioglasses in the Na 2 O – CaO – P 2 O 5 – SiO 2 system prepared via sol gel. May, 1–7. https://doi.org/10.1016/j.cherd.2013.05.017

Chen, X., Meng, Y., Li, Y., & Zhao, N. (2008). Investigation on bio-mineralization of melt and sol-gel derived bioactive glasses. *Applied Surface Science*, *255*(2), 562–564. https://doi.org/10.1016/j.apsusc.2008.06.101

Chen, Z., Li, Z., Li, J., Liu, C., Lao, C., Fu, Y., Liu, C., Li, Y., Wang, P., & He, Y. (2019). 3D printing of ceramics: A review. *Journal of the European Ceramic Society*, *39*(4), 661–687. https://doi.org/10.1016/j.jeurceramsoc.2018.11.013

Chong, S. F., Smith, A. A. A., & Zelikin, A. N. (2013). Microstructured, functional PVA hydrogels through bioconjugation with oligopeptides under physiological conditions. *Small*, *9*(6), 942–950. https://doi.org/10.1002/smll.201201774

Corrado, P. (2017). Bioinert ceramics: State-of-The-Art. *Key Engineering Materials, 758*, 3–13.

Croisier, F., & Jérôme, C. (2013). Chitosan-based biomaterials for tissue engineering. *European Polymer Journal, 49*(4), 780–792.

Crompton, K. E., Goud, J. D., Bellamkonda, R. V., Gengenbach, T. R., Finkelstein, D. I., Horne, M. K., & Forsythe, J. S. (2007). Polylysine-functionalised thermoresponsive chitosan hydrogel for neural tissue engineering. *Biomaterials, 28*(3), 441–449.

Culver, H. R., Clegg, J. R., & Peppas, N. A. (2017). Analyte-Responsive Hydrogels : Intelligent Materials for Biosensing and Drug Delivery. *Accounts of Chemical Research, 50*(2), 170–178.

Demir, A. G., Monguzzi, L., & Previtali, B. (2017). Selective laser melting of pure Zn with high density for biodegradable implant manufacturing. *Additive Manufacturing, 15*, 20–28.

Dhand, C., Ong, S. T., Dwivedi, N., Diaz, S. M., Venugopal, J. R., Navaneethan, B., Fazil, M. H. U. T., Liu, S., Seitz, V., Wintermantel, E., Beuerman, R. W., Ramakrishna, S., Verma, N. K., & Lakshminarayanan, R. (2016). Bio-inspired in situ crosslinking and mineralisation of electrospun collagen scaffolds for bone tissue engineering. *Biomaterials, 104*, 323–338.

Dong, L., & Jiang, H. (2007). Autonomous microfluidics with stimuli-responsive hydrogels. *Soft Matter, 3*(10), 1223–1230.

Doppalapudi, S., Jain, A., Khan, W., & Domb, A. J. (2014). Biodegradable polymers-an overview. *Polymers for Advanced Technologies, 25*(5), 427–435.

Drury, J. L., & Mooney, D. J. (2003). Hydrogels for tissue engineering: Scaffold design variables and applications. *Biomaterials, 24*(24), 4337–4351.

El-Ghannam, A., & Ducheyne, P. (2017). Bioactive ceramics. *Comprehensive Biomaterials II, 204–234.*

Feng, Q., Wei, K., Lin, S., Xu, Z., Sun, Y., Shi, P., Li, G., & Bian, L. (2016). Mechanically resilient, injectable, and bioadhesive supramolecular gelatin hydrogels crosslinked by weak host-guest interactions assist cell infiltration and in situ tissue regeneration. *Biomaterials, 101*, 217–228.

Fernández-Ferreiro, A., González Barcia, M., Gil-Martínez, M., Vieites-Prado, A., Lema, I., Argibay, B., Blanco Méndez, J., Lamas, M. J., & Otero-Espinar, F. J. (2015). In vitro and in vivo ocular safety and eye surface permanence determination by direct and Magnetic Resonance Imaging of ion-sensitive hydrogels based on gellan gum and kappa-carrageenan. *European Journal of Pharmaceutics and Biopharmaceutics, 94*, 342–351.

Francis, R., Joy, N., & Sivadas, A. (2016). Relevance of natural degradable polymers in the biomedical field. *Biomedical Applications of Polymeric Materials and Composites*, 303–360.

Gerlach, G., & Arndt, K.-F. (2009). *Hydrogel Sensors and Actuators: Engineering and Technology* (Vol. 6). Springer Science & Business Media, Berlin, Heidelberg, New York.

Groll, J., Burdick, J. A., Cho, D. W., Derby, B., Gelinsky, M., Heilshorn, S. C., & Woodfield, T. B. F. (2018). A definition of bioinks and their distinction from biomaterial inks. *Biofabrication, 11*(1), 013001.

Günay, K. A., Theato, P., & Klok, H. (2013). Standing on the shoulders of Hermann Staudinger: Post-polymerization modification from past to present. *Journal of Polymer Science Part A: Polymer Chemistry, 51*(1), 1–28.

Hamidi, M., Azadi, A., & Rafiei, P. (2008). Hydrogel nanoparticles in drug delivery. *Advanced Drug Delivery Reviews, 60*(15), 1638–1649.

Heilig, M. L. (1994). United States patent office. *ACM SIGGRAPH Computer Graphics, 28*(2), 131–134.

Highley, C. B., Prestwich, G. D., & Burdick, J. A. (2016). Recent advances in hyaluronic acid hydrogels for biomedical applications. *Current Opinion in Biotechnology, 40*, 35–40.

Hoffman, A. S. (2012). Hydrogels for biomedical applications. *Advanced Drug Delivery Reviews*, *64*, 18–23.

Hollander, D. A., Von Walter, M., Wirtz, T., Sellei, R., Schmidt-Rohlfing, B., Paar, O., & Erli, H. J. (2006). Structural, mechanical and in vitro characterisation of individually structured Ti-6Al-4V produced by direct laser forming. *Biomaterials*, *27*(7), 955–963.

Hsu, R. W. W., Yang, C. C., Huang, C. A., & Chen, Y. S. (2005). Electrochemical corrosion studies on Co-Cr-Mo implant alloy in biological solutions. *Materials Chemistry and Physics*, *93*(2–3), 531–538.

Hupa, L. (2011). Melt-derived bioactive glasses. In *Bioactive Glasses: Materials, Properties and Applications* (pp. 3–28), ed. Heimo O. Ylänen, Woodhead Publishing, Sawston, UK.

Jabbari, E., Leijten, J., Xu, Q., & Khademhosseini, A. (2016). The matrix reloaded: The evolution of regenerative hydrogels. *Materials Today*, *19*(4), 190–196.

Jayaswal, G. P., Dange, S. P., & Khalikar, A. N. (2010). Bioceramic in dental implants: A review. *Journal of Indian Prosthodontist Society*, *10*(1), 8–12.

Jones, J. R. (2007). Bioactive ceramics and glasses. In *Tissue Engineering Using Ceramics and Polymers* (pp. 52–71), eds. Aldo R. Boccaccini & Julie E. Gough, Woodhead Publishing, Sawston, UK.

Jones, R. G., Kahovec, J., Stepto, R., Wilks, E. S. Hess, M., & Tatsuki Kitayama, W. V. M. (2008). Compendium of polymer terminology and nomenclature *Pharmaceutical Technology*, *42*(6).

Juhasz, J. A., & Best, S. M. (2012). Bioactive ceramics: Processing, structures and properties. *Journal of Materials Science*, *47*(2), 610–624.

Jung, I. Y., Kim, J. S., Choi, B. R., Lee, K., & Lee, H. (2017). Hydrogel based biosensors for in vitro dia of biochemicals, *Proteins, and Genes 1601475*, 1–19.

Kharkar, P. M., Kiick, K. L., & Kloxin, A. M. (2013). Designing degradable hydrogels for orthogonal control of cell microenvironments. *Chemical Society Reviews*, *42*(17), 7335–7372.

Khorasani, A. M., Goldberg, M., Doeven, E. H., & Littlefair, G. (2015). Titanium in biomedical applications—properties and fabrication: A review. *Journal of Biomaterials and Tissue Engineering*, *5*(8), 593–619.

Kirchmajer, D. M., Gorkin, R., & In Het Panhuis, M. (2015). An overview of the suitability of hydrogel-forming polymers for extrusion-based 3D-printing. *Journal of Materials Chemistry B*, *3*(20), 4105–4117

Koch, K., Brave, D., & Nasseh, A. A. (2012). A review of bioceramic technology in endodontics. *CE Article*, *4*, 6–12.

Kumar, A. C., & Erothu, H. (2016). Synthetic Polymer Hydrogels. *Biomedical Applications of Polymeric Materials and Composites*, *6*, 141–162.

Kundu, B., Rajkhowa, R., Kundu, S. C., & Wang, X. (2013). Silk fibroin biomaterials for tissue regenerations. *Advanced Drug Delivery Reviews*, *65*(4), 457–470.

Lee, K. Y., & Mooney, D. J. (2001). Hydrogels for tissue engineering. *Chemical Reviews*, *101*(7), 1869–1879.

Li, J., Wu, C., Chu, P. K., & Gelinsky, M. (2020a). 3D printing of hydrogels: Rational design strategies and emerging biomedical applications. *Materials Science and Engineering R: Reports*, *140*(November 2019).

Li, J., Wu, C., Chu, P. K., & Gelinsky, M. (2020b). Materials Science & Engineering R 3D printing of hydrogels: Rational design strategies and emerging biomedical applications. *Materials Science & Engineering*, *100543*.

Li, N., & Zheng, Y. (2013). Novel magnesium alloys developed for biomedical application: A review. *Journal of Materials Science and Technology*, *29*(6), 489–502.

Li, T., Wang, J., Zhang, L., Yang, J., Yang, M., Zhu, D., Zhou, X., Handschuh-Wang, S., Liu, Y., & Zhou, X. (2017). 'Freezing', morphing, and folding of stretchy tough hydrogels. *Journal of Materials Chemistry B*, *5*(29), 5726–5732.

Liu, T., Jiao, C., Peng, X., Chen, Y. N., Chen, Y., He, C., Liu, R., & Wang, H. (2018). Super-strong and tough poly(vinyl alcohol)/poly(acrylic acid) hydrogels reinforced by hydrogen bonding. *Journal of Materials Chemistry B*, *6*(48), 8105–8114.

Mahan, G. D. (2019). *Crystal Structures: Condensed Matter in a Nutshell*, Princeton University Press, Princeton, NJ, 9–30.

Manavitehrani, I., Fathi, A., Badr, H., Daly, S., Negahi Shirazi, A., & Dehghani, F. (2016). Biomedical applications of biodegradable polyesters. *Polymers*, *8*(1), 20.

Mantovani, D. (2000). Shape memory alloys: Properties and biomedical applications. *JOM*, *52*(10), 36–44.

Mehl, R., Barrett, C., & Smith, D. (1938). *Greninger and Mooradian, Metals Technology (A.I.M.E.)*, December 1937.

Mironov, V. (2003). Printing technology to produce living tissue. *Expert Opinion on Biological Therapy*, *3*(5), 701–704.

Nair, L. S., & Laurencin, C. T. (2007). Biodegradable polymers as biomaterials. *Progress in Polymer Science (Oxford)*, *32*(8–9), 762–798.

Ni, J., Ling, H., Zhang, S., Wang, Z., Peng, Z., Benyshek, C., Zan, R., Miri, A. K., Li, Z., Zhang, X., Lee, J., Lee, K. J., Kim, H. J., Tebon, P., Hoffman, T., Dokmeci, M. R., Ashammakhi, N., Li, X., & Khademhosseini, A. (2019). Three-dimensional printing of metals for biomedical applications. *Materials Today Bio*, *3*(May).

Nigmatullin, R., Thomas, P., Lukasiewicz, B., Puthussery, H., & Roy, I. (2015). Polyhydroxyalkanoates, a family of natural polymers, and their applications in drug delivery. *Journal of Chemical Technology and Biotechnology*, *90*(7), 1209–1221.

Niinomi, M. (2007). Recent research and development in metallic materials for biomedical, dental and healthcare products applications. *Materials Science Forum*, *539–543* (PART 1), 193–200.

Niinomi, M., Narushima, T., & Nakai, M. (2015). *Advances in Metallic Biomaterials*. Springer, Berlin Heidelberg.

Pattanashetti, N. A., Heggannavar, G. B., & Kariduraganavar, M. Y. (2017). Smart biopolymers and their biomedical applications. *Procedia Manufacturing*, *12*(December 2016), 263–279.

Punyaratabandhu, T., Lohwongwatana, B., Puncreobutr, C., Kosiyatrakul, A., Veerapan, P., & Luenam, S. (2017). A patient-matched entire first metacarpal prosthesis in treatment of giant cell tumor of bone. *Case Reports in Orthopedics*, *2017*, 1–6.

Puppi, D., & Chiellini, F. (2020). Biodegradable polymers for biomedical additive manufacturing. *Applied Materials Today*, *20*, 100700.

Qin, Y., Wen, P., Guo, H., Xia, D., Zheng, Y., Jauer, L., Poprawe, R., Voshage, M., & Schleifenbaum, J. H. (2019). Additive manufacturing of biodegradable metals: Current research status and future perspectives. *Acta Biomaterialia*, *98*, 3–22.

Qu, J., Zhao, X., Ma, P. X., & Guo, B. (2017). pH-responsive self-healing injectable hydrogel based on N-carboxyethyl chitosan for hepatocellular carcinoma therapy. *Acta Biomaterialia*, *58*, 168–180.

Ratner, B. D., Hoffman, A. S., Schoen, F. J., & Lemons, J. E. (2004). *Biomaterials Science: An Introduction to Materials in Medicine*. Elsevier, San Diego, CA.

Sabahi, N., Chen, W., Wang, C. H., Kruzic, J. J., & Li, X. (2020). A review on additive manufacturing of shape-memory materials for biomedical applications. *JOM*, *72*(3), 1229–1253.

Schexnailder, P., & Schmidt, G. (2009). Nanocomposite polymer hydrogels. *Colloid and Polymer Science*, *287*(1), 1–11.

Schuurman, W., Khristov, V., Pot, M. W., Van Weeren, P. R., Dhert, W. J. A., & Malda, J. (2011). Bioprinting of hybrid tissue constructs with tailorable mechanical properties. *Biofabrication*, *3*(2), 5.

Seliktar, D. (2012). Designing cell-compatible hydrogels for biomedical applications. *Science*, *336*(6085), 1124–1128.

Senatov, F. S., Zadorozhnyy, M. Y., Niaza, K. V., Medvedev, V. V., Kaloshkin, S. D., Anisimova, N. Y., Kiselevskiy, M. V., & Yang, K. C. (2017). Shape memory effect in 3D-printed scaffolds for self-fitting implants. *European Polymer Journal*, *93*(May), 222–231.

Sinnett-Jones, P. E., Wharton, J. A., & Wood, R. J. K. (2005). Micro-abrasion-corrosion of a CoCrMo alloy in simulated artificial hip joint environments. *Wear*, *259*(7–12), 898–909.

Spotnitz, W. D. (2010). Fibrin sealant: Past, present, and future: A brief review. *World Journal of Surgery*, *34*(4), 632–634.

Stansbury, J. W., & Idacavage, M. J. (2016). 3D printing with polymers: Challenges among expanding options and opportunities. *Dental Materials*, *32*(1), 54–64.

Strittmatter, J., Gümpel, P., & Hiefer, M. (2019). Intelligent materials in modern production – Current trends for thermal shape memory alloys. *Procedia Manufacturing*, *30*, 347–356.

Sulaeva, I., Henniges, U., Rosenau, T., & Potthast, A. (2015). Bacterial cellulose as a material for wound treatment: Properties and modifications: A review. *Biotechnology Advances*, *33*(8), 1547–1571.

Tappa, K., & Jammalamadaka, U. (2018). Novel biomaterials used in medical 3D printing techniques. *Journal of Functional Biomaterials*, *9*(1).

Vorndran, E., Wunder, K., Moseke, C., Biermann, I., Müller, F. A., Zorn, K., & Gbureck, U. (2011). Hydraulic setting Mg 3(PO4) 2 powders for 3D printing technology. *Advances in Applied Ceramics*, *110*(8), 476–481.

Wang, S., Lee, J. M., & Yeong, W. Y. (2015). Smart Hydrogels for 3D Bioprinting. *International Journal of Bioprinting*, *1*(1).

Wauthle, R., Van Der Stok, J., Yavari, S. A., Van Humbeeck, J., Kruth, J. P., Zadpoor, A. A., Weinans, H., Mulier, M., & Schrooten, J. (2015). Additively manufactured porous tantalum implants. *Acta Biomaterialia*, *14*, 217–225.

Williams, D., Thayer, P., Martinez, H., Gatenholm, E., & Khademhosseini, A. (2018). A perspective on the physical, mechanical and biological specifications of bioinks and the development of functional tissues in 3D bioprinting. *Bioprinting*, *9*, 19–36.

Witte, F. (2010). The history of biodegradable magnesium implants: A review. *Acta Biomaterialia*, *6*(5), 1680–1692.

Wohlers, T. (2013). *Wohler's report 2013*. https://wohlersassociates.com/2013report.htm. Accessed: 24 November 2021.

Xiang, R., Ding, D., Fan, L., Huang, X., & Xia, K. (2014). Symbol Antibacterial mechanism and safety of zinc oxide. *Journal of Clinical Rehabilitative Tissue Engineering Research*, *18*(3), 470–475.

Yamada, K., Tabata, Y., Yamamoto, K., Miyamoto, S., Nagata, I., Kikuchi, H., & Ikada, Y. (1997). Potential efficacy of basic fibroblast growth factor incorporated in biodegradable hydrogels for skull bone regeneration. *Journal of Neurosurgery*, *86*(5), 871–875.

Yaszemski, M. J., Payne, R. G., Hayes, W. C., Langer, R. S., Aufdemorte, T. B., & Mikos, A. G. (1995). The ingrowth of new bone tissue and initial mechanical properties of a degrading polymeric composite scaffold. *Tissue Engineering*, *1*(1), 41–52.

Yi, L., & Liu, J. (2017). Liquid metal biomaterials: A newly emerging area to tackle modern biomedical challenges. *International Materials Reviews*, *62*(7), 415–440.

Zarek, M., Layani, M., Cooperstein, I., Sachyani, E., Cohn, D., & Magdassi, S. (2016). 3D printing of shape memory polymers for flexible electronic devices. *Advanced Materials*, *28*(22), 4449–4454.

Zheng, Y. F., Gu, X. N., & Witte, F. (2014). Biodegradable metals. *Materials Science and Engineering R: Reports*, *77*, 1–34.

6 Materials for 3D Printing in Medicine
Metals, Polymers, Ceramics, Hydrogels

Kritik Saxena
National Institute of Technology Calicut, Kerala, India

CONTENTS

6.1　INTRODUCTION

The increasing prevalence of bone fractures due to bruises, vitamin deficiency, surgical procedures in bone infections, abscission in bone tumours, and the like, has propounded immense stress on the medical management system globally. An observational study of 3 years from 2009 to 2011 was carried out on people of 18 to 49 years of age. It states that 1,447 out of 1,730 men and 1,035 out of 1,164 women were fractured due to road accidents needing transplants [1]. In 2000, 1.5 million cases were estimated affected by hip fractures worldwide. These cases were studied to be about 20 per cent of all fractures in people aged 50 or above. The fracture cases are expected to significantly increase by 2025 [2]. The fractures pose a risk of post-fall morbidity and mortality. Owing to such a high percentage of young adults and old people getting fractured, a significant exigency of scaffolds for transplantation is seen.

The implants for transplantation can be worked out with various materials available, but they should qualify specific properties such as alterable chemistry, befitting mechanical properties, structure, porous structure and other relevant aspects. On the other hand, irregular geometry defines bone defects. The defects need

DOI: 10.1201/9781003301066-6

counteracting with personalised solutions to design implants. The patient-specific implants are accurate and optimum for patients. These have individualised control of shape, porosity, organisation, surface characteristics, and mechanical properties that will suffice for bone tissue regeneration and support the medical systems' requirements [3].

A paradigm shift from conventional to additive manufacturing is about the development of new and novel materials developed. The range of raw materials for 3D printing incorporates polymers, ceramics, composite materials, and metals. Metal-based materials have properties like high strength, making them a perfect match for applications requiring load-bearing and high abrasion. These include applications such as the pelvis, tibia, thorax, spine and hip joints. Materials including polymers have high printability properties, which satiates the medical requirements of interactive cell coatings, drug delivery, tissue implant manufacturing and skin regeneration. The scaffold designing through additive manufacturing requires specific characteristic properties in the material [4]. Overall, an ideal bone scaffold has good biocompatible properties, excellent bioactivity, and appropriate structures with porosity. An ideal bone scaffold must also be having suitable mechanical properties similar to the actual bone tissue. AM is equipped with features that can achieve the objective as it can control the chemistry, porosity and intricacy of the part being prepared.

The focus of tissue engineering is the reconstruction, refurbishment or substitution of faulty or damaged effective biological organs and tissues. The scaffold design's more significant objective is to substitute or regenerate the original tissues with the same utilitarian attributes and are anatomically similar. The scaffolds substituted should have internal pathways for cell extension and relocation; they must convey numerous developmental factors, and unwanted products should pertain to their shape and size while the nearby cells are flourishing and should have requisite mechanical properties [5]. Recent years in the medical field have showed the use of colossal and strategic enhancement in certain aspects of human tissue regeneration.

List of materials commonly used in medical AM applications:

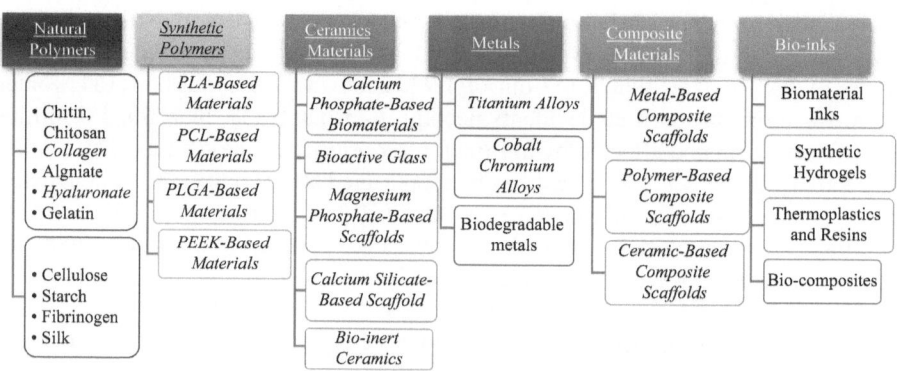

The various materials developed for 3D printing in medical applications are classified as follows:

6.1.1 Natural Polymer Materials

The materials which are seen to have applications in medical scenarios for decades are natural polymers. By 300 BC, ancient Egypt used natural sutures made of animal parts and coconut shells to repair the injured skulls. Countries like India and Greece were found to perform plastic surgery by the use of biomaterials made of natural elements. In 600 AD, the Mayan people reached complete bone unification by creating nacre teeth from seashells. Germany has a history of hip joint substitution for the first time executed in the year 1891. These implants employed ivory because of the enhanced biomechanical binding properties [6]. Natural biopolymers have attained their superior position as AM material over the past decade. The most common materials for 3D printing in natural polymers include chitin and chitosan, alginate, collagen, gelatin, Hyaluronate and fibrinogen. Due to natural polymers' various beneficial properties, they have been a research interest both in teaching and manufacturing for more than 50 years [7]. Basic biological materials are converted into natural polymers to be used as 3D-printing material. The following are the various natural polymers utilised in AM industry:

a. *Chitin/Chitosan*
   Chitin is derived from mushrooms, invertebrates, yeast and green algae. It is one of the most superabundant biopolymers available which is made of N-acetyl glucosamine and N-glucosamine monomer structures. While chitosan is derivative of chitin with N-deacetylate. Chitin and chitosan are known to possess an accelerating effect on the process of tissue restoration and obstruction to the development of scar tissue due to N-acetyl glucosamine presence in them. Since Chitosan is easily convertible into thin films and fibres, it is a distinguished candidate for tissue and bone scaffold manufacturing. Moreover, a product formed after the degradation of chitin and chitosan is M-glucosamine which is non-toxic and originally present in the extracellular matrix of the human body's eukaryotic cells. The prominent property of chitosan is the control over degradation rate, which is managed by changing the molecular weight of chitosan, ranging from 300 to 1000kDa [7].

b. *Collagen*
   Collagen is the most richly present natural protein in the human body and has been used in tissue production for decades. It has the property of being naturally non-immunogenic, and it has satisfactory strength, which helps in rebuilding tissue and its regeneration behaviour. It is built of a triple-helical architecture combined with hydrogen-bonding properties. These include major amino acid groups such as proline, glycine and hydroxy-proline. This architecture consisting of triple helices gives flexibility to the material. Though it is not strong enough, with crosslinking, the degradation can be controlled. Thus the mechanical properties are enhanced by making different types of collagen. The crucial properties of collagen being biodegradable and biocompatible make it appropriate for applications in 3D printing of medical parts. Collagen has been seen to remove osteochondral defects and prepare cartilage regeneration applications.

c. *Alginate*

This is another natural polymer that has enlarged its popularity in medical applications with its biocompatible effects and feasibility for gelation. Alginate is derived from polysaccharides and is found in algae's cell walls, brown seaweed and bacterial strains. Alginate is used as a solidifying and gel-developing mediator for medical usage due to its ease of gelation. Combinational form as alginate hydrogel, it grasped superiority due to the drug encapsulation feature. With 3D printing, alginate is used for bone cells and in vitro tumour model preparation.

d. *Hyaluronate*

Hyaluronate is formed from hyaluronic acid, a single chain polysaccharide made of glucuronic acid and N-acetyl glucosamine-related links from end to end alternate glycosidic bonds. Properties inherited by Hyaluronate are biocompatibility, biodegradability and viscoelasticity. Hyaluronate is widely used in tissue engineering. The amalgamation of Hyaluronate with other natural polymers such as chitosan has shown enhanced chondrocyte proliferation and cartilage ECM production. Hyaluronic acids are also utilised as a lubricant for parts and surfaces subjected to a lot of friction through movements [8].

e. *Gelatin*

Gelatin is obtained from the degradation of insoluble collagen after disintegration and denaturation. It is used in the medical field with interactive cell coatings, drug delivery, and tissue implant manufacturing applications. It is also utilised in fibre formation because of its secure hydrogen bonding and capacity for solidifying it at low temperatures. Recently, fruitful potentials have been seen in mixing alginate and gelatin having agents with mineralisation effects, thus improving the crosslinking property.

f. *Cellulose*

Cellulose is a single chain polysaccharide capable of making fundamental components of plant cell walls. Its major functions were seen in laceration dressing, tissue production, and administered drug delivery systems. The chemical arrangement of cellulose gives effects for dissolution familiar in diluents, which makes them hard to be utilised in tissue production applications [9].

g. *Starch*

Starch is synthesised from a blend of glycans. The major applications of starch in the medical industry are hydrogel and drug delivery. It is also beneficial in substantiating cell development at several progressive stages of the human body due to its highly organised architecture.

h. *Fibrinogen*

Another popular natural polymer used in medical industries is fibrinogen. It is a soluble plasma glycoprotein that is majorly produced in the human body, especially the liver. Fibrinogen permits the selection of cellular interactivities and tissue restoration, and thus it is one of the best materials for tissue scaffold, hemostatic, and lesion dressing application [9].

i. *Silk*
   Silk is obtained from silkworms, and it includes hydrophobic spheres comprised of undersized amino acid side connections that can wrap around into β-sheet arrangements. This feature allows a tight packing of sheets with hydrogen bonding of anti-parallel linkages of proteins in them. Silk has high strength, elasticity, biodegradability, controlled degradation rates, and biocompatibility due to the non-harmful byproducts that shed away on degradation, such as amino acids. These properties make it very useful for tissue engineering [10].

Overall, natural polymers are adapted to the biomedical community's market with the various feasible features they carry. New and more beneficial scaffolds can be developed shortly with natural polymers by controlling and improving specific properties like biocompatibility, biodegradability and bioresorbability. Many AM techniques are capable of working with natural polymers helping the creation of tissue implants and artificial bones. Chemical composition and stability, mechanical integrity, and enhanced biological properties are some characteristics that are further studied to achieve greater heights in the development of polymer-based AM medical products.

6.1.2 SYNTHETIC POLYMER MATERIALS

With many beneficial properties existing with polymers, they have captured the AM medical market at a greater level. The manufacturing of synthetic polymers has also found advancements in the field due to the feasibility in preparation, low-budget costing, biocompatibility, controllable degradation, mechanics and other beneficial properties. Countless synthetic polymers are prepared to produce tissue scaffolds. The polymers can be synthesised in laboratories into two significant categories: biodegradable and non-biodegradable. Biodegradable polymers include polystyrene, poly-L-lactic acid (PLLA), polyglycolic acid (PGA), polyphosphazene, polylactide, and its copolymer poly-lactic-co-glycolic acid (PLGA), polycaprolactone, polyanhydride, polyurethane, poly (propylene fumarate), etc. Despite the numerous properties inculcated by these synthetic polymers, there are chances that these materials are not accepted by the human body system due to their low bioactivity [11]. It has been found that a significant byproduct of synthetic polymer-based scaffolds is acidic solutions on degradation. Thus, the bodily pH will be decreased more than required, resulting in lower strength and cell-tissue necrosis (Figure 6.1).

Various synthetic polymers used in AM-based medical industries are:

a. *PLA-based materials*
   Polylactic acid (PLA) is a noticeable polymer for Fused Deposition Modelling (FDM). PLA has potential characteristics like biocompatibility, nontoxicity, biodegradability, continuous raw material, ease of sterilisation and ease of preparation. It is used in the AM industry due to its low coefficient of expansion, making it stable in shape for medical operations.

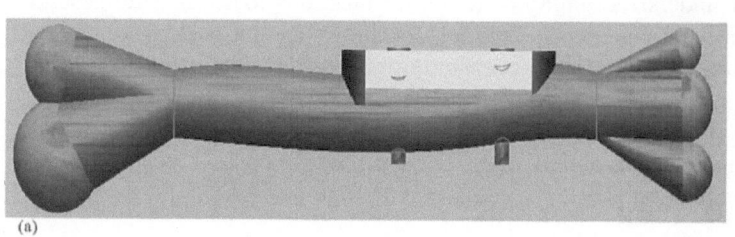
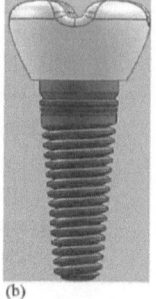

FIGURE 6.1   (a) Bone implant with fixture; (b) Dental implant.

b. *PCL-based materials*

Polycaprolactone (PCL) is a thermoplastic material used in FDM, the same as PLA. It has a low melting point and a high decomposition temperature of around 350°C. Its properties include biodegradability, economic costing, and astonishing viscoelastic and rheological behaviour upon heating. Thus it is best to use under extrusion printing method.

c. *PLGA-based materials*

Poly(lactic-co-glycolic acid) is a material having applications in bone reconstruction applications for its potential to tune degradation rate and mechanical properties. The degradation rate of PLGA can be controlled as per the copolymer from about a few weeks to several months, varying the LA/GA ratio.

d. *PEEK-based materials*

Polyether ether ketone (PEEK) is highly feasible for a craniofacial implant with AM methodologies. It has beneficial properties like admirable biocompatibility, low heat conductivity, elasticity, osteointegration and mechanical strength that match the bones, making it suitable for bone implants. PEEK scaffolds can have high porosity of around 38 per cent, and yield strength of about 30MPa by fabrication with FDM AM technology.

6.1.3 Ceramic Materials

Ceramics are materials with high hardness and brittleness, heat resistance and corrosion resistance. They can be easily shaped and hardened with high temperatures. They are highly used in bone scaffold fabrication with their capability of showing osteogenic behaviours. However, ceramics have narrow processability due to the high brittleness they acquire. Moreover, there are various challenges in choosing and developing suitable ceramic-based printing material for bone scaffold fabrication. The physicochemical and biological properties are majorly concerned before selecting a material for AM medical usage. The most common methods of 3D printing ceramic-based materials are 3DP, SLS and EB. With 3DP, SLS and EB methodologies of AM, the bone scaffolds are constructed with ceramic-based materials to achieve various performances. Ceramic-based biopolymers are highly in demand in

AM medical industry. However, due to the elevated production demand for materials for 3D printing with a limited number of ceramic biomaterials appropriate for 3D-printing applications [12].

The various ceramics involving materials used in medical AM industries are as follows:

a. *Calcium phosphate-based biomaterials*
   CaP-based biomaterials are supremely naturally used in bone repair due to calcium, which has similar properties to human bones. Extrusion-based 3D-printing methods are possible with calcium phosphate cement (CPC) since it is a low-temperature based application material. CaP-based scaffolds exhibit elevated mechanical strength and intricate pore architecture at a high-temperature range, making them a perfect fit for bone repair, especially in applications requiring high load-bearable parts.

b. *Bioactive glass*
   Bioactive glass is another ceramic-based material with exceptional bioactive capability and bone fixing properties, making it suitable to manufacture bone reconstruction scaffolds. The bioactive glass is made up of Na_2O, CaO, SiO_2 and P_2O_5. However, little resistance to fracture and inadequate mechanical reliance are seen, due to exceptionally high brittleness, and high degradation rates of bioactive glass result. Various studies have shown that bioactive glass can be fabricated with pre-designed porosity with regulation to the architecture, manufacturing and post-heating environments. Its strength is found to be similar to human bones in trabecular and cortical regions [13].

c. *Magnesium pho.sphate-based scaffolds*
   Uniquely as calcium phosphates, magnesium phosphate (MgP) implants are utilised in bone tissue healing having noble cell compatibility and osteogenic activity. However, it was found that MgP-based implants exhibit inadequate deprivation and bio-resorption after implantation in body regions such as calvarial defects. Moreover, in comparison to CaP powder, MgP powder works without any sort of binder [13].

d. *Calcium silicate-based scaffold*
   Another ceramic material that adds to the bone reconstruction process is calcium silicate-based materials. The silicon ions released through these scaffolds are proven to be efficient in regulating the cell behaviours and promoting bone conductivity of the implant prepared with them. Their implants are the most bioactive ceramics, and they have good biocompatibility combined with good osteogenic activity [14].

e. *Bio-inert ceramics*
   These ceramics have good cell compatibility features with low fracture toughness, corrosion resistance and structural stability and are thus slightly able to help in bone reconstruction. The two primary ceramic materials coming in this range of materials are alumina (Al_2O_3) and zirconia (ZrO_2), which are widely feasible in clinical applications, mainly bone and teeth repair. These materials are inert. Thus they do not form any chemical bond with the living tissues and maintain structural stability for a long time [13].

6.1.4 METALS

With high physical strength and other relevant properties, metals are well known for medical applications. The human body's majorly focused areas under metal-based implants are bone-related, dental and craniofacial usages. The traditional method of using metal for implants has used stainless steel, cobalt-chromium molybdenum, and titanium alloys using casting, forging and machining. Studies have shown that titanium (Ti) and tantalum (Ta)-based metals and their alloys are beneficial candidates for materials under medical applications out of the various metals available. Metals, proven to be the strongest of materials, have specific limitations such as (i) inadequate biological reactions on the material's external appearance, (ii) negligible degradability, (iii) low chemical integration response, (iv) toxic discharge naturally or through corrosion, and (v) unfeasibility to embrace/tolerate the structures of low-density metallic implants, which hinders the use of metals for scaffold manufacturing at a greater level (Figure 6.2).

The various metal-based materials used in AM under medical applications are as follows:

a. ***Titanium alloys***

Titanium (Ti) and its alloys are the most used metal category materials for their load-bearing capacity with excellent anticorrosion, mechanical and biological properties. The AM technologies mostly inherited for Ti and its alloy fabrication are electron beam melting (EBM) and selective laser melting (SLM). Stress shielding is one reason that can cause complications in such implants after long-term usage due to any severe incongruity in the toughness of scaffolds with help of host bone. Using open-cell structures is a cure to such difficulties. Ti-6Al-4V found a special place among Ti-alloys, as it has exceptional biocompatibility and developed physical characteristics over traditional stainless steel, cobalt-based alloys and pure titanium metal [15].

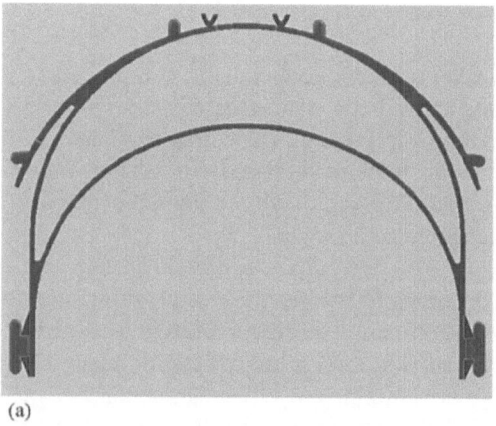
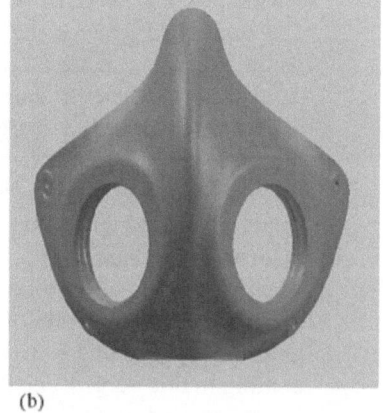

(a)   (b)

FIGURE 6.2   (a) CAD model of COVID-19 face shield for 3D printing; (b) CAD model of COVID-19 mask for 3D printing.

b. *Cobalt-chromium alloys*

These alloys have an impact in orthopaedic surgeries, specifically in hip bone replacement or knee arthroplasty, due to their excellent biocompatible properties and good physical and tear wear bearable characteristics [15].

c. *Biodegradable metals*

Recent studies have shown that biodegradable metals as scaffold materials can avoid second surgery and assuage patients' suffering. Iron-based and magnesium-based metals are common biodegradable metal materials used in AM technology. The inclusion of calcium in Fe-Mn alloy could also accelerate the degradation rate and enhance the cytocompatibility associated with simple Fe-Mn mixtures [16].

6.1.5 COMPOSITE MATERIALS WITH ENHANCED PERFORMANCES

The medical industry has understood that bone is a varied composition having various composite constituents (collagen, lipids, hydroxyapatite, and others) and porous microstructures with gradually varying mechanical strengths. Thus, AM's material should also be a composite to fulfil the matching criteria with the bone. Metals, having high printability, and ceramics being similar to bone characteristics can be combined to form composites beneficial in the AM industry for scaffold generation [17]. These composites will be hybrid materials, having the properties relevant to an ideal AM material such as physical strength, porousness, degradability and extraordinary osteogenic characteristics. It has been found that for a perfect material, the compressive strength should be within 10 to 100 MPa for cancellous and cortical bones, respectively. Porosity should be optimally controlled with an ordered porosity level (ranging from macropores with 100–500 μm, to micropores with<10 μm) and high porosity of 50–90 per cent to favour tissue development.

Moreover, the degradation rate should be controllable. All these properties can be obtained by considering a composite material of two or more phases to prepare the best-fit bone scaffold. The various composites known to AM market in the medical industry are:

a. *Metal-based composite scaffolds*

The mechanical strength similar to that of human bone can be obtained through magnesium titanium and its alloys. Compositing metals with other substitutes can provide better degradation rate control and sufficient osteogenic activities in the scaffold. The compressive yield strength and Young's modulus of 3D-printed Fe-based implants are found experimentally in human bone, with great porousness of about 68 per cent. Inhibition of Fe ion released by the nanostructured HA leads with HA coatings over them to make major enhancement of the scaffolds' biocompatibility. Moreover, the degradation rate was also influenced by modifying the magnesium alloy surfaces with materials such as CaP coatings [18].

b. *Polymer-based composite scaffolds*

The essential property needed in bone scaffolds is the osteogenic activity, which is impossible to get through a single material. PLA, PLGA, PCL, and PEEK are polymers known to have low osteogenic properties, and thus a combination of these polymers with other materials is a must to achieve the desired properties in them for bone reconstruction through AM.

i. *PLGA-based composite scaffolds*

Although PLGA is known to have a high melting point, using commonly available solvents can help get the desired shape out of the material through 3D printing. Thus using solvents over PLGA polymer can make it feasible to cast it into any required form with the AM methodologies.

ii. *PLA-based composite scaffolds*

PLA is a common material to be used in AM industries, but limitations due to its high brittle nature and low compressive strength compared to human bone make it incompatible with being used directly as a bone scaffold. PLA is made into composites with ceramic or natural polymers. These include majorly silk or chitosan, which can result in beneficial ways to increase the compressive strength of the implants.

iii. *PEEK-based composite scaffolds*

PEEK is known to have low osteointegration properties, resulting in insufficient feasibility of PEEK in bone reconstruction through AM. Getting composites of PEEK with organic ceramic results in improved mechanical qualities, and adding carbon to the composite can make it feasible for FDM techniques. Limiting compressive strength variations, increase in carbon content allows the bending and tensile strength enhancement, with no compressive strength variations. Silver nanoparticles are added to the composites to prevent the occurrence of postoperative infections.

iv. *Hydrogel-based composite scaffolds*

Hydrogel-based scaffolds have shown unique properties compared to other materials having polymers. Hydrogels have a channel formation with extraordinary water content, which makes them biocompatible, and support tissue repair activity. Only hydrogel-based materials are challenging to print through extrusion in AM facilities. To increase the feasibility, the hydrogel is mixed with several other materials such as alginate, polyvinyl alcohol, etc.

c. ***Ceramic-based composite scaffolds***

Ceramic materials have high brittleness, slow degradation rates, and poor customisable properties compared with polymers. Therefore, a combination of ceramics with polymers is beneficial to create a scaffold with enhanced properties. In such composites, polymers can exhibit dual forms: solvent binding and additive form. Printing HA or α/β-TCP powders, and polymers, in the binding document, can result in reinforced scaffolds by binding the particles altogether and thus reduces the brittleness of ceramics [19].

6.1.6 Bio-inks

Bioprinting with live cells called bio-inks is genuinely different from 3D printing an implant without cells from biomaterial ink and then seeding them into it for continuing the regeneration process of bone scaffolds. Bio-inks are mainly developed from hydrogels. Thus they are appropriate in 3D-printing applications for cell proliferation, possessing decent biocompatibility, and are greatly manageable for their physical, and natural properties. Hydrogels have the limitation of having low viscosities before crosslinking, and thus they form poor shapes on extrusion 3D printing, which makes them incapable of forming larger structures without collapsing features. Alginate is a hydrogel derived from brown algae, which is negatively charged and is the most common in tissue engineering and bioprinting. Alginate is generally amalgamated with biopolymers to control their printing and biological features. Gelatin is another natural polymer that is popular in cell culture preparation [20].

Various materials used in bioprinting are as follows:

a. **Biomaterial inks**
   Biomaterials have to be used inside the human body. Thus they are being prepared in cytotoxic situations such as extremely high temperatures and certain solvents, but these conditions are made possible using additives such as therapeutic molecules to make them withstand these processing conditions. Biomedical applications utilise thermoplastics, ceramics, composites and metals for additive manufacturing processing [12].

b. **Synthetic hydrogels**
   Synthetic hydrogels are superior to naturally obtained ones as they are modified under certain conditions to achieve the best qualities. One of the standard synthetic hydrogels is pluronic, which allows thermal linkages or is maintained with chemical bindings for UV linkages. 3D printing for structures involving overhangs can be made using the pluronic as a support material. These act as a material sacrificed after 3D printing to produce intricate and hollow objects. Other such materials are elastomers that provide features to be used in bioprinting due to their excellent mechanical properties and ability to mimic host tissues' viscoelasticity [20].

c. **Thermoplastics and resins**
   Thermoplastics are materials well known to all industries and are commonly used by hobbyists for model making. Their feasibility in bioprinting is because of the critical advantage with which we can manage and undertake numerous heating successions to integrate various factors and quickly form filaments for 3D printing through extrusion-based methods. Thermoplastics such as PLA, PCL, PVA, etc., are generally used to support cell-seeded hydrogels and direct implantation in the human body. High resolution in structures and excellent shape formations are produced with 3D printing. This results in superior control over porosity and mechanical properties. Resins are polymers that are easy to be processed with photolithography.

d. **Bio-composites**
   Ceramics are calcium and phosphate-based and have mineral salts, which aid bone and dental reconstruction with osteoconductivity properties. But due to the high brittleness, ceramics are difficult to 3D for implant fabrication. Therefore, they are mixed with polymers to enhance their extrusion properties. Commonly used bio-ceramics are tricalcium phosphate, hydroxyapatite, biphasic calcium phosphate, bioglass and polymethyl methacrylate. The

composite scaffolds by ceramics and polymers show slow degradation, non-cytotoxicity, non-antigenic, non-immunogenic, non-mutagenic actions and cell biocompatibility feasibility. Studies have shown that around 30 per cent of the biomaterials used in 3D printing are composite materials due to the enhanced properties one can achieve by amalgamating different materials. Ceramic materials are made for load-bearing orthopaedic usages (like hip acetabular cups with coatings), bone grafts/cement, and dental applications [21].

6.2   CONCLUSION

Additive manufacturing (AM) is emerging in society with its features facilitating designing different models, high precision of produced parts, and customisation possible with manufacturing methodologies' production rate. AM, also known as 3D printing or rapid prototyping, can make complex geometries, high porosity manipulations, the heterogeneous formation of cell cultures, and control mechanical properties of the part produced. Conventional autogenous bone grafts, allogenic grafts, and deal with tissue manufacturing scaffolds are already used in medical industries. Still, AM technology gives extra support to define the part properties effusively and control various parameters for the customisation of products for individual patients.

Orthopaedic applications are easily meant with titanium and its alloys with their excellent physical properties and outstanding biocompatibility. However, Vanadium and Aluminium ions released from Ti-alloys are harmful to the living beings, and thus, they possessed a vital hazard of toxic and unattached implants. Moreover, there are complications due to the stress shielding in the implant affected by the enhanced titanium stiffness than bone. Peek is found to have additional compatibility than metal materials as it possesses excellent biologically inertness and properties comparable to human bone. However, PEEK has a risk factor due to the lack of bioactivity of PEEK in clinical practices. Bioprinting is known to be present in past decades to have small functional units called organoids and body organs with quite good complexity. The bioprinting successfully transplanted the produced body part as a properly active part into patients suffering from various diseases. This has lowered the wait time for donor organs for transplantation, especially crucial in emergency cases. However, several situations have made it clear that the current range of materials available with the 3D-printing process is insufficient to suffice the need for medical applications. Thus, more research is to be done to produce new and novel materials with the characteristics required for organ transplantation and scaffold making.

REFERENCES

1. Farr, J. N., Melton, L. J., Achenbach, S. J., Atkinson, E. J., Khosla, S., Amin, S., Clinic, M., Clinic, M., & Clinic, M. (n.d.). *Original Article*. https://doi.org/10.1002/jbmr.3228
2. Rapp, K., Büchele, G., Dreinhöfer, K., Bücking, B., Becker, C., & Benzinger, P. (2019). Epidemiology of hip fractures Systematic literature review of German data and an overview of the international. January 2018, 10–16. https://doi.org/10.1007/s00391-018-1382-z
3. Banga, H. K., Kumar, P., & Kumar, H. (2021). Utilization of Additive Manufacturing in Orthotics and Prosthetic Devices Development. *IOP Conference Series: Materials Science and Engineering (MSE)*. https://doi.org/10.1088/1757-899X/1033/1/012083

4. Banga, H. K., Kalra, P., Belokar, R.M., & Kumar, R. (2020). Customized design and additive manufacturing of kids ankle foot orthosis. *Rapid Prototyping Journal*, 26(10). https://doi.org/10.1108/RPJ-07-2019-0194

5. Banga, H. K., Kalra, P., Belokar, R.M., & Kumar, R. (2020). Design and fabrication of prosthetic and orthotic product by 3D printing online first. *IntechOpen*. https://doi.org/10.5772/intechopen.94846. Available from: https://www.intechopen.com/online-first/design-and-fabrication-of-prosthetic-and-orthotic-product-by-3d-printing

6. Banga, H. K., Kalra, P., Belokar, R. M., & Kumar, R. (2020). Effect of 3D-printed ankle foot orthosis during walking of foot deformities patients. In: Kumar H., Jain P. (eds) *Recent Advances in Mechanical Engineering*. Lecture Notes in Mechanical Engineering. Springer, Singapore, pp. 275–288.

7. Chen, Y., Li, W., Zhang, C., Wu, Z., & Liu, J. (2020). Recent developments of biomaterials for additive manufacturing of bone scaffolds. 2000724, 1–28. https://doi.org/10.1002/adhm.202000724

8. Wang, C., Huang, W., Zhou, Y., He, L., He, Z., Chen, Z., He, X., Tian, S., Liao, J., Lu, B., Wei, Y., & Wang, M. (2020). Bioactive materials 3D printing of bone tissue engineering scaffolds. 5 (July 2019), 82–91. https://doi.org/10.1016/j.bioactmat.2020.01.004

9. Brien, F. J. O. (2011). Biomaterials & scaffolds Every day, thousands of surgical procedures are performed to replace. *Materials Today*, 14(3), 88–95. https://doi.org/10.1016/S1369-7021(11)70058-X

10. Manuscript, A. (2020). Materials horizons. https://doi.org/10.1039/D0MH00277A

11. Javaid, M., & Haleem, A. (2018). Additive manufacturing applications in medical cases: A literature-based review. *Alexandria Journal of Medicine*, 54(4), 411–422. https://doi.org/10.1016/j.ajme.2017.09.003

12. Soori, M. (2019). Applications of additive manufacturing to tissue engineering. *Materials Today*. May.

13. Ahangar, P., Cooke, M. E., Weber, M. H., & Rosenzweig, D. H. (2019). Additive manufacturing in medical applications. *Applied Sciences: Current Biomedical Applications of 3D Printing and Additive Manufacturing*.

14. Sinha, S. K. (2020). Additive manufacturing (AM) of medical devices and scaffolds for tissue engineering based on 3D and 4D printing.

15. Li, J. J., & Dunstan, C. R. In sheep tibiae Additive manufacturing of polymer melts for implantable medical devices and scaffolds.

16. Gleadall, A., Visscher, D., Yang, J., Thomas, D., & Segal, J. (2018). Review of additive manufactured tissue engineering scaffolds: Relationship between geometry and performance. 1–16.

17. Bahraminasab, M. (2020). Challenges on optimization of 3D-printed bone scaffolds. *BioMedical Engineering OnLine*, 1–33. https://doi.org/10.1186/s12938-020-00810-2

18. Liu, J., & Yan, C. (n.d.). 3D Printing of scaffolds scaffolds for tissue tissue engineering engineering. https://doi.org/10.5772/intechopen.78145

19. Baino, F., & Fiume, E. (2020). 3D printing of hierarchical scaffolds based on mesoporous bioactive glasses (MBGs)—Fundamentals and applications. *Materials*, 10(3), 1–5.

20. Pensa, N. W., Curry, A. S., Bonvallet, P. P., Bellis, N. F., Rettig, K. M., Reddy, M. S., Eberhardt, A. W., & Bellis, S. L. (2019). 3D printed mesh reinforcements enhance the mechanical properties of electrospun scaffolds. *Tissue Engineering*, 23(3), 1–7.

21. Liu, M., Yin, Y., Fan, Z., Zheng, X., Shen, S., Deng, P., Zheng, C., Teng, H., & Zhang, W. (2012). Nuclear instruments and methods in physics research B The effects of gamma-irradiation on the structure, thermal resistance, and mechanical properties of the PLA/EVOH blends. *Nuclear Inst. and Methods in Physics Research B*, 274, 139–144. https://doi.org/10.1016/j.nimb.2011.12.020

22. Singh, D., Singh, D., & Han, S. S. (2016). 3D printing of scaffold for cells delivery: Advances in skin. *Tissue Engineering* 1–17. https://doi.org/10.3390/polym8010019

23. Kuznetsov, V. E., Solonin, A., Urzhumtsev, O. D., & Schilling, R. (2018). Strength of PLA components fabricated with fused deposition technology using a desktop 3D printer as a function of geometrical parameters of the process. January. https://doi.org/10.3390/polym10030313

24. Cubo-Mateo, N. (2020). Design of thermoplastic 3D-printed scaff olds for bone tissue engineering: Influence of parameters of 'hidden' importance in the physical properties of scaffolds. *Material Sience and Engineering*, 4(1), 1–20.

25. Idris, M., Ismail, S., Mohamed, S. B., Sultan, U., & Abidin, Z. (2018). Mechanical properties of bone scaffold prototypes fabricated by 3D printer. November.

26. Yang, Y., Wang, G., Liang, H., Gao, C., Shen, L., & Shuai, C. (2019). Mechanics behind additive manufactured scaffolds. *International Journal of Bioprinting*, 5(1).

27. You, A., Be, M. A. Y., & In, I. (2020). Design of 3D scaffold geometries for optimal biodegradation of poly (lactic acid) -based bone tissue. *International Journal of Bioprinting*, 020062 (January), 3–8.

7 Materials for 3D Printing in Medicine
Metals, Polymers, Ceramics and Hydrogels

Sümeyra Ayan
Yildiz Technical University, Istanbul, Turkey
TUBITAK, Gebze, Turkey

Fatih Ciftci
Yildiz Technical University, Istanbul, Turkey
Fatih Sultan Mehmet Vakif University, Istanbul, Turkey

Mustafa Sengor
Marmara University, Istanbul, Turkey

Muhammet Emin Cam
Marmara University, Istanbul, Turkey
University College London, London, UK

Nazmi Ekren
Marmara University, Istanbul, Turkey

Oguzhan Gündüz
Marmara University, Istanbul, Turkey

Cem Bülent Üstündag
Yildiz Technical University, Istanbul, Turkey

CONTENTS

DOI: 10.1201/9781003301066-7

7.1   INTRODUCTION

3D printing, also known as additive manufacturing (AM), is a method of building 3D objects using computer-aided design (CAD) tools (i. e. Blender, SolidWorks, SketchUp, AutoCAD, Brush, Free CAD, and Meshmixer) (Tappa & Jammalamadaka, 2018; Yan et al., 2018). 3D printing is based on the layer by layer manufacturing (Yan et al., 2018). 3D printing enables the flexible preparation of highly complex and delicate structures that are difficult to achieve using traditional manufacturing techniques (e.g. casting) (Z. Chen et al., 2019b). The 3D-printing technology in medical applications can be classified into four main areas as follows; (i) manufacturing pathological organ models to aid preoperative planning and surgical treatment analysis, (ii) the production of personalised permanent non-bioactive implants, (iii) fabricating scaffolds that are used in tissue engineering, and (iv) direct printing of tissues and organs with complete life functions (Yan et al., 2018). The ability to produce neither low-volume nor one-of-a-kind parts on-demand based on patient (Bandyopadhyay et al., 2015), cost-effectiveness and speed are significant advantages of 3D printing as compared with injection moulding and machining (Berman, 2012).3D biomaterial printing is widely used for regenerative medicine and tissue engineering (Cornelissen et al., 2017). Two important components are usually needed to obtain biological implants. The first component is a bioprinter, which has materials like living cells (e.g. stem cells/tissue spheroids) and biodegradable scaffolds/matrices (e.g hydrogels and polymers). The second component is a bioreactor that is used to produce organs for the maturation of mimic organs *in vitro* (Ho et al., 2015). Although polymers are frequently used in temporary medical implants (e.g. implants and

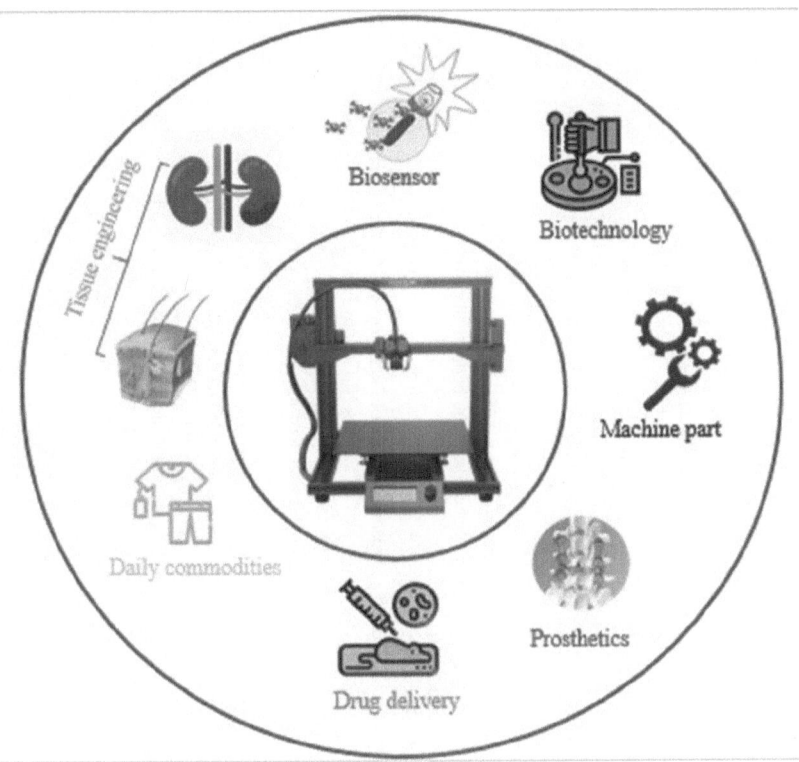

FIGURE 7.1   The biomedical application of the 3D printing technology.

stents), they have some disadvantages like having low mechanical strength, hardness and wear resistance. Metallic biodegradable materials are widely used in medical implants due to their higher yield, ultimate strength, toughness, hardness, wear resistance (Vojtěch et al., 2014), orthopaedic implants, bone fixators, and artificial joints (Hanawa, 2012). Applications of 3D-printing technology are illustrated in Figure 7.1.

7.2   METALS USED IN 3D BIOPRINTING

Metal biomaterials are generally 3D-printed in powder form by focusing high energy (i.e. laser) or by adhering to a binder polymer (Ho et al., 2015). Some metals are quite difficult to 3D print as the metals are usually solid at ambient temperature (Visser et al., 2015). The formation of a surface oxide layer on the low-viscosity liquid metal balances the shape of the 3D-printed metal (Parekh et al., 2016). Among various biodegradable metals, magnesium (Mg), zinc and iron (Fe) indicate good biocompatibility (Vojtěch et al., 2014). Applications of metal biomaterials generally target bone tissues. Key properties of human bone tissue are pore size, percentage of pores, interpore connection, mechanical properties, and bone surface. The synthetic bone tissue with these properties can best meet the need (Ho et al., 2015). Applications of metals in medicine produced via 3D printing are shown in Table 7.1.

TABLE 7.1

Applications of Metals that Are Produced Via 3D Printing

Metal	Side Material	Structure	Method	Application	Result	References
Ni	Polyaniline	Nanocages	3D-printing technology	Capacitor	Gives better performance than traditional porous structures.	Lu et al. (2018)
Fe	-	Scaffold	3D-printing technology	Bone tissue engineering	When corrosion rate, weight loss and reduction in cell viability increase, porosity is reduced.	Sharma et al. (2020)
Co-Cr alloys	3% calcium phosphate	Stent	3D-printing technology	Stent design	The corrosion of the alloy decreased by four times.	Sahasrabudhe et al. (2018)
Co-Cr alloys	MoW	Microstructures	The SLM method	Tissue engineering	Both alloys exhibited structures with relative density exceeding 99.5%.	Hitzler et al. (2018)
Co-Cr alloys	-	Scaffold	AMCasting	Making comparison production methods between the AM method and casting	AM produced parts fare better than casting.	Hong & Yeoh (2020)
Co-Cr alloy and Ni-Cr alloy	hADSC	Scaffold	SLM method Casting method	Dental prosthetics	The biocompatibility of the 3D-printed Co-Cr alloys was better than Ni-Cr alloys and Co-Cr with produced via casting.	Ganbold et al. (2019)
WE43	Rare elements	Scaffold	Laser melting	Mimic bone	The samples produced maintained the same mechanical properties as the bone even after 4 weeks in the degradation tests, and there was a 20% volume loss. Cell tests show that Mg alloys have a promising future.	Y. Li et al. (2018)
MKPC	Silica fume	Scaffold	3D printing	Tissue engineering	The 20-layer sample demonstrated the feasibility of the adopted mixture.	Weng et al. (2019)
Ti alloy	-	Hexagonal inner structure	3D printing	Bone scaffold	The requirement that the holes drilled in the fixation plates should be at the same angle as the intact bone on the opposite side made the 3D manufacturing method much more effective.	Cronskär et al. (2015)
316L stainless steel	-	Implant	The SLM method	Biomedical implant devices	0° building orientation exhibited the lowest dimensional accuracy.	

Laser powder bed fusion (LPBF) is a 3D technique to print metal parts. The creation of porous materials does not have constraints of traditional manufacturing routes in the LPBF method (Hojjatzadeh et al., 2019). Selective laser melting (SLM) is a type of LPBF that uses high-energy laser beams to melt powders together (Hitzler et al., 2018). This method starts with laying a thin layer of metal powder on a substrate plate, and the printing is continued until all systems are built up (Yap et al., 2015).

Binder jet printing (BJP) is a technique where a liquid binder is jetted on layers of powdered materials. The powdered material is spread out in a layer and combined with the binder into the printed layer shape. The BJP method is compatible with virtually any powdered material and has real potential to overcome powder bed fusion. This process has the widest choice of materials of whole AM methods. Some heat is used in the BJP method, nevertheless, this heating is minimal (Mostafaei et al., 2020).

7.2.1 Fe Alloys

Fe alloys possess the highest strength in comparison with hard bone tissue and are very useful for creating implants (Vojtěch et al., 2014). Iron manganate (FeMn) alloys are preferred because they corrode more slowly in the body electrochemically than pure Fe. Ho and co-workers were able to print a scaffold with 30 per cent porosity by using the inkjet 3D-printing method that would show the same mechanical properties as bone (Ho et al., 2015). Sharma and co-workers (Sharma et al., 2020) produced Fe scaffolds using both the 3D-printing method and pressureless microwave sintering for bone tissue engineering. They examined cytocompatibility, hem compatibility, and *in vitro* degradation behaviour. Fe scaffold has interconnected porosity varying from 50.70 to 80.97 per cent. The interconnected porosity plays a significant role in degradation properties and cytocompatibility. When corrosion rate, weight loss and reduction in cell viability are increased, porosity is reduced.

7.2.2 Cobalt-chrome Alloys

Cobalt-chromium (Co-Cr) alloys have corrosion resistance, high strength, and biocompatibility (Demir & Previtali, 2017). Although Co-Cr is an inert material, it can be corroded in environments under load and the residues left on the body can create toxic effects (Demir & Previtali, 2017). The use of the high power energy source can cause residual stresses, defects in the underlying surfaces, and bend the part during printing. For this reason, supports should be added to the part geometry by the user or the software. In some cases, it may be necessary to pre-sinter the layer being printed. These processes are often expensive and time-consuming. Alternatively, some metals are pressed in their oxide form and then subjected to the reduction reaction with hydrogen. Metal oxide powder is cheaper than metal powder, does not show carcinogenic effects, and the explosion risk is low (Williams et al., 2011). Hong and Yeoh (2020) examined corrosion resistance and mechanical properties (hardness, tensile strength, and yield strength) of the produced Co-Cr alloys via the AM method and casting. The grain size for the AM method and casting were 30 μm and 4000 μm, respectively. The corrosion resistance for AM sample was at 6.21 ± 3.91 MU cm^{-2}

while for the cast sample was at 3.74 ± 1.86 MU cm^{-2}. For tensile strength, the value was 1070 MPa for AM, while for cast samples, the value was at 655 MPa. The yield strength values decreased to 622 MPa for AM. The hardness value was 38 for AM, and 30 for casting. According to the results, AM produced parts fare better than casting.

7.2.3 NICKEL

Nickel (Ni)-based superalloys are widely used in spacecraft, gas turbine discs and rocket motors because of their good hot resistance to wear resistance, oxidation, and high strength (Xia et al., 2016). Lu and co-workers (Lu et al., 2018) synthesised porous Ni/polyaniline nanocages of battery electrodes via 3D-printing technology. The 3D-printed electrode plays better performance than a traditional porous structure for the application and the loaded electrode material. Ganbold and co-workers (Ganbold et al., 2019) compared human adipose-derived stem cell (hADSC) behaviour between the 3D-printed Co-Cr alloy and Ni-Cr alloy for dental prosthetics. Co-Cr discs were manufactured via casting method, a metal milling method and the SLM method. On the other side, Ni-Cr discs were manufactured via the casting method. The cell proliferation and viability of the Ni-Cr discs with hADSCs were lower than the other specimens. Nevertheless, the Co-Cr discs illustrated no differences in their different fabricating methods. To sum up, the 3D-printed Co-Cr alloys were more biocompatible than Ni-Cr alloys and Co-Cr alloys that are produced via the casting method.

7.2.4 MG

Mg, which is a good alternative to existing implant material, can be absorbed in the body and dissolve over time. Due to its light weight and biomechanical compatibility, it does not cause problems (i.e. abrasion in the host or adjacent tissue). Corrosions are positive for Mg. It does not require a secondary operation and does not cause complications as it degrades over time. Mg ions direct the growth and proliferation of bone cells. Calming with another metal, polishing its surface by electrolysis, shot-peening methods are among the most preferred methods to prevent corrosion. In 2016, the first Mg-based biological scaffold was introduced to the market as clinical studies were conducted (Karunakaran et al., 2020). Mg alloys are used in screw implants, bone plates, stents, wound closure, and biodegradable batteries (Yin et al., 2014). WE43 is an alloy of Mg with rare elements, and it is one of the most used types in the implant field. AZ91D is one of the most commonly used Mg-aluminium (Al) alloys and has high corrosion resistance. Li and his colleagues (Y. Li et al., 2018) were able to simulate bone, both mechanically and in terms of connecting the pores with each other, by pressing the WE43 alloy from the powder state by laser melting. They carried out the corrosion and toxicity tests of the scaffolds they produced in an environment with an oxygen rate of less than 10 ppm under argon gas. The size of the powders is between 25 and 40 microns. The samples produced maintained the same mechanical properties as the bone even after four weeks in the degradation tests, and there was a 20 per cent volume loss. Cell tests show that Mg alloys have a promising future. Weng and co-worker's study (Weng et al., 2019) proposes a 3D-printable cementitious material involving the use of Mg potassium phosphate cement (MKPC) with multiple ratios ranging from 0 to 60 wt% for using various applications. The optimal MKPC formulation including 60 wt% fly ash and 10 wt% silica fume with a borax-to-magnesia ratio of 1: 4 was printed for the 20-layered sample, and it showed good mechanical and rheological properties.

7.2.5 Titanium Alloys

Titanium (Ti) and stainless steel-based implants do not integrate with the body after they enter the body in their lean form (Karunakaran et al., 2020). Ti alloys are widely preferred in the biomedical field such as orthopaedic implants, bone screws, pacemakers and stents due to their inert nature. The most used types are Ti6Al4V (Ti-64) (which contains 6% Al and 4% vanadium) and commercial pure titanium. Although its thermal conductivity is low compared to other types, it is enormous in terms of strength, corrosion resistance, resource and manufacturability. Considering these properties, Ti-64 powder particles can be transformed into complex structures by the solid powder pressing technique (Khorasani et al., 2015). Ti implants imprinted with electron or laser-induced melting methods have different pros and cons in themselves. Samples produced in the electron method have much less residual stress, resistance corrosion, and surface roughness (Popov et al., 2018). When the need for a conventional TiAMimplant occurs, the damaged area is first detected with medical imaging devices and a 3D image is taken. Then, after calculating from which points the implant will be integrated into the body, the 3D Ti-64 implant is printed. Ti-64 implants usually go through a few more processes to adjust the pore degree and increase fatigue strength after they are manufactured with the AM method. Processes such as hot isostatic pressing and heat treatment are among the techniques commonly used to increase the strength of implants and eliminate residual stresses. If the expansion coefficient of Ti is taken as $9-10 \times 10^{-6}$ ($1/°C$), its elastic modulus is ~450 MPa at ~400°C, while the residual stress due to expansion around 800°C is ~150 MPa. As the temperature increases, the material is ductile and the expansion coefficient also increases (Saini et al., 2016). Cronskär and co-workers (Cronskär et al., 2015) tested the fixation plate by modelling it from Ti alloy on three patients with a collarbone injury. Using computed tomography (CT) based design, the plate contour and screw positioning can be optimised to the actual case. The topography of the damaged bone was obtained by the medical imaging method. The model of the implant to be placed in place was first removed from a conventional 3D filament printer with a hexagonal inner structure and tried by the surgeon. Post-processing was initially evaluated through three case studies, and the plate fit on the reduced fracture was tested during surgery (then replaced by commercial plates). In all three cases, the plates had an adequate fit on the reduced fracture. The time from the CT scan of the fracture to the final implant was two days. Especially in normal surgical operations, the requirement that the holes drilled in the fixation plates should be at the same angle as the intact bone on the opposite side made the 3D manufacturing method much more effective. Because dealing with adjusting the angle and position of the hole on the plate again, while the implant is being performed means a waste of time.

7.2.6 STAINLESS STEEL

The SLM steel material is used in various applications, with respect to the properties like biocompatibility, strength, and ductility. Kozior and co-workers (Kozior et al., 2020) studied 316L steel-based powder surface with high corrosion resistance using bed fusion technology. The samples were placed at 0°, 45°, and 90° angles in the plane. According to their examination, samples can be stated that the orientation of arrangement plays a significant role in the quality of the technological surface texture. 0° building orientation exhibited the lowest dimensional accuracy comparison with other specimens, which are contributed by the deformation that occurs during sample fabrication. Godec and co-workers (Godec et al., 2020) combined compounding, filament making and fused filament fabrication, which is a type of 3D printing of metal parts, processing of feedstock material with 55 per cent volume of 17-4PH stainless steel powder. They examined the most suitable optimisation parameters (i.e. extrusion layer thickness, environmental conditions, and flow rate multiplier), in order to obtain the maximum tensile strength of the 3D-printed samples. Their results examined that flow rate was the biggest factor that affected the tensile properties.

7.3 POLYMERS USED IN 3D BIOPRINTING

Polymer chains can be in linear or branched structures. Branching consists of side chains attached to the main chain. The resulting side branches are connected to the main part of the other chain and cross-linked polymers are formed. While branching of polymers complicates solubility, cross-linked structures are insoluble, absorb solvent into their structure and swell (Katti, 2004; Wheeler, 1994). Polymers have a very common usage area in the field of biomaterials thanks to their structures resembling soft tissues. Cotton, wood, and leather are types of natural polymers (Callister, 1991). The 3D-printed structures can be embedded in a variety of soft (e.g. elastomeric) and rigid (e.g. thermoset) polymers (Parekh et al., 2016). Examples of polymers used in medical applications are poly (lactic acid) (PLA), polyurethane (PU), poly (tetra-fluoroethylene), poly (ethylene) (PE), polysulfone, polyacetal, poly (methyl methacrylate) (PMMA), poly(glycolic acid) (PGA), silicone rubber and poly(ethylene thaphthalate). The use of polymeric materials in lenses, medical devices, vascular applications, orthopaedic applications (i.e. hip slots), and catheter applications has a wide place (Donaruma, 1990; Ratner et al., 2013). The polymer used on the surfaces of artificial joints should have a low wear rate and a low coefficient of friction. Today, ultra-high molecular weight polyethylene (UHMWPE), Teflon, nylon, silicone and similar materials are used in artificial blood vessels, sutures used in surgery, and hip socket implants (Donaruma, 1990; Ratner et al., 2013).

Polymers used as bone mortars are used to fix the implant and natural bone tissue superficially with each other. PMMA is widely used as bone mortar (Donaruma, 1990; Ratner et al., 2013). Polymers have high resilience and low strength and are easy to manufacture, deform, and deteriorate over time (Hench, 1998). Biodegradable polymers placed in the body allow it to replace the natural bone tissue regenerated, which reduces the 'strain relief' condition. These implants do not need to be removed from the body with their deterioration, which is an important advantage as a second surgery will not be required. Small molecules released from implants that degrade in the body can cause toxic effects in the body. Therefore, the biocompatibility of bio-degradable polymers is very important. Polymers used as biomaterials are grouped as natural and synthetic (artificial) (Raghavendra et al., 2015).

7.3.1 NATURAL POLYMERS

Natural polymers, which are indispensable resources in the field of biomaterials, do not cause reactions such as toxic effects and infections, since they are the same or similar to the structure of the molecules in the biological locations where they are applied. Biodegradable polymers have unique functional properties and are classified as natural polymers. Proteins (i.e. elastin, collagen, actin, gelatin), polynucleotides (i.e. starch, cellulose, dextran, chitin), and polynucleotides (i.e. deoxyribonucleic acid and ribonucleic acid) are mainly natural polymers. When the temperature is high, deterioration may occur in their structures. The disadvantages of natural polymers are that their composition changes depending on the source used and that they are immu-nogenic apart from these, the costs of manufacturing are high due to the complex structures of living organisms, and there is not enough production. Biodegradable polymers can be used in many different areas such as lubricant, gel builder, binder, thickener, implant material, and adhesive (Hickok et al., 2018; Park & Lakes, 2007).

7.3.2 SYNTHETIC (ARTIFICIAL) POLYMERS

The monomers of artificial polymers have a long hydrocarbon chain, consisting of carbon and hydrogen. The simplest artificial monomers are 'ethylene', and by polymerisation reaction, PE is formed. When polymers consist of other atoms (i.e. nitrogen, silicon or phosphorus) they are called 'inorganic polymers' (Katti, 2004; Wheeler, 1994). PMMA is a linear, hydrophobic chain polymer with a glassy struc-ture at ambient temperature. Trade names are Lucite and Plexiglas. Their structure is rigid and has good light transmittance and stability. For this reason, they are used in the production of intraocular lenses and hard contact lenses. Soft contact lenses are synthesised by adding the methylol ($-CH_2OH$) group to hydroxyethyl methacrylate (HEMA) methyl methacrylate.

Poly (HEMA) and a small amount of ethylene glycol methacrylate are mutually opposed to prevent dissolution of the polymer for contact lens preparation (Hickok et al., 2018; Wheeler, 1994). High-density PE is used in medical applications, while low-density ones cannot withstand the sterilisation temperature. If PE is evaluated in terms of its properties, its hardness is good and it is resistant to oils. While it is used in catheters and tubular studies, UHMWPE can be used in artificial hip implants. Polypropylene (PP), which is similar to PE, is harder in structure compared to PE. It has high chemical resistance. It has high tensile strength. PP can also be used in appli-cations where polyethylene is used. Another polymer is poly(tetrafluoroethylene) (PTFE) known as Teflon. It has a structure similar to PE. It is synthesised by replacing hydrogen atoms in PE with fluorine atoms. PTFE, which is difficult to process, is a hydrophobic, excellent lubricity, heat and chemically stable polymer. A form known as Gore-Tex is used in vascular prostheses (Donaruma, 1990; Pollard & Kitchen, 2017).

Another polymer used in tube form in medical applications is poly (vinyl chloride) (PVC). It can be used for nutrition, blood transfusion and dialysis. Although PVC is hard and fragile, with the addition of plasticiser a flexible and soft structure is formed. It can cause various problems when used for long-term applications. For example, PVC may lose its flexibility with the leakage of plasticiser from the structure and may also create toxic effects (Hickok et al., 2018). Poly (methyl siloxane) (PDMS) is another type of polymer, and it has a silium-oxygen base chain instead of the carbon base chain. They are used in catheters, vascular prostheses, drainage pipes and membranes in respiratory devices due to their high oxygen permeability. Moreover, they are used in finger joints, heart valves, external ear, jaw and nasal implants, blood vessels and breast implants due to their flexibility and stability in structure (Pollard & Kitchen, 2017). Polycarbonate is a hard material in terms of structure and has high impact resistance. It is synthesised by the polymerisation of bisphenol A and phosgene. Thanks to high impact resistance, it is used in eyeglasses/safety glasses, respiratory devices and heart-lung pumps. Polyamides (i.e. nylons) are formed as a result of the reaction of dibasic acids and diamines. Surgical thread can be given as an example of the usage area of nylons (Katti, 2004; Pollard & Kitchen, 2017). Block copolymers consisting of soft and hard segments are called PU. Its compatibility with blood is very good, therefore, it is a preferred material, especially in cardiovascular applications (Katti, 2004; Pollard & Kitchen, 2017). A material with suitable physical and chemical properties can also cause various unexpected damage if not designed correctly. Considering this situation, making the most suitable design for the material is one of the most important situations (Zhu et al., 2018).

7.3.3 APPLICATION OF 3D POLYMER BIOMATERIALS

Since the early 2000s, interest in the use of 3D printing for the production of soft tissues (organs and skin) and hard tissues (bones, teeth, and cartilage) has increased (Lee Ventola, 2014; Ligon et al., 2017; Stansbury & Idacavage, 2016; Xiaohong Wang et al., 2016; Xin Wang et al., 2017). Polymers have become consumer items. Because these are used in the production of bottles, transportation components, toys, phones, computers, tools, mattresses, bags, and electronics (Andrady & Neal, 2009; Muskovich & Bettinger, 2012). Organ damage or organ loss due to accident, trauma or disease is a health problem that negatively affects many people all over the world (R. K. Chen et al., 2016; Park & Kon Kim, 2002). Prosthetics of organs such as the chin and face are defined as the art of restoring the problematic part of the human body (Watson & Hatamleh, 2014). Soft tissue prostheses (i.e. artificial nose, eyes and ears) are widely used in maxillofacial treatments (He et al., 2014). The production stages of classical soft tissue implants consist of laborious, expensive and long steps such as impression, plaster reproduction, base plate manufacturing, mould manufacturing and external surface processes. However, the 3D-printing method is cheaper, easier and allows for implant production in a short time compared to conventional methods. In addition to all these, they can be used in many areas thanks to their bleaching and stain removal, acidity and alkalinity balancing, high conductivity, neutron absorption capacities, antiseptic, antibacterial properties, and flame retardant and anticorrosive properties. The printed interconnected porous scaffold is implanted in the sick and acts as a template. Biomaterials used in medicine should provide cell differentiation, adhesion and growth. The main challenge with natural polymers (e.g. fibrin, collagen, chitosan, and gelatin) is their low mechanical strength (Xiaohong Wang et al., 2016). Polymers can be used for both tissue and organ production (Hull, 1984) for allowing cell attachment, migration (Xin Wang et al., 2017), transferring growth factors (Ligon et al., 2017), and maintaining shape as cells grow (Stansbury & Idacavage, 2016). It is reported that chitosan dissolved in citric acid, acetic acid and lactic acid used the biofluid printing technique. They illustrated good cell proliferation, adhesion and growth as characterised by using SEM, the Live-Dead assay, and fluorescence microscope (Q. Wu et al., 2017). Lewis's team 3D-printed a scaffold of PCL, PDMS, and PLA-based materials (E.D. et al., 2016). They showed that it is possible to design and produce 3D-printed grafts. High-frequency displacement and acoustics were arranged by concentric rings, and the 3D-printed specimens were characterised by using dynamic mechanical analysis, digital opto-electronic holography, and laser Doppler vibrometry. In another examination, Suntornnond and co-workers (Suntornnond et al., 2017) 3D printed cellular materials with vascular networks for flowing were manufactured using Pluronic F-127, GelMA, and fibroblast cell culture as an ink. After that, Pluronic F-127 was removed by cooling to 4°C, providing open channels representing vascular networks. This examination showed that other cellular fluids and blood can flow through ducts with minimal cell death.

Skin burn patients and chronic wounds often suffer from long-term healing and haste high cost treatment process. Autologous split-thickness skin graft (ASSG) is utilised to cure large wounds. The injured area is placed in skin tissue and helps the healing and wound closure. The ASSG technique has disadvantages such as being limited to the size of donor areas and creating different injury sites (Min et al., 2014). The 3D-printed biomaterials will solve these mentioned problems by using the ASSG technique. Skin cells are cultured *in vitro* and biocompatible polymers are added to the culture.

The dental industry benefits from 3D-printing technologies for the production of crowns, braces, aligners, and dental implants (Dawood et al., 2015). Biocompatible materials, such as PLA, PCL, polyglycolide, and acrylates, are used for manufacturing dental parts using the 3D-printing technique (Ligon et al., 2017). With the inclusion of additives (e.g. quaternary ammonium salts), it was possible to manufacture antibacterial dental implants (Ge et al., 2015; Grischke et al., 2016; Yue et al., 2015). One of the other important areas of polymer is the pharmaceutical industry (Nokhodchi et al., 2015). Research and developments focus on 3D-printed materials that allow rapid production (Tetsuka & Shin, 2020). A product made from the 3D-printing technology has poor mechanical properties and anisotropic behaviour (De Schutter et al., 2018). The quality of the printed specimen depends on the accuracy of the 3D-printing technique and the printing scale (Ngo et al., 2018). Microscale 3D printing can sometimes present challenges with resolution, surface quality, and layer bonding that require post-processing techniques (e.g. sintering) (Z. Chen et al., 2019b). The 3D-printer focused CAD systems with easy usage are design instruments (Jaakma & Kiviluoma, 2019). The 3D printer is suitable for the production of several personalised products. In addition, with the use of CAD, additional costs (i.e. mould making and machining) are avoided in the case of a personalised

TABLE 7.2

Polymers Used in 3D-printing Technology-based Drug Delivery Systems

Polymers	Drug Delivery Systems	References
Ethylcellulose (EC)	Tablets	Yang et al. (2018)
Hydroxypropyl methylcellulose	Matrix tablets	Zhang et al. (2017)
PVA	Tablets, capsule	Goyanes et al. (2015); Xu et al. (2019)
Poly(lactic-co-glycolic acid)	Microsphere, capsule, tablet, nanosphere	Naseri et al. (2020); Tetsuka & Shin (2020); Wang et al. (2020); Zhang et al. (2019)
PMMA	Tablets	Chen et al. (2019b)
Poly(methacrylates) (Eudragit)	Nanocapsule, tablets	Azad et al. (2020); Beck et al. (2017)
PU	Tablets, hydrogel	C. T. Huang et al. (2017b), B. J. Park et al. (2019)
Poly(ethylene glycol) diacrylate	Hydrogel	Joas et al. (2018)
PLA	Nanofiber	Alam et al. (2020)
PCL	Tablets, carbon nanotubes	Beck et al. (2017), Ho et al. (2017)
Pluronic	Hydrogel	Müller et al. (2015)
Poly(vinyl pyrrolidone) (PVP or Kollidon®)	Tablet	Solanki et al. (2018)
Poly(N-(2-hydroxypropyl)-methacrylamide-mono/dilactate)-PEG-triblock-co-polymer (M15P10)	Hydrogel	Abbadessa et al. (2016)

product containing complex geometries such as mesh structures (Zhakeyev et al., 2017). Given these advantages, the US Food and Drug Administration approved the first 3D-printed tablet SPRITAM® in order to use in the treatment of epilepsy in July 2015 (Konta et al., 2017). However, there are still possibilities to improve manufacturing speed and reduce total production costs thanks to advances in machine design (Thomas, 2016). Table 7.2 shows the polymers used in the 3D-printing technology-based drug delivery systems.

7.4   CERAMICS USED IN 3D BIOPRINTING

Bone and cartilage tissue is one of the ceramic-based tissues of our body. Natural bone is an innate example of organic-inorganic biocomposites with a composition of 70 per cent by weight of inorganic crystals of calcium phosphate [$Ca_{10}(PO_4)_6.2H_2O$], which is itself a ceramic, and 30% by weight of organic compounds (including collagen, glycosaminoglycan, elastin, etc). $Ca_{10}(PO_4)_6.2H_2O$ are frequently used as bioceramics due to their properties such as bioactive, biodegradable, biocompatible, osteoconductive, osteo-integrated and osteo-inductive. Due to its excellent interaction with natural bone, it can be used frequently in bone patches, dental conditions, and cartilage tissue patches (Rho et al., 1998; Weiner & Traub, 1986). Application of ceramics that are produced via the 3D-printing method as shown in Table 7.3

TABLE 7.3

Applications of Ceramics Produced Via the 3D-printing Method

Ceramic	Side Material	Structure	Method	Application	Result	References
TCP, HA, Bio-Oss or DCB	PCL	Scaffold	Filament printing method	Tissue engineering	Scaffolds with 60% pore volume are produced.	Nyberg et al. (2017)
HA	Polymer	Scaffold	3D-printing technology	Tissue engineering	The pore percentage of the bone scaffolds they press at a layer thickness of 100 microns is 55%.	Cox et al. (2015)
TCP	PVA and graphene oxide	Scaffold	3D-printing technology	Tissue engineering Mimic bone	Micropores of 2 μm diameter were also formed on the walls of the scaffolds with 500 μm diameter pores.	Wu et al. (2015)
Bone powders	Polymer	Scaffold	Laser beam method	Tissue engineering	They were able to produce macropores between 20 and 1000 μm and micropores below 5 μm.	Li et al. (2020)
Silicon-based bioglass	Mg and calcium	Implant	3D-printing technology	Bone implants	The bioglass particles are very hard so stress build-up and naturally crack formation can occur.	Zhang et al. (2017)
TiO$_2$	MC3T3-E1 cell line	Scaffold	3D-printing technology	Bone tissue engineering	3D TiO$_2$ ceramic scaffolds showed good viability for cell growth and attachment.	Wang et al. (2018)
HA/TCP	-	Scaffold	DLP 3D printing	Bone tissue engineering	HA/TCP scaffolds can be produced with different pore architectures.	Lim et al. (2020)
HA	-	Scaffold	3D-printing technology	Bone tissue engineering	Mechanical properties are effected from the printing ink formulation.	Zhang et al. (2018)

Tricalcium phosphate (TCP) is used in the manufacturing of medical tools like neither calcium fortifiers nor artificial bones. Printing TCP has some disadvantages because TCP has strong interactions between the particles and it solidifies easily after mixing with hydrogel (Lee et al., 2017). Nyberg and co-workers (Nyberg et al., 2017) using the filament printing method, placed hydroxyapatite (HA) powders into a polymer and pressed them as a composite. They incorporated ceramic powders [TCP, HA, Bio-Oss or decellularised bone matrix (DCB)], into PCL. The composite materials are transformed into a molten form by applying heat. They were able to print scaffolds with 60 per cent pore volume with the help of pneumatic pressure from a 460 μm nozzle tip. The HA sample printed with the powder pressing method is studied in Cox and co-workers' examination (Cox et al., 2015). In the classical powder the AM method, a polymer that binds ceramic powders sprinkled into the bed is used. However, Cox and co-workers also threw bone powder into the binding polymer to make a denser scaffold. The pore percentage of the bone scaffolds they press at a layer thickness of 100 microns is 55 per cent.

The liquid injection method is one of the most commonly used techniques. In this technique, components such as bone powders (HA and TCP) are placed in a temporary polymer and pressed into paste form. Wu and co-workers (C. Wu et al., 2015) were able to print the chemically synthesised TCP by mixing it with a 6 per cent poly (vinyl alcohol) (PVA) solution and graphene oxide. Then they removed the binding polymer by keeping it at 1100°C for 3 h and sintered the powders. Micropores of 2 μm diameter were also formed on the walls of the scaffolds with 500 μm diameter pores, so they could imitate the bone structure thoroughly. Bone has a hierarchical pore structure. In other words, there are micro-scale pores inside the macro-scale pores. To obtain this shaped scaffold, controlled macro and microporous structure, Li and co-workers (X. Li et al., 2020) used the production technique of curing the resin in liquid form with the laser beam method. They were able to produce macropores between 20 and 1000 μm, and macropores below 5 μm. They used the bone powders first after mixing them with the light-cured liquid and grinding them well at 200 rpm. The polymer used has to be dissolved sequentially. The reason for this is to prevent the gases that can be released by thermal melting (pyrolysis) from damaging the ceramic tissue. At this stage, when the polymer, which is the binding tissue, is gone, it leaves pores in its place. Then the powders are sintered by heating up to 1200°C. During this process, contraction occurs in the sample. This method seems to be a good method for the need for a bone patch that will not work under load. They reported the compression strength as 15 MPa. Their cell studies and animal studies also support this. The inclusion of some metals and bioglasses in the structure of the scaffold can be very effective on factors such as vascularisation, dissolution and cell differentiation.

Zhang and co-workers (2017b), by adding metals such as Mg and calcium into scaffolds containing silicon-based bioglass, solved the problem of slow vascular development and the release of bioactive agents in bone implants with hollow cylindrical fibres and reached a strength of up to 26 MPa. This can be obtained from the relatively high strength bioglass, however, because the bioglass particles are very hard, stress build-up and naturally crack formation can occur (W. Zhang et al., 2017a). Wang and co-workers (2018) studied 3D periodic titanium dioxide (TiO_2) bioceramic scaffolds with TiO_2 sol-gel ink followed by sintering for bone tissue engineering.

Interconnectivity, structure and pore sizes were able to be controlled through 3D structure design and printing process. In order to determine the potential of these 3D TiO_2 bioceramic scaffolds, the mouse osteoblastic cell line MC3T3-E1 was cultured on the ink. According to the result of Wang and co-workers' examination, 3D TiO_2 bioceramic scaffolds showed good viability for cell growth and attachment.

A digital light processing (DLP) is a type of 3D printer that is used in many other areas containing computational imaging, microneedle-mediated drug delivery systems, wavelength multiplexing hyperspectral imaging and medical devices (Kadry et al., 2019). Lim and co-workers (Lim et al., 2020) produced pure ceramic scaffolds with variable pore architectures. They examined the mechanical properties and bone regeneration ability of the 3D-printed pure HA/TCP using a DLP 3D printer. The porosity and the compressive strength of the blocks with different specimens were studied *in vivo*. Larger scaffold pore sizes resulted in increased bone formation after four weeks ($p < 0.05$) shown as *in vivo* examination. According to their examination, different pore architectures of HA/TCP scaffolds can be produced via DLP 3D printing. Zhang and co-workers (2018) produced scaffolds using HA powders of spherical powder with diameters ranging from 10 to 50 μm, nano-sized grains with diameters ranging from 30 to 50 nm, and air-jet milling powders with diameters ranging from 10 to 30 μm. According to their study, both the air-jet milling powders and spherical powder inks might print porous scaffolds successfully. The ceramic micro and macro porous architectures and mechanical properties are effected from the printing ink formulation. The maximum compressive strength of spherical powder was 0.9 MPa, 5.5 MPa, and 3.2 MPa with porosities of 80, 60 and 70 per cent, respectively. With the same porosities, the compressive strength of air-jet milling powders specimens was slightly higher than that of the spherical powder specimens.

7.5   HYDROGELS USED IN 3D BIOPRINTING

Lee, Kwon, and Park first coined the term hydrogel in 1894 (Yahia, 2015). A hydrogel is a form of colloidal gel derived from inorganic salts, and they are used for matrix cell encapsulation, soft tissue, repair and replacement of organs. They are polymeric based materials that are compatible with body tissues, have high hydrophobicity, and can carry materials with various functions (Yahia, 2015; Zhao et al., 2013). According to their structure, they are divided into two main groups: natural and synthetic hydrogels. There are 3D-printing works such as alginate, chitosan, fibrin, PVA, PHEMA and poly (ethylene glycol) (PEG). Both advantages and disadvantages of hydrogels are shown in Table 7.4.

7.5.1   Natural Hydrogels

7.5.1.1   Alginate Hydrogels

Alginates, which are derived from brown algae (Figure 7.2), are a kind of polysaccharide composed of beta D-mannuronate and α-L-guluronate units (Ozbolat, 2016). The higher number of β-D-mannuronates means the higher the gel formability (degree of gelation). Alginate hydrogels are shape memory, cytocompatible, supporting cell proliferation, superior biocompatibility, degradation, non-immunological

TABLE 7.4

Advantages and Disadvantages of Hydrogel

Advantages	Disadvantages
Cell tissues and compounds can be changed	Mechanical properties are poor
They can protect cells from external factors	Difficult to synthesise
They can transport nutrients to cell tissue	Difficult to sterilise

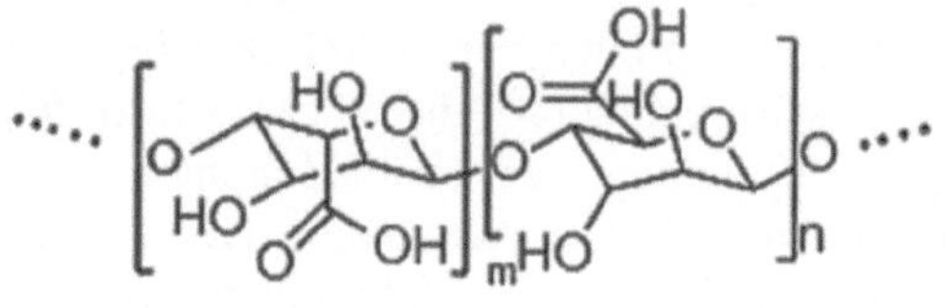

α-L-guluronate   β-D-mannuronates

FIGURE 7.2   The chemical structure of alginate.

effects, enhanced porosity, and mechanical strength (Jang et al., 2014; Zhao et al., 2013). Hydrogels derived from alginates are used in tissue engineering as scaffolds (Holland et al., 1998), biological structures (i.e. protein, enzyme or cell distribution), cartilage engineering (Alsberg et al., 2002), and as some matrix elements for *in vitro* studies of embryos (Tomei et al., 2014). The viscosity, porosity and cross-linking time of the alginate-based hydrogel are determined by the alginate concentration. Alginates used in tissue engineering have lower compressive strength than natural joint tissues (Zhao et al., 2013). Depending on the purpose of the 3D biomaterial printing process, bioprinted structures can be reinforced with other functional materials (i.e. crosslinkers) (Blaeser et al., 2013), 3 per cent by weight fluorocarbon, low melting point agarose, and 3 per cent added viscose. Concentration, viscosity, surface tension, gelation times, wettability, and addition of functional materials are important parameters for successful 3D biomaterial printing with alginate-based hydrogels (Gudapati et al., 2014).

7.5.1.2   Chitosan Hydrogels

Linear and randomly distributed β-(1→4)-bound D-glucosamine (de-acetylated unit) and N-acetyl-D-glucosamine (acetylated unit) known as chitosan is another type of polysaccharide with glucosamine structures as shown in as Figure 7.3. Chitosan is

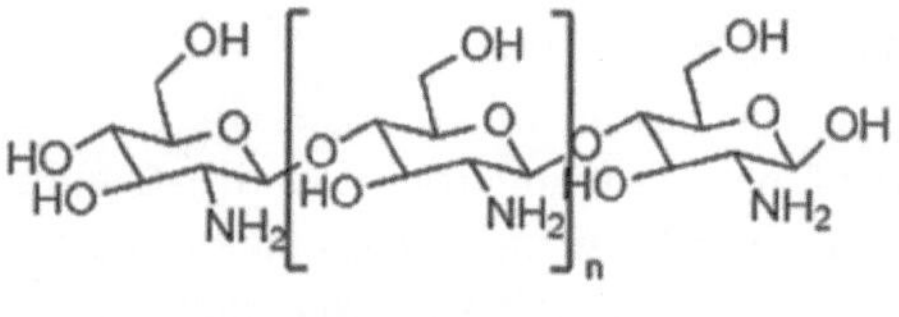

FIGURE 7.3   The chemical structure of chitosan.

usually made by processing chitin shells of seafood such as shrimp and other crustaceans with the aid of an alkaline substance such as sodium hydroxide. High bioactivity, biofunctionalities in glucosamine groups, and chemical differences may be obtained. For example, cell adhesion properties can be controlled by N-acetylation groups (Freier et al., 2005). Chitosan is one of the most important materials generally used as a biomaterial because of its many advantages such as high biodegradability, non-toxic response, biocompatibility, antibacterial ability and non-immunological properties (Kumar et al., 2004). Chitosan has a wide range of uses in cartilage, scaffolding and wound healing (Croisier & Jérôme, 2013). Nevertheless, chitosan is not suitable for scaffold synthesis for cell support as hydrogels, due to its poor mechanical strength and limited 3D bio-printability (Geng et al., 2005). The mechanical strength of chitosan can be increased by the mechanism of cross-linking through ionic or covalent agents after dissolution in acidic solutions (Ozbolat & Hospodiuk, 2016). B. Huang et al. (2017a, 2017b) studied the addition of halloysite nanotubes (HNT) to the strength and storage modulus of chitosan hydrogels and showed that the addition of HNT or regeneration in ethanol solution resulted in an extraordinary increase in the mechanical hardness of chitosan hydrogels.

7.5.1.3 Fibrin Hydrogels

Fibrin is a biological structure with a fibrous shape and non-spherical protein located in blood cells, and it is one of the key proteins that also stop blood clotting. Fibrins support enhanced cell proliferation (Cui & Boland, 2009), and play an important role in wound healing. Their natural cell adhesion abilities and high cell seeding have been used in the modifications and fabrication of skin grafts (Skardal et al., 2012; Yanez et al., 2015).

Fibrin hydrogels are often used in cardiovascular therapies, different muscle types, liver proliferation, skin replacements, cartilage engineering, and bone tissue regeneration (Ahmed et al., 2008). The mechanical stability of fibrin hydrogels depends on the amount of fibrinogen and the pH of the environment (Eyrich et al., 2007). The biggest disadvantages of these are both poor mechanical strength and rapid fragmentation (Zhao et al., 2013). Since the degradation times of fibrin hydrogels are very fast, they are not suitable for prolonged encapsulation inside the cell. Fibrin structure cutting and thinning capabilities are used in 3D biomaterial printing processes, especially in the extrusion process (Ozbolat & Hospodiuk, 2016). However, some work has been done to optimise these disadvantages of fibrins. In the extrusion process, the mechanical weakness of fibrins can be overcome by the photocrosslinking technique (Gruene et al., 2011).

7.5.2 SYNTHETIC HYDROGELS

7.5.2.1 Poly(HEMA) Hydrogels

Poly(HEMA), which is the chemical structure as shown in Figure 7.4, is a type of polymeric compound that can hydrogelise in water. Poly(HEMA) can be seen in many medical fields such as contact lenses (Ratner & Hoffman, 1976), artificial skin manufacturing, and dressings (particularly burn wounds) (Gibas & Janik, 2010). The use of different chemicals such as ammonium persulfate and sodium pyrosulfite (catalyst

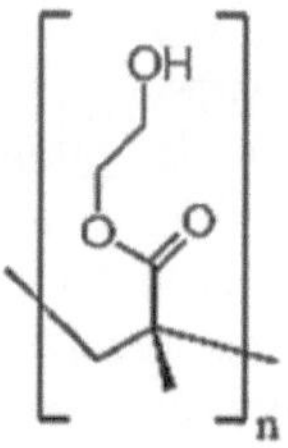

FIGURE 7.4   The chemical structure of poly (HEMA).

chemicals), and tri-ethylene glycol di-methacrylate (cross-linking agents) can be used as additives. Poly(HEMA) was first prepared by DuPont™ scientists (Ratner & Hoffman, 1976). Poly(HEMA) synthesis can be performed by simultaneous cross-linking with UV radiation. The properties of poly(HEMA) depend on many factors, including synthesis methods, polymer content, degree of cross-linking, and environmental conditions (Gibas & Janik, 2010). The wide range of stiffness values of these hydrogels can broaden their use for higher mechanical properties (Cretu et al., 2004).

7.5.2.2   PVA Hydrogels

PVA (Figure 7.5), which is a type of synthetic polymer, is soluble in water. It is frequently used in papermaking, textile, various coating industries, biomedical field, (i.e. contact lenses, cartilage regeneration applications, synthetic organs and wound healing). It is unique due to being a colourless and odourless polymer (Ratner & Hoffman, 1976).

Unlike the advantages of hydrogels, it has properties such as water absorbability, permeability, texture imitation, soft behaviour (high elasticity or elastic stretch), and high biocompatibility (Gibas & Janik, 2010). Due to their improved mechanical stiffness and ability to reshape their original form in water, providing improved volume properties in all environments. Hydrogel forms of PVA polymers can be obtained by various methods as neither freezing nor thawing. These methods have superior mechanical stiffness to other methods such as using UV light sources for the cross-linking process (M. Wu et al., 2001).

7.5.3   PEG Hydrogels

PEG (Figure 7.6), is a soluble type of polyether alcohol and can be mixed with water. Thanks to the solubility in alcohol and methylene chloride, it can be polymerised in

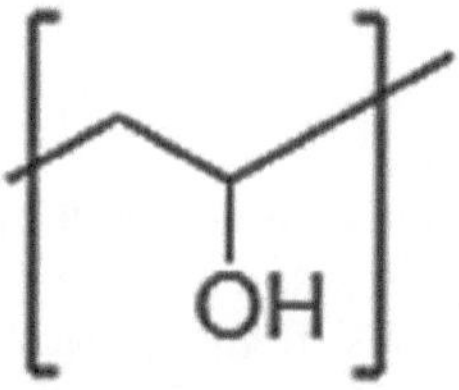

FIGURE 7.5   The chemical structure of PVA.

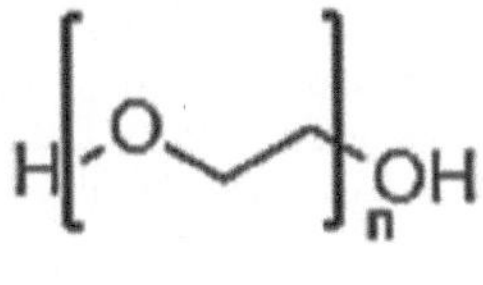

FIGURE 7.6 The chemical structure of PEG.

solution forms with UV light. However, the addition of a UV photo cross-linkable photo initiator can damage cell viability. PEGs are areas of use such as mineral oils, emulsifiers, moisturisers, alcohol compounds, chromatic pigments, abrasives, hydraulic fluids, organic synthesisers, office products, cell culture studies, wound healing, and medical fields (i.e. regenerative medicine). Due to the hydrophilic nature of PEG, it has adsorption resistance for proteins. One of the biggest drawbacks is low mechanical strength. To overcome this limitation, adding other compounds such as other photo starters or reinforcement materials is very useful (Ozbolat & Hospodiuk, 2016).

7.6 FUTURE ASPECTS AND STUDIES

3D biomaterial printing has made rapid progress in tissue engineering and regenerative medicine (Cornelissen et al., 2017). The biomaterial market is expected to reach 1.82 billion dollars in 2022 (Jessop et al., 2017). Therefore, future research aims to develop new biomaterials in the field of 3D biomaterials for use in tissue engineering applications and focus on printable biomaterials (Cornelissen et al., 2017). The 3D-printing technology is widely used for the production and transplantation of tracheal splints, skin, heart tissue, bone, vascular grafts, cartilaginous structures, toxicology, and drug discovery (Murphy & Atala, 2014). In comparison with conventional printers, the 3D-printing technology has the potential to allow mass customisation of goods and has potential in medicine including ophthalmology (Schubert et al., 2014). Although the scope of this script limits us, a 3D-printed food industry with rebuilt flavour, shape and altered substances is emerging (Piyush et al., 2020).

REFERENCES

Abbadessa, A., Blokzijl, M. M., Mouser, V. H. M., Marica, P., Malda, J., Hennink, W. E., & Vermonden, T. (2016). A thermo-responsive and photo-polymerizable chondroitin sulfate-based hydrogel for 3D printing applications. *Carbohydrate Polymers*, 149, 163–174.

Ahmed, T. A. E., Dare, E. V., & Hincke, M. (2008). Fibrin: A versatile scaffold for tissue engineering applications. *Tissue Engineering-Part B: Reviews*, 14(2), 199–215.

Alam, F., Shukla, V. R., Varadarajan, K. M., & Kumar, S. (2020). Microarchitected 3D printed polylactic acid (PLA) nanocomposite scaffolds for biomedical applications. *Journal of the Mechanical Behavior of Biomedical Materials*, 103, 103576.

Alsberg, E., Anderson, K. W., Albeiruti, A., Rowley, J. A., & Mooney, D. J. (2002). Engineering growing tissues. *Proceedings of the National Academy of Sciences of the United States of America*, 99(19), 12025–12030.

Andrady, A. L., & Neal, M. A. (2009). Applications and societal benefits of plastics. *Philosophical Transactions of the Royal Society B: Biological Sciences*, 364(1526), 1977–1984.

Azad, M. A., Olawuni, D., Kimbell, G., Badruddoza, A. Z. M., Hossain, M. S., & Sultana, T. (2020). Polymers for extrusion-based 3D printing of pharmaceuticals: A holistic materials–process perspective. *Pharmaceutics*, 12(2), 124.

Bandyopadhyay, A., Bose, S., & Das, S. (2015). 3D printing of biomaterials. *MRS Bulletin*, 40, 108–115.

Banga, H. K., Kalra, P., Belokar, R. M., & Kumar, R. (2020a). Customized design and additive manufacturing of kids' ankle foot orthosis. *Rapid Prototyping Journal*, 26(10). https://doi.org/10.1108/RPJ-07-2019-0194

Banga, H. K., Kalra, P., Belokar, R. M., & Kumar, R. (2020b). Design and fabrication of prosthetic and orthotic product by 3D printing [Online First]. *IntechOpen*. https://doi.org/10.5772/intechopen.94846. Available from: https://www.intechopen.com/online-first/design-and-fabrication-of-prosthetic-and-orthotic-product-by-3d-printing

Banga, H. K., Kalra, P., Belokar, R. M., & Kumar, R. (2020c). Effect of 3D-printed ankle foot orthosis during walking of foot deformities patients. In: Kumar H., Jain P. (eds) *Recent Advances in Mechanical Engineering*. Lecture Notes in Mechanical Engineering. Springer, Singapore, pp. 275–288.

Banga, H. K., Kumar, P., & Kumar, H. (2021). Utilization of additive manufacturing in orthotics and prosthetic devices development. *IOP Conference Series: Materials Science and Engineering (MSE)*. https://doi.org/10.1088/1757-899X/1033/1/012083

Beck, R. C. R., Chaves, P. S., Goyanes, A., Vukosavljevic, B., Buanz, A., Windbergs, M., Basit, A. W., & Gaisford, S. (2017). 3D printed tablets loaded with polymeric nanocapsules: An innovative approach to produce customized drug delivery systems. *International Journal of Pharmaceutics*, 528(1–2), 268–279.

Berman, B. (2012). 3-D printing: The new industrial revolution. *Business Horizons*, 55(2), 155–162.

Blaeser, A., Duarte Campos, D. F., Weber, M., Neuss, S., Theek, B., Fischer, H., & Jahnen-Dechent, W. (2013). Biofabrication under fluorocarbon: a novel freeform fabrication technique to generate high aspect ratio tissue-engineered constructs. *BioResearch Open Access*, 2(5), 374–384.

Callister, W. D. (1991). *Materials Science and Engineering: An Introduction* (2nd edition). Materials & Design, New York.

Chen, R. K., Jin, Y., Wensman, J., & Shih, A. (2016). Additive manufacturing of custom orthoses and prostheses-A review. *Additive Manufacturing*, 12, 77–89.

Chen, S. G., Yang, J., Jia, Y. G., Lu, B., & Ren, L. (2019a). Tio_2 and PEEK reinforced 3d printing pmma composite resin for dental denture base applications. *Nanomaterials*, 9(7), 1049.

Chen, Z., Li, Z., Li, J., Liu, C., Lao, C., Fu, Y., Liu, C., Li, Y., Wang, P., & He, Y. (2019b). 3D printing of ceramics: A review. *Journal of the European Ceramic Society*, 39(4), 661–687.

Cornelissen, D. J., Faulkner-Jones, A., & Shu, W. (2017). Current developments in 3D bioprinting for tissue engineering. *Current Opinion in Biomedical Engineering*, 2, 76–82.

Cox, S. C., Thornby, J. A., Gibbons, G. J., Williams, M. A., & Mallick, K. K. (2015). 3D printing of porous hydroxyapatite scaffolds intended for use in bone tissue engineering applications. *Materials Science and Engineering C* doi:10.1016/j.msec.2014.11.024

Cretu, A., Gattin, R., Brachais, L., & Barbier-Baudry, D. (2004). Synthesis and degradation of poly (2-hydroxyethyl methacrylate)-graft-poly (ε-caprolactone) copolymers. *Polymer Degradation and Stability*, 83(3), 399–404.

Croisier, F., & Jérôme, C. (2013). Chitosan-based biomaterials for tissue engineering. In *European Polymer Journal*, 49(4), 780–792.

Cronskär, M., Rännar, L. E., Bäckström, M., Nilsson, K. G., & Samuelsson, B. (2015). Patient-specific clavicle reconstruction using digital design and additive manufacturing. *Journal of Mechanical Design, Transactions of the ASME*, 137(11).

Cui, X., & Boland, T. (2009). Human microvasculature fabrication using thermal inkjet printing technology. *Biomaterials*, 30(31), 6221–6227

Dawood, A., Marti, B. M., Sauret-Jackson, V., & Darwood, A. (2015). 3D printing in dentistry. *British Dental Journal*, 219(11), 521–529.

De Schutter, G., Lesage, K., Mechtcherine, V., Nerella, V. N., Habert, G., & Agusti-Juan, I. (2018). Vision of 3D printing with concrete: Technical, economic and environmental potentials. *Cement and Concrete Research*, 112, 25–36.

Demir, A. G., & Previtali, B. (2017). Additive manufacturing of cardiovascular CoCr stents by selective laser melting. *Materials and Design*, 119, 338–350.

Donaruma, L. G. (1990). Biocompatibility—interactions of biological and implantable materials, volume 1: Polymers, by Frederick Silver and Charles Doillon, V. C. H. Publishers, Inc, New York, 1989, 306 pp. Price: $45.00. *Journal of Polymer Science Part C: Polymer Letters*, 28(9), 295–296.

Eyrich, D., Brandl, F., Appel, B., Wiese, H., Maier, G., Wenzel, M., Staudenmaier, R., Goepferich, A., & Blunk, T. (2007). Long-term stable fibrin gels for cartilage engineering. *Biomaterials*, 28(1), 55–65.

Freier, T., Koh, H. S., Kazazian, K., & Shoichet, M. S. (2005). Controlling cell adhesion and degradation of chitosan films by N-acetylation. *Biomaterials*, 26(29), 5872–5878.

Ganbold, B., Heo, S. J., Koak, J. Y., Kim, S. K., & Cho, J. (2019). Human stem cell responses and surface characteristics of 3D printing Co-Cr dental material. *Materials*, 12(20), 3419.

Ge, Y., Wang, S., Zhou, X., Wang, H., Xu, H. H. K., & Cheng, L. (2015). The use of quaternary ammonium to combat dental caries. *Materials*, 8(6), 3532–3549.

Geng, L., Feng, W., Hutmacher, D. W., Wong, Y. S., Loh, H. T., & Fuh, J. Y. H. (2005). Direct writing of chitosan scaffolds using a robotic system. *Rapid Prototyping Journal*, 11(2), 90–97.

Gibas, I., & Janik, H. (2010). Synthetic polymer hydrogels for biomedical applications. *Chemistry and Chemical Technology*, 4(4), 297–298.

Godec, D., Cano, S., Holzer, C., & Gonzalez-Gutierrez, J. (2020). Optimization of the 3D printing parameters for tensile properties of specimens produced by fused filament fabrication of 17-4PH stainless steel. *Materials*, 13(3), 774.

Goyanes, A., Wang, J., Buanz, A., Martínez-Pacheco, R., Telford, R., Gaisford, S., & Basit, A. W. (2015). 3D printing of medicines: engineering novel oral devices with unique design and drug release characteristics. *Molecular Pharmaceutics*, 2(11), 4077–4084.

Grischke, J., Eberhard, J., & Stiesch, M. (2016). Antimicrobial dental implant functionalization strategies: A systematic review. *Dental Materials Journal*, 35(4), 545–558.

Gruene, M., Pflaum, M., Deiwick, A., Koch, L., Schlie, S., Unger, C., Wilhelmi, M., Haverich, A., & Chichkov, B. N. (2011). Adipogenic differentiation of laser-printed 3D tissue grafts consisting of human adipose-derived stem cells. *Biofabrication*, 3(1), 015005.

Gudapati, H., Yan, J., Huang, Y., & Chrisey, D. B. (2014). Alginate gelation-induced cell death during laser-assisted cell printing. *Biofabrication*, 6(3), 035022.

Hanawa, T. (2012). Research and development of metals for medical devices based on clinical needs. *Science and Technology of Advanced Materials*, 13(6), 64102.

He, Y., Xue, G. H., & Fu, J. Z. (2014). Fabrication of low cost soft tissue prostheses with the desktop 3D printer. *Scientific Reports*, 4(1), 1–7.

Hench, L. L. (1998). Biomaterials: A forecast for the future. *Biomaterials*, 19(16), 1419–1423.

Hickok, N. J., Shapiro, I. M., & Chen, A. F. (2018). The Impact of Incorporating Antimicrobials into Implant Surfaces. *Journal of Dental Research*, 97(1), 14–22.

Hitzler, L., Alifui-Segbaya, F., Williams, P., Heine, B., Heitzmann, M., Hall, W., Merkel, M., & Öchsner, A. (2018). Additive manufacturing of cobalt-based dental alloys: Analysis of microstructure and physicomechanical properties. *Advances in Materials Science and Engineering*, 2018, 12.

Ho, C. M. B., Mishra, A., Lin, P. T. P., Ng, S. H., Yeong, W. Y., Kim, Y. J., & Yoon, Y. J. (2017). 3D printed polycaprolactone carbon nanotube composite scaffolds for cardiac tissue engineering. *Macromolecular Bioscience*, 17(4), 1600250.

Ho, C. M. B., Ng, S. H., & Yoon, Y. J. (2015). A review on 3D printed bioimplants. *International Journal of Precision Engineering and Manufacturing*, 16(5), 1035–1046.

Hojjatzadeh, S. M. H., Parab, N. D., Yan, W., Guo, Q., Xiong, L., Zhao, C., Qu, M., Escano, L. I., Xiao, X., Fezzaa, K., Everhart, W., Sun, T., & Chen, L. (2019). Pore elimination mechanisms during 3D printing of metals. *Nature Communications*, 10(1), 3088.

Holland, N. B., Qiu, Y., Ruegsegger, M., & Marchant, R. E. (1998). Biomimetic engineering of non-adhesive glycocalyx-like surfaces using oligosaccharide surfactant polymers. *Nature*, 392(6678), 799–801.

Hong, J. H., & Yeoh, F. Y. (2020). Mechanical properties and corrosion resistance of cobalt-chrome alloy fabricated using additive manufacturing. *Materials Today: Proceedings*, 29, 196–201.

Huang, B., Liu, M., & Zhou, C. (2017b). Chitosan composite hydrogels reinforced with natural clay nanotubes. *Carbohydrate Polymers*, 175, 689–698.

Huang, C. T., Kumar Shrestha, L., Ariga, K., & Hsu, S. H. (2017a). A graphene-polyurethane composite hydrogel as a potential bioink for 3D bioprinting and differentiation of neural stem cells. *Journal of Materials Chemistry B*, 5(44), 8854–8864.

Hull, C. W. (1984). Apparatus for production of three-dmensonal objects by stereo thography. United States Patent, Appl., No. 638905, Filed.

Islam, N. K. M. S., Harun, W. S. W., Ghani, S. A. C., Ghazalli, Z., Shri, D. N. A., Adib, M. A. H. M., & Sahat, I. M. (2017). Manufacture by selective laser melting & physical behaviour of commercial 316L stainless steel. *International Medical Device and Technology Conference, Malaysia*, 2017, 87–89).

Jaakma, K., & Kiviluoma, P. (2019). Auto-assessment tools for mechanical computer aided design education. *Heliyon*, 5(10), e02622.

Jang, J., Seol, Y. J., Kim, H. J., Kundu, J., Kim, S. W., & Cho, D. W. (2014). Effects of alginate hydrogel cross-linking density on mechanical and biological behaviors for tissue engineering. *Journal of the Mechanical Behavior of Biomedical Materials*, 37(2014), 69–77.

Jessop, Z. M., Al-Sabah, A., Gardiner, M. D., Combellack, E., Hawkins, K., & Whitaker, I. S. (2017). 3D bioprinting for reconstructive surgery: Principles, applications and challenges. *Journal of Plastic, Reconstructive and Aesthetic Surgery*, 70(9), 1155–1170.

Joas, S., Tovar, G., Celik, O., Bonten, C., & Southan, A. (2018). Extrusion-based 3D printing of Poly(ethylene glycol) diacrylate hydrogels containing positively and negatively charged groups. *Gels*, 4(3), 69.

Kadry, H., Wadnap, S., Xu, C., & Ahsan, F. (2019). Digital light processing (DLP)3D-printing technology and photoreactive polymers in fabrication of modified-release tablets. *European Journal of Pharmaceutical Sciences*, 135, 60–67.

Karunakaran, R., Ortgies, S., Tamayol, A., Bobaru, F., & Sealy, M. P. (2020). Additive manufacturing of magnesium alloys. *Bioactive Materials*, 5(1), 44–54.

Katti, K. S. (2004). Biomaterials in total joint replacement. *Colloids and Surfaces B: Biointerfaces*, 39(3), 133–142.

Khorasani, A. M., Goldberg, M., Doeven, E. H., & Littlefair, G. (2015). Titanium in biomedical applications—properties and fabrication: A review. *Journal of Biomaterials and Tissue Engineering*, 5(8), 593–619.

Koch, L., Deiwick, A., Schlie, S., Michael, S., Gruene, M., Coger, V., Zychlinski, D., Schambach, A., Reimers, K., Vogt, P. M., & Chichkov, B. (2012). Skin tissue generation by laser cell printing. *Biotechnology and Bioengineering*, 109(7), 1855–1863.

Konta, A. A., García-Piña, M., & Serrano, D. R. (2017). Personalised 3D printed medicines: Which techniques and polymers are more successful? *Bioengineering*, 4(4), 79.

Kozin, E. D., Black, N. L., Cheng, J. T., Cotler, M. J., McKenna, M. J., Lee, D. J., Lewis, J. A., Rosowski, J. J., & Remenschneider, A. K. (2016). Design, fabrication, and in vitro testing of novel three-dimensionally printed tympanic membrane grafts. *Hearing Research*, 340, 191–203.

Kozior, T., Bochnia, J., Zmarzły, P., Gogolewski, D., & Mathia, T. G. (2020). Waviness of freeform surface characterizations from austenitic stainless steel (316l) manufactured by 3d printing-selective laser melting (slm) technology. *Materials*, 13(19), 4372.

Kumar, M. N. V. R., Muzzarelli, R. A. A., Muzzarelli, C., Sashiwa, H., & Domb, A. J. (2004). Chitosan chemistry and pharmaceutical perspectives. *Chemical Reviews*, 104(12), 6017–6084.

Lee, J., Kim, K. E., Bang, S., Noh, I., & Lee, C. (2017). A desktop multi-material 3D bio-printing system with open-source hardware and software. *International Journal of Precision Engineering and Manufacturing*, 18(4), 605–612.

Lee Ventola, C. (2014). Medical applications for 3D printing: Current and projected uses. *P and T*, 9(10), 704.

Li, X., Yuan, Y., Liu, L., Leung, Y.-S., Chen, Y., Guo, Y., Chai, Y., & Chen, Y. (2020). 3D printing of hydroxyapatite/tricalcium phosphate scaffold with hierarchical porous structure for bone regeneration. *Bio-Design and Manufacturing*, 3(1), 15–29.

Li, Y., Zhou, J., Pavanram, P., Leeflang, M. A., Fockaert, L. I., Pouran, B., Tümer, N., Schröder, K. U., Mol, J. M. C., Weinans, H., Jahr, H., & Zadpoor, A. A. (2018). Additively manufactured biodegradable porous magnesium. *Acta Biomaterialia*, 67, 378–439.

Ligon, S. C., Liska, R., Stampfl, J., Gurr, M., & Mülhaupt, R. (2017). Polymers for 3D printing and customized additive manufacturing. *Chemical Reviews*, 117(15), 10212–10290

Lim, H. K., Hong, S. J., Byeon, S. J., Chung, S. M., On, S. W., Yang, B. E., Lee, J. H., & Byun, S. H. (2020). 3D-printed ceramic bone scaffolds with variable pore architectures. *International Journal of Molecular Sciences*, 21(18), 6942.

Lu, X., Zhao, T., Ji, X., Hu, J., Li, T., Lin, X., & Huang, W. (2018). 3D printing well organized porous iron-nickel/polyaniline nanocages multiscale supercapacitor. *Journal of Alloys and Compounds*, 760, 78–83.

Min, J. H., Yun, I. S., Lew, D. H., Roh, T. S., & Lee, W. J. (2014). The use of Matriderm and autologous skin graft in the treatment of full thickness skin defects. *Archives of Plastic Surgery*, 41(04), 330–336.

Mostafaei, A., Elliott, A. M., Barnes, J. E., Li, F., Tan, W., Cramer, C. L., Nandwana, P., & Chmielus, M. (2020). Binder jet 3D printing – Process parameters, materials, properties, and challenges. *Progress in Materials Science*, 19, 100707.

Müller, M., Becher, J., Schnabelrauch, M., & Zenobi-Wong, M. (2015). Nanostructured Pluronic hydrogels as bioinks for 3D bioprinting. *Biofabrication*, 7(3), 035006.

Murphy, S. V., & Atala, A. (2014). 3D bioprinting of tissues and organs. *Nature Biotechnology*, 32(8), 773–785.

Muskovich, M., & Bettinger, C. J. (2012). Biomaterials-Based electronics: Polymers and interfaces for biology and medicine. *Advanced Healthcare Materials*, 1(3), 248–266.

Naseri, E., Butler, H., MacNevin, W., Ahmed, M., & Ahmadi, A. (2020). Low-temperature solvent-based 3D printing of PLGA: A parametric printability study. *Drug Development and Industrial Pharmacy*, 46(2), 173–178.

Ngo, T. D., Kashani, A., Imbalzano, G., Nguyen, K. T. Q., & Hui, D. (2018). Additive manufacturing (3D printing): A review of materials, methods, applications and challenges. *Composites Part B: Engineering*, 143, 172–196.

Nokhodchi, A., Palmer, D., Asare-Addo, K., Levina, M., & Rajabi-Siahboomi, A. (2015). Application of polymer combinations in extended release hydrophilic matrices. In: *Handbook of Polymers for Pharmaceutical Technologies*, Wiley, pp. 23–50. ISBN 978-1-119-04134-4

Nyberg, E., Rindone, A., Dorafshar, A., & Grayson, W. L. (2017). Comparison of 3D-Printed Poly-ε-Caprolactone scaffolds functionalized with tricalcium phosphate, hydroxyapatite, Bio-Oss, or decellularized bone matrix. *Tissue Engineering-Part A*, 23(11–12), 503–514.

Ozbolat, I. T. (2016). *3D Bioprinting: Fundamentals, Principles and Applications: 3D Bioprinting: Fundamentals, Principles and Applications*. Elsevier Inc, Amsterdam.

Ozbolat, I. T., & Hospodiuk, M. (2016). Current advances and future perspectives in extrusion-based bioprinting. *Biomaterials*, 76, 321–343.

Parekh, D. P., Ladd, C., Panich, L., Moussa, K., & Dickey, M. D. (2016). 3D printing of liquid metals as fugitive inks for fabrication of 3D microfluidic channels. *Lab on a Chip*, 16(10), 1812–1820.

Park, B. J., Choi, H. J., Moon, S. J., Kim, S. J., Bajracharya, R., Min, J. Y., & Han, H. K. (2019). Pharmaceutical applications of 3D printing technology: Current understanding and future perspectives. *Journal of Pharmaceutical Investigation*, 49(6), 575–585.

Park, J., & Lakes, R. S. (2007). *Biomaterials: An Introduction*: 3rd edition, Springer, New York.

Park, J. B., & Kon Kim, Y. (2002). *Metallic biomaterials. Biomaterials: Principles and Applications*. Marcel Dekker, New York.

Pollard, B. J., & Kitchen, G. (2017). Plastic surgery. In: *Handbook of Clinical Anaesthesia*, Fourth Edition.

Popov, V. V., Muller-Kamskii, G., Kovalevsky, A., Dzhenzhera, G., Strokin, E., Kolomiets, A., & Ramon, J. (2018). Design and 3D-printing of titanium bone implants: Brief review of approach and clinical cases. *Biomedical Engineering Letters*, 8(4), 337–344

Piyush, Kumar, R., & Kumar, R. (2020). 3D printing of food materials: A state of art review and future applications. *Materials Today: Proceedings*, 33, 1463–1467.

Raghavendra, G. M., Varaprasad, K., & Jayaramudu, T. (2015). *Biomaterials: Design, Development and Biomedical Applications* (pp. 21–44).

Ratner, B. D., & Hoffman, A. S. (1976). Synthetic hydrogels for biomedical applications. In *Hydrogels for Medical and Related Applications*, J. D. Andrade, ed. ACS Symposium Series, American Society, Washington, DC, Vol. 31, pp. 1–36.

Ratner, B. D., Hoffman, A. S., Schoen, F. J., & Lemons, J. E. (2013). *Biomaterials Science: An Introduction to Materials*, 3rd edition.

Rho, J. Y., Kuhn-Spearing, L., & Zioupos, P. (1998). Mechanical properties and the hierarchical structure of bone. *Medical Engineering and Physics*, 20(2), 92–102.

Sahasrabudhe, H., Bose, S., & Bandyopadhyay, A. (2018). Laser processed calcium phosphate reinforced CoCrMo for load-bearing applications: Processing and wear induced damage evaluation. *Acta Biomaterialia*, 66, 118–128

Saini, A., Pabla, B. S., & Dhami, S. S. (2016). Developments in cutting tool technology in improving machinability of Ti6Al4V alloy: A review. *Proceedings of the Institution of Mechanical Engineers, Part B: Journal of Engineering Manufacture*, 230(11), 1977–1989.

Schubert, C., Van Langeveld, M. C., & Donoso, L. A. (2014). Innovations in 3D printing: A 3D overview from optics to organs. *British Journal of Ophthalmology*, 98(2), 159–161.

Sharma, P., Jain, K. G., Pandey, P. M., & Mohanty, S. (2020). In vitro degradation behaviour, cytocompatibility and hemocompatibility of topologically ordered porous iron scaffold prepared using 3D printing and pressureless microwave sintering. *Materials Science and Engineering: C*, 106, 110247.

Skardal, A., Mack, D., Kapetanovic, E., Atala, A., Jackson, J. D., Yoo, J., & Soker, S. (2012). Bioprinted amniotic fluid-derived stem cells accelerate healing of large skin wounds. *STEM CELLS Translational Medicine*, 1(11), 792–802.

Solanki, N. G., Tahsin, M., Shah, A. V., & Serajuddin, A. T. M. (2018). Formulation of 3D printed tablet for rapid drug release by fused deposition modeling: screening polymers for drug release, drug-polymer miscibility and printability. *Journal of Pharmaceutical Sciences*, 107(1), 390–401.

Stansbury, J. W., & Idacavage, M. J. (2016). 3D printing with polymers: Challenges among expanding options and opportunities. *Dental Materials*, 32(1), 54–64.

Suntornnond, R., Tan, E. Y. S., An, J., & Chua, C. K. (2017). A highly printable and biocompatible hydrogel composite for direct printing of soft and perfusable vasculature-like structures. *Scientific Reports*, 7(1), 1–11.

Tappa, K., & Jammalamadaka, U. (2018). Novel biomaterials used in medical 3D printing techniques. *Journal of Functional Biomaterials*, 9(1), 17.

Tetsuka, H., & Shin, S. R. (2020). Materials and technical innovations in 3D printing in biomedical applications. *Journal of Materials Chemistry B*, 8(15), 2930–2950.

Thomas, D. (2016). Costs, benefits, and adoption of additive manufacturing: A supply chain perspective. *International Journal of Advanced Manufacturing Technology*, 100(1192), 485–488.

Tomei, A. A., Manzoli, V., Fraker, C. A., Giraldo, J., Velluto, D., Najjar, M., Pileggi, A., Molano, R. D., Ricordi, C., Stabler, C. L., & Hubbell, J. A. (2014). Device design and materials optimization of conformal coating for islets of Langerhans. *Proceedings of the National Academy of Sciences of the United States of America*, 111(29), 10514–10519.

Visser, C. W., Pohl, R., Sun, C., Römer, G.-W., Huis in 't Veld, B., & Lohse, D. (2015). Toward 3D printing of pure metals by laser-induced forward transfer. *Advanced Materials*, 27(27), 4087–4092.

Vojtěch, D., Kubásek, J., Čapek, J., & Pospíšilová, I. (2014). Magnesium, zinc and iron alloys for medical applications in biodegradable implants. *METAL 2014 - 23rd International Conference on Metallurgy and Materials, Conference Proceedings*, 1092–1096.

Wang, R., Zhu, P., Yang, W., Gao, S., Li, B., & Li, Q. (2018). Direct-writing of 3D periodic TiO_2 bio-ceramic scaffolds with a sol-gel ink for in vitro cell growth. *Materials and Design*, 144(2018), 304–309.

Wang, X., Ao, Q., Tian, X., Fan, J., Wei, Y., Hou, W., Tong, H., & Bai, S. (2016). 3D bioprinting technologies for hard tissue and organ engineering. *Materials*, 9(10), 802.

Wang, X., Jiang, M., Zhou, Z., Gou, J., & Hui, D. (2017). 3D printing of polymer matrix composites: A review and prospective. *Composites Part B: Engineering*, 110, 442–458.

Wang, Y., Qiao, X., Yang, X., Yuan, M., Xian, S., Zhang, L., Yang, D., Liu, S., Dai, F., Tan, Z., & Cheng, Y. (2020). The role of a drug-loaded poly (lactic co-glycolic acid) (PLGA) copolymer stent in the treatment of ovarian cancer. *Cancer Biology and Medicine*, 17(1), 237.

Watson, J., & Hatamleh, M. M. (2014). Complete integration of technology for improved reproduction of auricular prostheses. *Journal of Prosthetic Dentistry*, 111(5), 430–436.

Weiner, S., & Traub, W. (1986). Organization of hydroxyapatite crystals within collagen fibrils. *FEBS Letters*, 206(2), 262–266.

Weng, Y., Ruan, S., Li, M., Mo, L., Unluer, C., Tan, M. J., & Qian, S. (2019). Feasibility study on sustainable magnesium potassium phosphate cement paste for 3D printing. *Construction and Building Materials*, 221, 595–603.

Wheeler, P. (1994). Plastic surgery. *Ground Engineering*, 27(8), 24.

Williams, C. B., Cochran, J. K., & Rosen, D. W. (2011). Additive manufacturing of metallic cellular materials via three-dimensional printing. *International Journal of Advanced Manufacturing Technology*, 53(1), 231–239.

Wu, C., Xia, L., Han, P., Xu, M., Fang, B., Wang, J., Chang, J., & Xiao, Y. (2015). Graphene-oxide-modified β-tricalcium phosphate bioceramics stimulate in vitro and in vivo osteogenesis. *Carbon*, 93(2015): 116–129.

Wu, M., Bao, B., Yoshii, F., & Makuuchi, K. (2001). Irradiation of crosslinked, poly(vinyl alcohol) blended hydrogel for wound dressing. *Journal of Radioanalytical and Nuclear Chemistry*, 250(2), 391–395.

Wu, Q., Maire, M., Lerouge, S., Therriault, D., & Heuzey, M.-C. (2017). 3D printing of microstructured and stretchable chitosan hydrogel for guided cell growth. *Advanced Biosystems*, 1(6), 1700058.

Xia, M., Gu, D., Yu, G., Dai, D., Chen, H., & Shi, Q. (2016). Selective laser melting 3D printing of Ni-based superalloy: Understanding thermodynamic mechanisms. *Science Bulletin*, 61(13), 1013–1022.

Xu, X., Zhao, J., Wang, M., Wang, L., & Yang, J. (2019). 3D Printed Polyvinyl Alcohol Tablets with Multiple Release Profiles. *Scientific Reports*, 9(1), 1–8.

Yahia, Lh. (2015). History and applications of hydrogels. *Journal of Biomedical Sciencies*, 4(2), 0–0.

Yan, Q., Dong, H., Su, J., Han, J., Song, B., Wei, Q., & Shi, Y. (2018). A review of 3D printing technology for medical applications. *Engineering*, 4(5), 729–742.

Yanez, M., Rincon, J., Dones, A., De Maria, C., Gonzales, R., & Boland, T. (2015). In vivo assessment of printed microvasculature in a bilayer skin graft to treat full-thickness wounds. *Tissue Engineering - Part A*, 21(1–2), 224–233.

Yang, Y., Wang, H., Li, H., Ou, Z., & Yang, G. (2018). 3D printed tablets with internal scaffold structure using ethyl cellulose to achieve sustained ibuprofen release. *European Journal of Pharmaceutical Sciences*, 115, 11–18.

Yap, C. Y., Chua, C., Dong, Z., Liu, Z., Zhang, D., Loh, L. E., & Sing, S. L. (2015). Review of selective laser melting: Materials and applications. *Applied Physics Reviews*, 2, 41101.

Yin, L., Huang, X., Xu, H., Zhang, Y., Lam, J., Cheng, J., & Rogers, J. A. (2014). Materials, designs, and operational characteristics for fully biodegradable primary batteries. *Advanced Materials*, 26(23), 3879–3884.

Yue, J., Zhao, P., Gerasimov, J. Y., Van De Lagemaat, M., Grotenhuis, A., Rustema-Abbing, M., Van Der Mei, H. C., Busscher, H. J., Herrmann, A., & Ren, Y. (2015). 3D-printable antimicrobial composite resins. *Advanced Functional Materials*, 25(43), 6756–6767.

Zhakeyev, A., Wang, P., Zhang, L., Shu, W., Wang, H., & Xuan, J. (2017). Additive manufacturing: Unlocking the evolution of energy materials. *Advanced Science*, 4(10), 1700187.

Zhang, B., Pei, X., Song, P., Sun, H., Li, H., Fan, Y., Jiang, Q., Zhou, C., & Zhang, X. (2018). Porous bioceramics produced by inkjet 3D printing: Effect of printing ink formulation on the ceramic macro and micro porous architectures control. *Composites Part B: Engineering*, 155, 112–121.

Zhang, J., Yang, W., Vo, A. Q., Feng, X., Ye, X., Kim, D. W., & Repka, M. A. (2017b). Hydroxypropyl methylcellulose-based controlled release dosage by melt extrusion and 3D printing: Structure and drug release correlation. *Carbohydrate Polymers*, 177(2017), 49–57.

Zhang, W., Feng, C., Yang, G., Li, G., Ding, X., Wang, S., Dou, Y., Zhang, Z., Chang, J., Wu, C., & Jiang, X. (2017a). 3D-printed scaffolds with synergistic effect of hollow-pipe structure and bioactive ions for vascularized bone regeneration. *Biomaterials*, 135, 85–95.

Zhang, Z. Z., Zhang, H. Z., & Zhang, Z. Y. (2019). 3D printed poly(ε-caprolactone) scaffolds function with simvastatin-loaded poly(lactic-co-glycolic acid) microspheres to repair load-bearing segmental bone defects. *Experimental and Therapeutic Medicine*, 17(1), 79–90.

Zhao, W., Jin, X., Cong, Y., Liu, Y., & Fu, J. (2013). Degradable natural polymer hydrogels for articular cartilage tissue engineering. *Journal of Chemical Technology and Biotechnology*, 88(3), 327–339.

Zhu, Z., Guo, S. Z., Hirdler, T., Eide, C., Fan, X., Tolar, J., & McAlpine, M. C. (2018). 3D printed functional and biological materials on moving freeform surfaces. *Advanced Materials*, 30(23), 1707495.

8 Recent Advances and Developments in the Field of Rapid Prototyping for Clinical Applications

Navdeep Singh and Parnika Shrivastava
National Institute of Technology Hamirpur, Hamirpur, India

CONTENTS

8.1 INTRODUCTION

The medical industry is recognising the benefits of 3D printing, also known as additive manufacturing (AM), for a wide variety of medical applications at an increasing pace. This manufacturing strategy has emerged in the last decade as an alternative and efficient method of producing goods quickly and easily (Matsumoto et al., 2016). 3D printing began mostly as a commercial tool to facilitate concept-to-physical product manufacturing. It has now become a widely used technology that has an impact on many facets of our society. AM is also being used to create patient-specific replicas of bones, organs and blood vessels, as well as new surgical cutting and drill manuals, orthopaedic implants, and prosthetics (Nadagouda et al., 2020; Tack et al., 2016).

These advances demonstrate the value of AM in the medical field, where personalised products tailored to each individual can be created. Medical professionals gain a better understanding of their patients' comfort levels as they gain access to objects designed specifically for their anatomy (Abed et al., 2020; McMenamin et al., 2014). Pre-surgical preparation, intraoperative guidance, and custom implant development are the immediate clinical applications of 3D printing (Sousa et al., 2020; Wang & Boyle, 1994). Treatment planning, customised prostheses, bioprinting, medical-patient education and radiology resources are only a few of the topics discussed. Medical practitioners are in charge of proper image evaluation and possession; they also have the ability to lead rapid prototyping and use it in care planning (Attaran, 2017; Banga et al., 2017, 2020a).

Preliminary investigation reported that a few pieces of research have been dedicated to rapid prototyping for clinical applications. To encourage this technology's continued growth, the National Additive Manufacturing Innovation Institute was established in 2012. The use of this technology in medicine has been advocated by many professional societies. A 3D-Printing Special Interest Group was formed in 2016 in the Radiological Society of North America. This organisation has organised several meetings and workshops in the past. It is even looking at how the procedure could be developed for medical purposes (Banga et al., 2018; Belokar et al., 2017). Even in dental care industries, due to the improvement in manufacturing processes and materials, orthodontic appliances and equipment have seen an increased use over the past few decades. Still, for successful patient acceptability understanding the mechanical, geometric and physical properties of dental products is imperative (Jindal et al., 2020). This subject has undoubtedly grown in prominence as a result of its enormous potential for medical practitioners, researchers and patients. If properly implemented, AM has the potential to strengthen patient safety while also increasing the relative contribution of radiologists' care (Banga et al., 2020a). Radiologists, in particular, may use this approach to provide personalised medicine based on anatomic data. Providing such a service allows you to engage with referring doctors differently and more effectively (Lal & Patralekh, 2018).

The present work is an effort to report and highlight the current developments related to the use of 3D printing in clinical applications. In today's world, it is essential to realise the benefits that the medical industry can get from 3D printing. In the following sections, the manuscript provides an organised representation of challenges faced by medical practitioners followed by the solutions provided by 3D-printing techniques. It can be ensured that this will facilitate medical professionals globally to increase life expectancy.

8.2   CLINICAL COMPLICATIONS

The following subsections categorise major clinical complications that can be addressed and cured by rapid prototyping techniques.

8.2.1 Issues During Clinical Training

Traditionally, animal models, mannequins and human cadavers have been used in clinical training, education and device testing to provide hands-on experience.

Ishii et al. (2006) show the surface of the mummified body conventionally used for clinical training purposes (Figure 8.1).

However, the use of animal models, mannequins and human cadavers is unapproachable, unrealistic, expensive and inconsistent with human anatomy when compared to the digital and physical 3D models. Conventional methods like the use of human cadavers for training added high costs to the institutions. Each human cadaver can cost as high as $1,000 (Malik et al., 2015). Besides, storage of cadavers demands proper facilities in an academic institution. The use of animal models often results in differences in drug dosing schedules and regimens that are not always relevant to human health. Because of differences in metabolic pathways and drug metabolites, different animal species and strains have different efficacy and toxicity.

8.2.2 Designing of Implants

Medical implants are instruments or tissues that are implanted into or on the body's surface. Some implants help organs and tissues by delivering drugs, monitoring body functions or providing support. Medical conditions that can be cured with the placement of implants are discussed as follows:

- Hydrocephalus: Implants along with the shunt system are used for the treatment
- Profound deafness: A small, complex electronic device called a Cochlear implant is used to help severely hard-of-hearing people

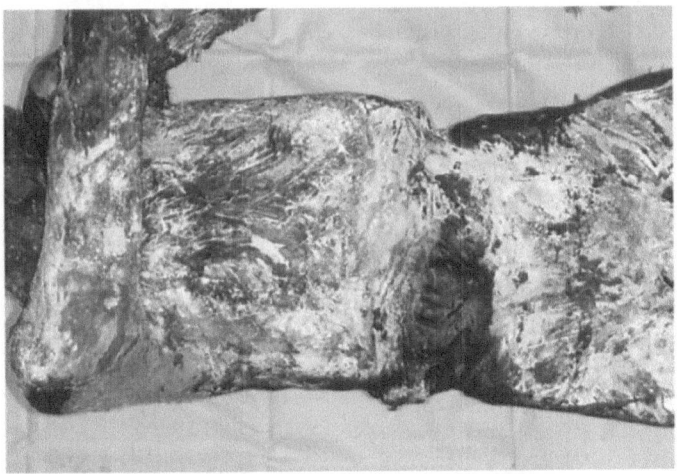

FIGURE 8.1 Human cadaver (Ishii et al., 2006).

- Hernia: Implants are used to provide permanent reinforcement to the repaired hernia
- Arthritis or fracture.

Metallic implants made of tantalum, gold, stainless steel, titanium alloys, cobalt-chromium alloy and shape memory alloy were conventionally used. These implants have favourable mechanical strength and excellent friction-resistance properties. Prosthetic loosening can happen due to the stress shielding effect, which is a result of a mismatch between the mechanical properties of these implants and normal human tissue. In addition, the presence of a metallic implant in the body limits the diagnosis when the patient is required to undergo magnetic resonance imaging (MRI) (Diment et al., 2017).

8.2.3 Accuracy and Efficiency of Prosthetics

Prosthetics are artificial devices used to replace a body part lost due to disease, trauma, accidents or any other medical condition. Prosthetic implants can replace body parts such as arms, legs, bone plates, etc. Strait (2006) provides the idea of the conventional leg prosthetics made up of different materials which are shown in Figure 8.2. Some of the materials used to produce prosthetics are plastic, wood, composites and rubber. Computer numerical control (CNC) machining, micromachining methods, and investment casting produced conventional prosthetics and implants. The disadvantages of these methods are wastage and longer operation time (which is crucial in the case of a medical emergency). Therefore, it can be reported as these manufacturing processes are incapable of producing an efficient product as per the application (Jin et al., 2015).

8.2.4 Cardiovascular Diseases

Cardiovascular disease (CVD) includes coronary artery diseases (CAD) such as angina, myocardial infarction, stroke and heart failure. Cardiovascular disease (CVD) broadly involves the ailment in the heart or blood vessels. As the issues pertaining to the increase in the number of patients with CVDs, doctors need to

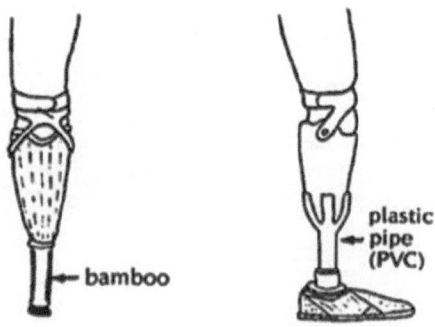

FIGURE 8.2 Conventional prosthetics (Strait, 2006).

do preoperative, intraoperative and postoperative evaluations. There are many life-threatening risks involved during the treatment of CVDs. An increasing number of cases calls for the development of patient-specific treatment models to eliminate these risks (Lim et al., 2016).

8.2.5 COMPLICATIONS IN HEARING

A hearing aid is a device designed to improve hearing by making sound audible to a person with hearing problems. Various challenges are faced by users while using hearing aids such as issues due to earwax, moisture content and improper fitting of the hearing aid. Hearing aids are required by the customers suffering from tinnitus, hyperacusis, single-sided deafness and ear infections (Banga et al., 2020b, 2020c, 2020d).

8.3 RAPID PROTOTYPING FOR CLINICAL APPLICATIONS

The recent advances have facilitated that the issues addressed in the previous sections can be cured with the help of rapid prototyping techniques. The recent and notable advances related to the use of 3D printing in clinical applications are provided in the following sections.

8.3.1 USE OF 3D PRINTING IN CLINICAL TRAINING

3D printing enables the building of realistic, polymer-based, 3D clinical prototypes. Medical professionals and students can practice critical surgical steps on these 3D-printed prototypes before treating the patients (Andolfi et al., 2017). This significantly increases the knowledge of medical students. George et al. (2017) show an ultra-realistic 3D-printed model scapula, and the same is shown in Figure 8.3.

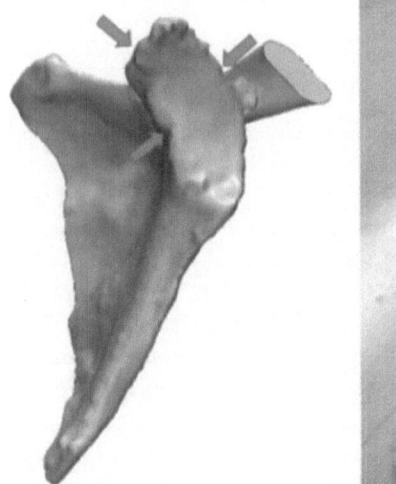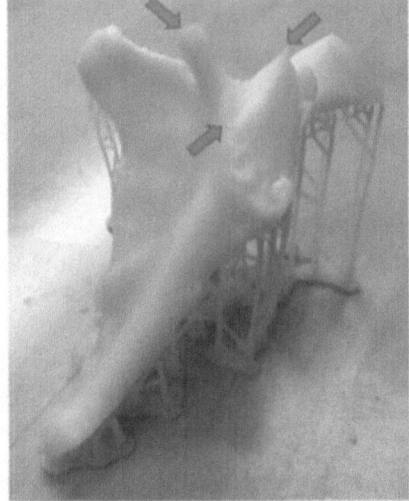

FIGURE 8.3 3D-printed model scapula (George et al., 2017).

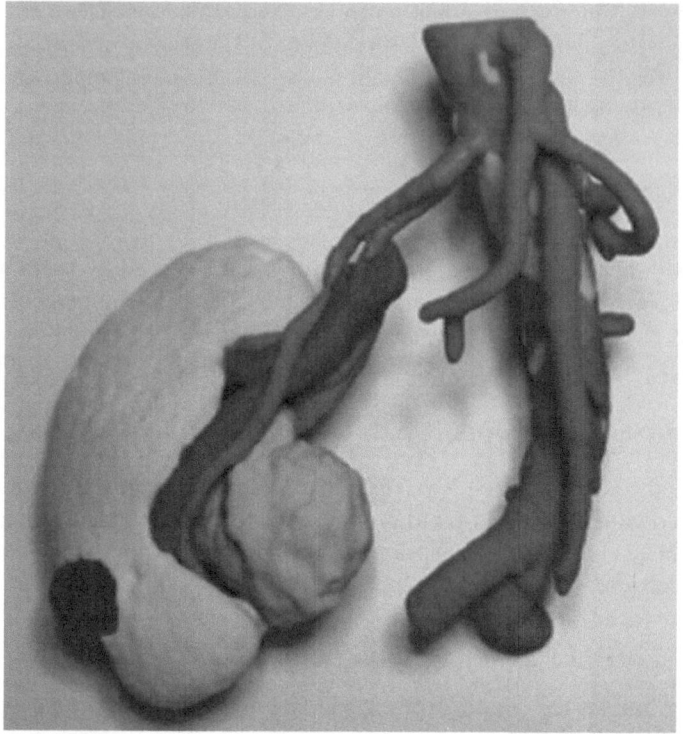

FIGURE 8.4   3D-printed model of kidney (Pugliese et al., 2018).

Pugliese et al. (2018) show a 3D-printed model of a kidney with a small cortical tumour of the lower pole (black) and a para pelvic cyst (green) made of plaster, using a binder jetting printer (Figure 8.4).

8.3.2   3D-Printed Implants and Fracture Fixers

3D printing makes it possible to create haptic models to plan the surgical approach. Based on patient-specific anatomy, the process facilitates creating custom prosthetics along with cross-sectional imaging. Medical professionals and researchers can thoroughly study cases as per the individual patients' requirements and problems. A 3D-printing service's versatility allows medical professionals to develop patient-specific implants at a low cost (Banga et al., 2021; Zuniga et al., 2015). AM is capable of producing very fine mesh and lattice structures that help in producing high-quality implants. When opposed to conventional implants, AM implants have twice the survival rate due to their superior surface geometry.AM techniques ensure that the produced implants are customised and rapidly produced at an affordable cost. It can produce replicas with tolerance in microns. Any 3D-printing materials can be sterilised using a steam autoclave or gamma radiation. Perfectly fit implants result in the speedy recovery of the patient (Upex et al., 2017; Vosselman et al., 2020).

The drawbacks of metallic and ceramic implants lead to the development of polymer-based implants. AM facilitates the production of biocompatible polymeric implants made from ultrahigh molecular weight polyethylene (UHMWPE), polymethyl methacrylate (PMMA), polylactide (PLA), polyglycolide (PGA), and polyhydroxy butyrate (PHB). Among the alloplastic materials, polyetheretherketone (PEEK) has emerged as an attractive option for patient-specific implants (Banga et al., 2017a, 2017b; Honigmann et al., 2018).

3D modelling allows surgeons to mould malleable plates to the configuration of the fracture before the operation process and ultimately improve outcomes in complex bone fractures eventually reducing operative time. Over the years, the use of 3D printing for fracture fixation has been an area of research and development. Many studies have resulted in promising outcomes. 3D-printing technique covers a range of fractures from head to toe, such as acromion, clavicle fractures in upper limbs, acetabulum, pelvis fractures in lower limbs, elbow fractures, osteotomies for distal radial malunion.

External fractures can be treated with 3D-printing techniques to assist fracture reduction, in association with computer-assisted reduction techniques, 3D-printing techniques are used to develop a customised external fixator (Qiao et al., 2015). The bone clip shaves made from 3D-printed PLA/silk composite are relatively non-invasive, biocompatible, and have a patient-specific design that is mechanically stable. Chana-Rodríguez et al. (2016) show definitive pre-contoured plates on the plastic model of the segmented left hemipelvis (Figure 8.5).

3D-printed scaffoldings for bone and cartilage have found innumerable and transformative applications in the field of orthopaedic trauma. A study found that exoskeletons produced using the process provide high power to mass ratio and enough stroke that can be used during bracing (Upex et al., 2017).

8.3.3   3D-PRINTED PROSTHETICS

Patient-specific prosthetics are in high demand all over the world. Each one must be made to order to meet the needs of the wearer. The development of prosthetic hands has been aided by the integration of rapid prototyping and robotic technologies (Xia et al., 2019). This enables the development of low-cost, personalised, lightweight and well-fitting prosthetics for infants. AM is also commonly used to create prosthetic parts that are tailored to the user's anatomy (Fuller et al., 2014; Jin et al., 2015).

Anything from prosthetic leg connections that fit easily in the individual to a complex and highly personalised facial prosthetic for a cancer patient has been made with AM technology (Banga et al., 2018). It is also used to make prosthetics with lifelike organic outer shells that conceal their mechanical appearance. This allows the user to personalise their prosthetics according to their needs. Dodziuk (2016) shows one such customised prosthetic design in which the mechanical appearance of the prosthetic is not visible, the same is shown in Figure 8.6.

Prosthetics can now be manufactured at a very low cost, thanks to the collaborative nature of AM and the widespread use of the internet. The number of peer-reviewed items that can be printed on desktop AM printers continues to increase (Auricchio & Marconi, 2016). These prototypes can be easily scaled or adjusted to suit the needs of the consumer. 3D-printed prosthetics are particularly useful for

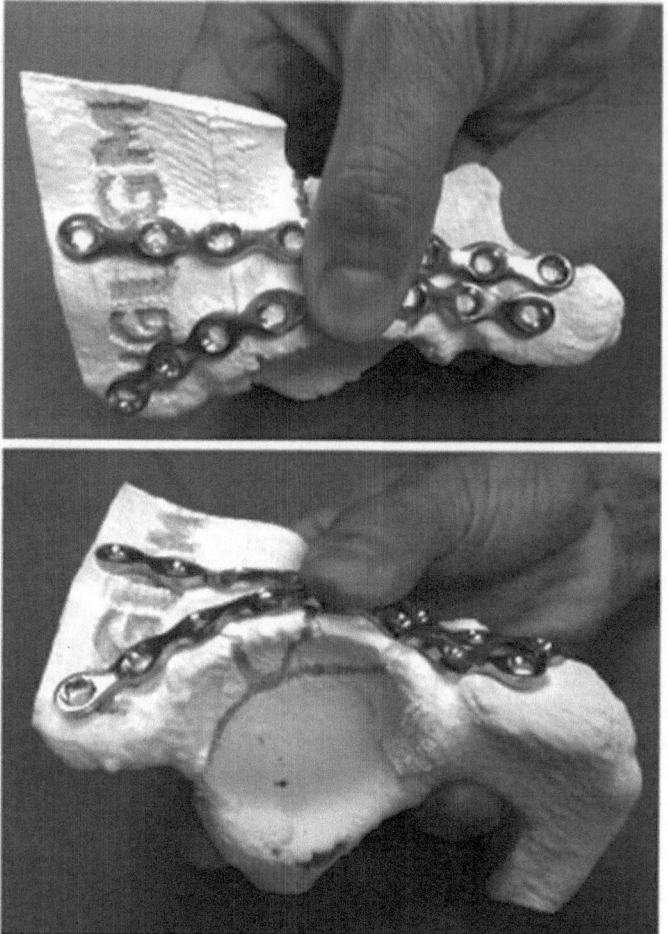

FIGURE 8.5 Contoured plates (Chana-Rodríguez et al., 2016).

children because they have a lifetime of more than five years. As a result, 3D-printed prosthetics, which are much easier to produce, are able to meet the demand for frequent prosthetic adjustments (Haleem et al., 2020).

8.3.4 3D Printing in Treatment of Cardiovascular Diseases

According to reports, quicker and less expensive 3D printers have entered the market, and as a result, more hospitals and universities would set aside funds to build the facility at the centre (Hoch et al., 2014). This would necessitate multidisciplinary teamwork in the broadest sense, including radiologists, clinical cardiologists, cardiac catheterisation experts, and surgeons, as well as, most importantly, the inclusion of engineers in a clinical team.

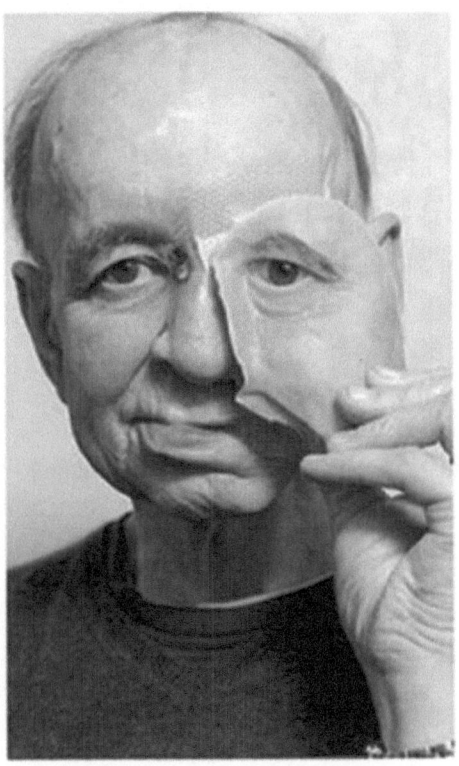

FIGURE 8.6   3D-printed prosthetic face (Dodziuk, 2016).

3D printing, without a doubt, is an extremely promising technique that has the potential to revolutionise the treatment of congenital and structural heart disorders in particular. The widespread use of 3D printing would be a significant benefit in addressing new diagnostic and therapeutic challenges. Schmauss et al. (2014) show a 3D-printing model of a porcelain aorta including the ascending aorta (1), the coronary arteries (2) and the aortic leaflets (3) occlusion (Figure 8.7).

8.3.5   3D-PRINTED HEARING AIDS

Making hearing aids used to be a nine-step procedure that included everything from making a cast mould to turning them into ear impressions and finally trimming the final cover. To complete the process, which took more than a week, hearing aid manufacturers hired artisans and set up hand shops. Hearing aid production has become much easier and more convenient as a result of the increased use of 3D printing. A previously nine-step method has been reduced to three: (1) scanning (2) modelling (3) printing. The approach decreases the amount of time and money it takes to make hearing aids. The technique has resulted in the development of hearing aids that are more comfortable and effective (Mannoor et al., 2013).

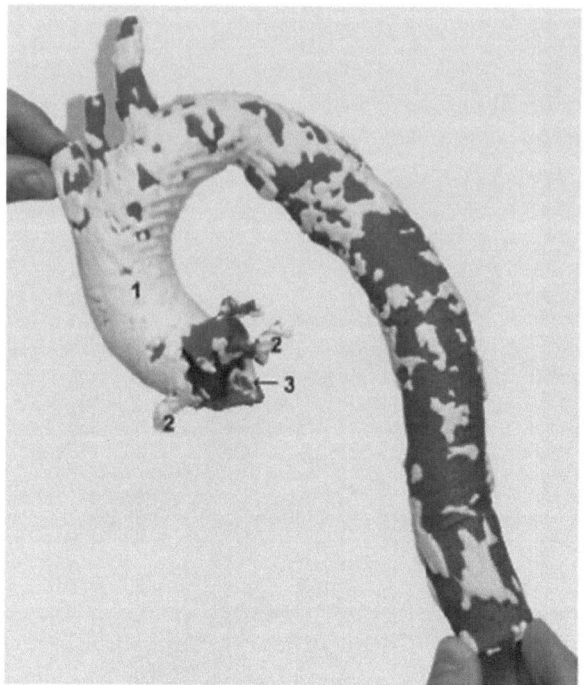

FIGURE 8.7   3D-printed model of aorta (Schmauss et al., 2014).

8.4   CONCLUSION

Rapid prototyping techniques are playing a vital role in the medical industry fulfilling its requirements in a fast and rapidly changing world. In today's times, it is crucial to establish a full potential usage of 3D-printing techniques for clinical applications. Rapid prototyping by 3D-printing techniques guarantees the fast and reliable treatment of various diseases. For clinical training, an exact anatomical specimen of the complex human body can be created with the help of the 3D-printing technique. Manufacturing biodegradable prostheses is now fast and easy with the help of rapid prototyping, especially for disabled children and the elderly. Complex, customised and biocompatible prostheses developed by rapid prototyping techniques are acting as a lifesaver for millions. It can be concluded that the technique can be utilised to develop the antidote to coronavirus disease (COVID-19) vaccine in a much lesser time as compared to the other vaccines developed in the history of the medical industry. There is still a vast area and the same is needed to be explored and practised to utilise 3D-printing techniques in clinical applications.

ANNEXURE FOR ABBREVIATIONS

AM	Additive manufacturing
CVD	Cardiovascular diseases
CNC	Computer numerical control

CAD	Coronary artery diseases
MRI	Magnetic resonance imaging
PMMA	Polymethyl methacrylate
PLA	Polylactide
PGA	Polyglycolide
PHB	Polyhydroxy butyrate
PEEK	Polyetheretherketone
TCP	Twisted coiled polymer
UHMWPE	Ultrahigh molecular weight polyethylene

REFERENCES

Abed, H., Burke, M., Fenlon, M. R., Scambler, S., & Scott, S. E. (2020). Denture use and dental risk factors associated developing osteoradionecrosis after head and neck radiotherapy: A retrospective analysis of hospital records. *Journal of Dentistry*, *99* (June), 103410. https://doi.org/10.1016/j.jdent.2020.103410

Andolfi, C., Plana, A., Kania, P., Banerjee, P. P., & Small, S. (2017). Usefulness of three-dimensional modeling in surgical planning, resident training, and patient education. *Journal of Laparoendoscopic and Advanced Surgical Techniques*, *27*(5), 512–515. https://doi.org/10.1089/lap.2016.0421

Attaran, M. (2017). The rise of 3-D printing: The advantages of additive manufacturing over traditional manufacturing. *Business Horizons*, *60*(5), 677–688. https://doi.org/10.1016/j.bushor.2017.05.011

Auricchio, F., & Marconi, S. (2016). 3D printing: Clinical applications in orthopaedics and traumatology. *EFORT Open Reviews*, *1*(5), 121–127. https://doi.org/10.1302/2058-5241.1.000012

Banga, H.K., Belokar, R.M., & Kumar, R., (2017b). A Novel Approach For Ankle Foot Orthosis Developed By Three Dimensional Technologies. *3rd International Conference on Mechanical Engineering and Automation Science (ICMEAS 2017)*, University of Birmingham, UK Vol. 8 No. 10, pp. 141–145.

Banga, H.K., Belokar, R.M., Madan, R., & Dhole, S. (2017a). Three dimensional Gait assessments during walking of healthy people and drop foot patients. *Defence Life Science Journal*, 2, 14–20.

Banga, H.K., Parveen, K., Belokar, R.M., & Kumar, R., (2018). Fabrication and stress analysis of ankle foot orthosis with additive manufacturing. *Rapid Prototyping Journal Emerald Publishing*, 24(2), 300–312.

Banga, H.K., Parveen, K., Belokar, R.M., & Kumar, R. (2020a). Customized design and additive manufacturing of kids' ankle foot orthosis. *Rapid Prototyping Journal*, 26(10). https://doi.org/10.1108/RPJ-07-2019-0194

Banga, H.K., Parveen, K., Belokar, R.M., & Kumar, R. (2020b). Design and fabrication of prosthetic and orthotic product by 3D printing [Online First], *Intech Open*. https://doi.org/10.5772/intechopen.94846. Available from: https://www.intechopen.com/online-first/design-and-fabrication-of-prosthetic-and-orthotic-product-by-3d-printing.

Banga, H.K., Parveen, K., Belokar, R.M., & Kumar R. (2020c). Effect of 3D-printed ankle foot orthosis during walking of foot deformities patients. In: Kumar H., Jain P. (eds) *Recent Advances in Mechanical Engineering*. Lecture Notes in Mechanical Engineering. Springer, Singapore, pp. 275–288.

Banga, H.K., Parveen, K., Belokar, R.M., & Kumar, R. (2020d) Role of finite element analysis in customized design of kids' orthotic product. In: Singh S., Prakash C., Singh R. (eds) *Characterization, Testing, Measurement, and Metrology*, pp. 139–159 CRC Press Taylor & Francis Group, USA.

Banga, H.K., Parveen, K., Belokar, R.M., & Kumar, R. (2020e). Improvement of human gait in foot deformities patients by 3D printed ankle–foot orthosis. In: Singh S., Prakash C., Singh R. (eds) *3D Printing in Biomedical Engineering*. Materials Horizons: From Nature to Nanomaterials. Springer, Singapore.

Banga, H.K., Parveen, K., & Kumar, H. (2021). Utilization of additive manufacturing in orthotics and prosthetic devices development. *IOP Conference Series: Materials Science and Engineering*. https://doi.org/10.1088/1757-899X/1033/1/012083

George, E., Liacouras, P., Rybicki, F. J., & Mitsouras, D. (2017). Measuring and establishing the accuracy and reproducibility of 3D printed medical models. *Radiographics*, *37*(5), 1424–1450. https://doi.org/10.1148/rg.2017160165

Haleem, A., Javaid, M., Khan, R. H., & Suman, R. (2020). 3D printing applications in bone tissue engineering. *Journal of Clinical Orthopaedics and Trauma*, *11*, S118–S124. https://doi.org/10.1016/j.jcot.2019.12.002

Honigmann, P., Sharma, N., Okolo, B., Popp, U., Msallem, B., & Thieringer, F. M. (2018). Patient-specific surgical implants made of 3D printed PEEK: Material, technology, and scope of surgical application. *BioMed Research International*, *2018*. https://doi.org/10.1155/2018/4520636

Ishii, K., Hitosugi, M., Kido, M., Yaguchi, T., Nishimura, K., Hosoya, T., & Tokudome, S. (2006). Analysis of fungi detected in human cadavers. *Legal Medicine*, *8*(3), 188–190. https://doi.org/10.1016/j.legalmed.2005.12.006

Jin, Y. A., Plott, J., Chen, R., Wensman, J., & Shih, A. (2015). Additive manufacturing of custom orthoses and prostheses – A review. *Procedia CIRP*, *36*, 199–204. https://doi.org/10.1016/j.procir.2015.02.125

Jindal, P., Worcester, F., Siena, F. L., Forbes, C., Juneja, M., & Breedon, P. (2020). Mechanical behaviour of 3D printed vs thermoformed clear dental aligner materials under non-linear compressive loading using FEM. *Journal of the Mechanical Behavior of Biomedical Materials*, *112*(June), 104045. https://doi.org/10.1016/j.jmbbm.2020.104045

Lal, H., & Patralekh, M. K. (2018). 3D printing and its applications in orthopaedic trauma: A technological marvel. *Journal of Clinical Orthopaedics and Trauma*, *9*(3), 260–268. https://doi.org/10.1016/j.jcot.2018.07.022

Lim, K. H. A., Loo, Z. Y., Goldie, S. J., Adams, J. W., & McMenamin, P. G. (2016). Use of 3D printed models in medical education: A randomized control trial comparing 3D prints versus cadaveric materials for learning external cardiac anatomy. *Anatomical Sciences Education*, *9*(3), 213–221. https://doi.org/10.1002/ase.1573

Malik, H. H., Darwood, A. R. J., Shaunak, S., Kulatilake, P., El-Hilly, A. A., Mulki, O., & Baskaradas, A. (2015). Three-dimensional printing in surgery: A review of current surgical applications. *Journal of Surgical Research*, *199*(2), 512–522. https://doi.org/10.1016/j.jss.2015.06.051

Mannoor, M. S., Jiang, Z., James, T., Kong, Y. L., Malatesta, K. A., Soboyejo, W. O., Verma, N., Gracias, D. H., & McAlpine, M. C. (2013). 3D printed bionic ears. *Nano Letters*, *13*(6), 2634–2639. https://doi.org/10.1021/nl4007744

Matsumoto, J. S., Morris, J. M., & Rose, P. S. (2016). 3-Dimensional printed anatomic models as planning aids in complex oncology surgery. *JAMA Oncology*, *2*(9), 1121–1122. https://doi.org/10.1001/jamaoncol.2016.2469

McMenamin, P. G., Quayle, M. R., McHenry, C. R., & Adams, J. W. (2014). The production of anatomical teaching resources using three-dimensional (3D) printing technology. *Anatomical Sciences Education*, *7*(6), 479–486. https://doi.org/10.1002/ase.1475

Nadagouda, M. N., Rastogi, V., & Ginn, M. (2020). A review on 3D printing techniques for medical applications. *Current Opinion in Chemical Engineering*, *28*, 152–157. https://doi.org/10.1016/j.coche.2020.05.007

Pugliese, L., Marconi, S., Negrello, E., Mauri, V., Peri, A., Gallo, V., Auricchio, F., & Pietrabissa, A. (2018). The clinical use of 3D printing in surgery. *Updates in Surgery*, *70*(3), 381–388. https://doi.org/10.1007/s13304-018-0586-5

Qiao, F., Li, D., Jin, Z., Gao, Y., Zhou, T., He, J., & Cheng, L. (2015). Application of 3D printed customized external fixator in fracture reduction. *Injury, 46*(6), 1150–1155. https://doi.org/10.1016/j.injury.2015.01.020

Schmauss, D., Haeberle, S., Hagl, C., & Sodian, R. (2014). Three-dimensional printing in cardiac surgery and interventional cardiology: A single-centre experience. *European Journal of Cardio-Thoracic Surgery, 47*(6), 1044–1052. https://doi.org/10.1093/ejcts/ezu310

Sousa, A. M., Pinho, A. C., Messias, A., & Piedade, A. P. (2020). Present status in polymeric mouthguards. A future area for additive manufacturing? *Polymers, 12*(7), 1–18. https://doi.org/10.3390/polym12071490

Strait, E. (2006). Prosthetics in developing countries. *White Paper*, January, 1–35. http://www.glb.nist.gov/tip/wp/pswp/upload/239_limb_prosthetics_services_devices.pdf

Tack, P., Victor, J., Gemmel, P., & Annemans, L. (2016). 3D-printing techniques in a medical setting: A systematic literature review. *BioMedical Engineering Online, 15*(1), 1–21. https://doi.org/10.1186/s12938-016-0236-4

Upex, P., Jouffroy, P., & Riouallon, G. (2017). Application of 3D printing for treating fractures of both columns of the acetabulum: Benefit of pre-contouring plates on the mirrored healthy pelvis. *Orthopaedics and Traumatology: Surgery and Research, 103*(3), 331–334. https://doi.org/10.1016/j.otsr.2016.11.021

Vosselman, N., Alberga, J., Witjes, M. H. J., Raghoebar, G. M., Reintsema, H., Vissink, A., & Korfage, A. (2020). Prosthodontic rehabilitation of head and neck cancer patients: Challenges and new developments. *Oral Diseases*, April, 1–9. https://doi.org/10.1111/odi.13374

Wang, R., & Boyle, A. (1994). A convenient method for guarding against localized mucositis during radiation therapy. *Journal of Prosthodontics, 3*(4), 198–201. https://doi.org/10.1111/j.1532-849X.1994.tb00155.x

Xia, R.Z., Zhai, Z.J., Chang, Y.Y., & Li, H.W. (2019). Clinical applications of 3-dimensional printing technology in hip joint. *Orthopaedic Surgery, 11*(4), 533–544. https://doi.org/10.1111/os.12468

Zuniga, J., Katsavelis, D., Peck, J., Stollberg, J., Petrykowski, M., Carson, A., & Fernandez, C. (2015). Cyborg beast: A low-cost 3d-printed prosthetic hand for children with upper-limb differences. *BMC Research Notes, 8*(1). https://doi.org/10.1186/s13104-015-0971-9

9 Surgery Planning and Tool Selection Using 3D Printing
Application to Neurosurgery

Shagun Sharma
Punjab Engineering College, Chandigarh, India

Chirag Ahuja
PGIMER, Chandigarh, India

Parveen Kalra
Punjab Engineering College, Chandigarh, India

Manarshhjot Singh
University Lille, CNRS, Centrale Lille, UMR 9189 –
CRIStAL – Centre de Recherche en Informatique
Signal et Automatique de Lille, Lille, France

Ashish Aggarwal
Post Graduate Institute of Medical Education & Research
(PGIMER), Chandigarh, India

Jagjit Singh Randhawa
Punjab Engineering College, Chandigarh, India

CONTENTS

DOI: 10.1201/9781003301066-9

9.1 INTRODUCTION

Accurate assessment of brain aneurysms is a necessary condition to be followed pre-surgically. An aneurysm is a focal outpouching in the vessel wall appearing as a balloon-shaped structure with a high propensity for rupture. These aneurysms may present with symptoms of rupture or may be an incidental detection during imaging of other brain pathologies. The former requires emergent surgical treatment while the latter may be followed or treated depending on the current management guidelines. Its detection involves vascular imaging with computed tomography (CT) angiography, magnetic resonance (MR) angiography or digital subtraction angiography (DSA). This helps in localisation of the aneurysm as well as defining its morphological characteristics. Depending on its location, a ruptured aneurysm may cause subarachnoid haemorrhage in the cistern where it projects or diffusely along the CSF spaces in the brain (Szmidt et al., 2007; Frego M et al., 2007) A ruptured aneurysm, as has been highlighted, requires immediate treatment to prevent its rupture, which can be potentially fatal. The most commonly used treatment modalities are clipping and coiling to seal the aneurysm. Both procedures pose potential risks, particularly bleeding in the brain or loss of blood flow to the brain. In either case, planning has to be accurate and well-rehearsed for beginners and experts.

The most accurate preoperative planning assessment is done by specialised neuroimaging techniques such as 3CT and magnetic resonance imaging (MRI) (Vannier et al., 1988; Wielopolski et al., 1992; Banga et al., 2017). Being variably used in data acquisition and evaluation of aneurysms these techniques provide an aid in determining the anatomical details of the surrounding vessels and making virtual views of surgical approaches. However, there are certain limitations as the interpretation of the shape and composition is viewed in 2D space or 3D volume in 2D slices. The data is a stack of images ranging from 600 to 1000 and helps in only screening the aneurysm. The observation of the anatomy is also dependent on the skills of the operator and the experience of the surgeon thus making the planning procedure an imaginary approach (Vieco et al., 1995; Casey et al., 1997).

With the advent of CAD/CAM surgeons can now view 3D visual representation of the vascular ring situated anywhere in the brain (Chong et al., 1999; Govsa et al., 2017; Banga et al., 2017). Various image processing software programs are used for pre-surgical planning of reconstruction and rehabilitation of anatomical defects. Frequently known as virtual surgical planning, the applications of CAD/CAM have helped surgeons to paw, pitch and roll the positions of the anatomy and manipulate the model to achieve anatomical balance. It segments the region of interest from CT and MRI with the assistance of image filtering tools and thresholding and converts images into 3D virtual models (Swann, 1996; Banga et al., 2020). The ROI can be segregated to get dimensions in terms of area and volume which further assists in the selection of clip for the aneurysm.

The complete branching structure can be converted into physical replicas with the help of another revolutionary technology known as 3D printing or rapid prototyping (Markl et al., 2005). They are obtained through patients' imaging data (CT and MRI) and fabricated using FDM and inkjet 3D-printing technology in a plethora of biocompatible and non-biocompatible materials (Naftulin et al., 2015; Sugawara et al., 2013; Ryan et al., 2015; Waran et al., 2014). These models are used as templates for pre-surgical planning and rehearsals as they are substantially held in the hands and analysed from a perception of the surgery. Its major advantage in the field of medicine is acknowledged by surgeons and physicians as an essential step for surgical planning (Arvier et al., 1994; D'Urso et al., 1998).

Surgical planning can be impromptu in terms of knowing the exact location of the aneurysm and its form and structure. This leads to longer planning time, patient wound exposure and post-operative complications. On the other hand, the use of prototypes allows the surgeons to plan procedures pre-surgically, thereby making the surgery predictive. The models provide more intuitive information in the selection of operational approaches such as clip selection and treating multiple and giant aneurysms (Knox et al., 2005; Banga et al., 2018). Visualisation of the 3D structure is a difficult affair for novice trainees as well as experienced surgeons. Therefore these can be also used for training and rehearsal of surgeries and clip selection techniques.

3D-printed models can be implanted in cadavers to create a real-time scenario for replicating clip techniques and practise certain approaches for patient-specific aneurysms. This aids in gaining experience for trainees and further enhances surgical skills even for the experienced surgeon. Pre-operative planning by using replicas is beneficial in stent grafting for aortic aneurysms by assisting surgeons to know about the location. Comparing the outcome of the surgery between 3D models and 3D CT resulted in significant improvement in the ability of trainees to plan the EVAR with the help of 3D models. Majorly used 3D-printing technologies like FDM and PolyJet can print models with high accuracy proving it vital to be used for emergency cases. The models used as templates make the approach predicative during the execution of the surgery thereby giving a high success rate.

9.2   METHODOLOGY OF OBTAINING A 3D MODEL FROM CT/MRI SCANS

The methodology of obtaining the 3D model of the aneurysm is based on logic derived from the principle of image processing, i.e. thresholding. Thresholding is the process of extraction of a portion of an image based on a range of intensity of pixels. For MRI/CT data the thresholding is performed on a stack of images captured from the equipment using Hounsfield units for setting up the limits of thresholding. Two approaches can be adapted to successfully extract the desired geometry from the MRI scan. These approaches are:

1. Top-down approach
2. Bottom-up approach.

The overview of the approaches is given in Figure 9.1.

The approaches detailed below are explained in the MIMICS software environment; however, the approaches themselves are software-independent and can be applied using other similar software tools.

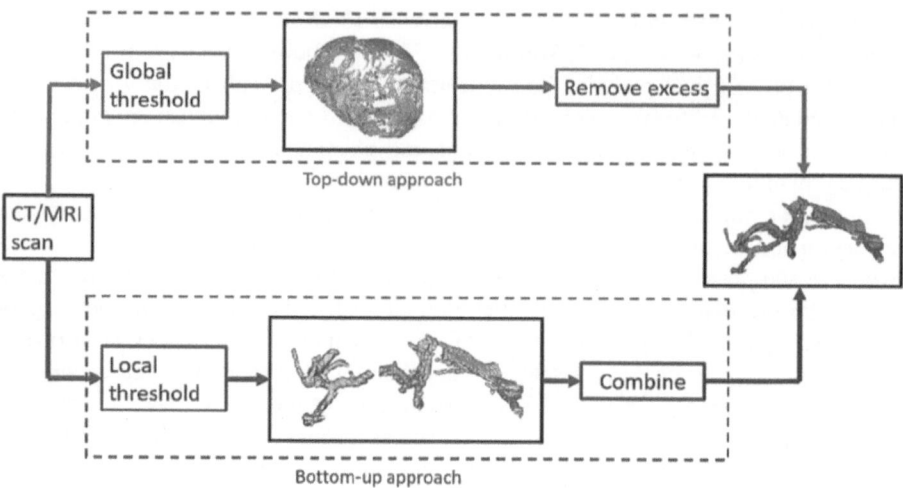

FIGURE 9.1   Overview of approaches.

9.2.1   TOP-DOWN APPROACH

In the top-down approach, initially a wider threshold is selected, resulting in a 3D geometry that is much more than that of interest. The excessive 3D structures are then removed selectively till only the geometry of interest remains.

In MIMICS the top-down approach is applied as follows:

1. Selection of global thresholds.
2. Creation of the mask.
3. Sculpting the mask to the region of interest.

The first step is to create a global threshold, i.e. define a lower and an upper threshold for the entire scan. To obtain these thresholds, the image histogram is used. The brightness and contrast of the image are set so that soft tissues close to the region of interest are not visible. This adjustment is shown in Figure 9.2.

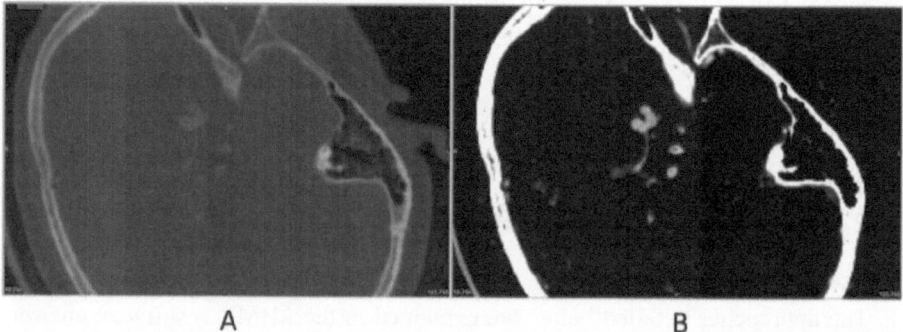

FIGURE 9.2   Brightness adjustment for global thresholds. (A) Actual image (B) Image after brightness and contrast adjustment.

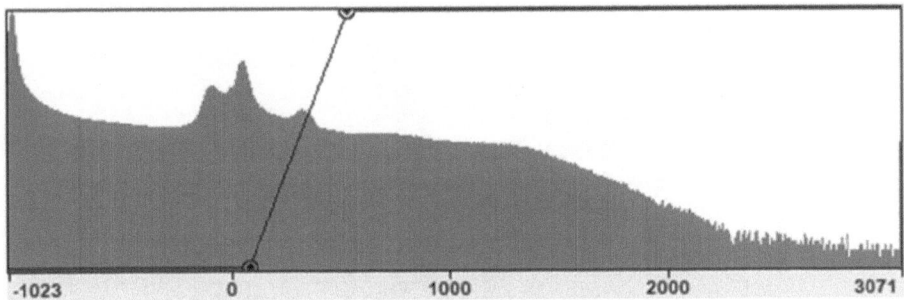

FIGURE 9.3 Image histogram.

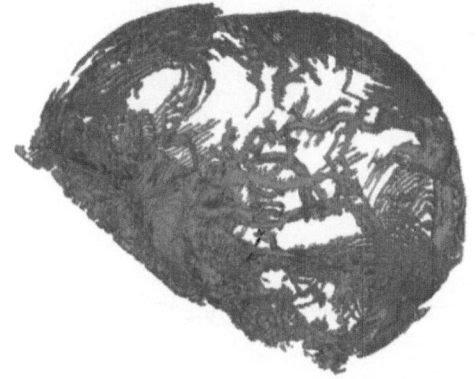

FIGURE 9.4 Volumetric representation of mask.

The image histogram corresponding to the brightness and contrast adjustment is observed. The histogram corresponds to the adjustment in Figure 9.2 as shown in Figure 9.3. It is observed that for voxels below ~50 HU, the pixel intensity is 0 and for all voxels above ~450 HU, the pixel intensity is maximum. Therefore, the lower threshold is set to 70 and the upper threshold is set to 450.

The volumetric representation of the image mask obtained using the above thresholds is given in Figure 9.4.

The global mask created is edited manually to selectively remove the excessive geometry that is not of interest. The final geometry obtained is shown in Figure 9.5.

9.2.2 BOTTOM-UP APPROACH

In the bottom-up approach, initially a narrower threshold range is selected, resulting in a 3D geometry that is a sub-portion of the geometry of interest. Multiple such sub-portions are then combined to create the final geometry.

In MIMICS the bottom-up approach is applied as follows:

1. Select a new local threshold and seed point.

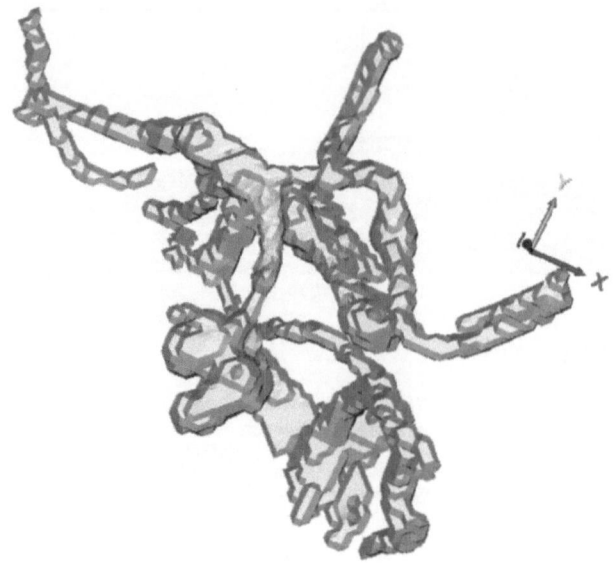

FIGURE 9.5   Geometry of interest using the top-down approach.

2. Create a new mask.
3. Is the whole geometry of interest captured?
   a. If yes, continue.
   b. If no, go to step 1.
4. Combine all the created masks to form new geometry

In MIMICS the definition of local threshold limits and seed points is done in a single step using the 'Dynamic region growing' command. The user defines a seed point and a lower and upper deviation. The software reads the image intensity at the seed point and adds it to an image mask. The points adjacent to the mask whose intensity deviates from that of the seed point within the user-defined range are also added. The process is repeated to till all the points adjacent to the mask deviate more than the prescribed deviation.

The selection of seed point is easy. The aneurysm under consideration is located on the MRI scan and any point on the aneurysm is selected as the seed point. In order to properly define the deviation, the 'Profile Line' tool is used. This tool is used to check the local threshold variation in any direction of the MRI scan. The variation of intensity along the length of the defined line is plotted.

The profile line is drawn on the aneurysm located on the scan. The profile line is drawn in the image and the image intensity variation along the line is checked. The profile line analysis is shown in Figure 9.6. From the figure, it is observed that the intensity rises twice corresponding to the image. The seed point is selected at a pixel with the highest intensity on the line. The lower deviation is set to 250 and the upper deviation is set to 10. The upper deviation is just to incorporate for human error in selecting the point of highest intensity.

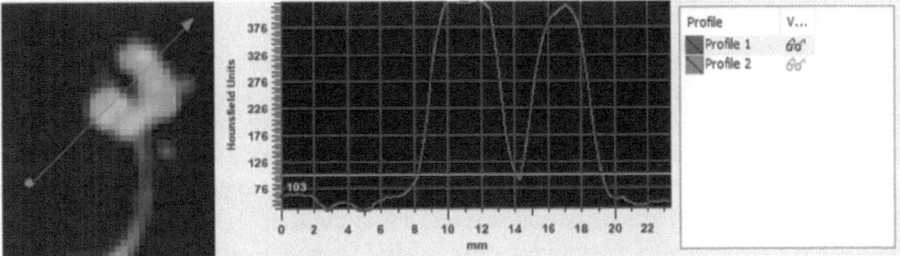

FIGURE 9.6   Profile line analysis.

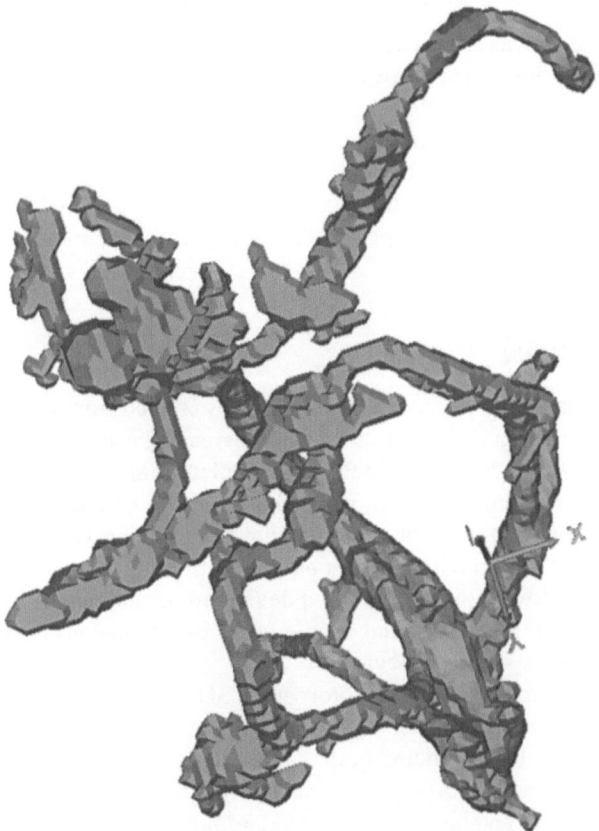

FIGURE 9.7   Geometry of interest using the bottom-up approach.

The volumetric representation of the mask can be checked if all the required geometries are included in the mask. For the current work, all the required geometries were modelled in a single iteration as shown in Figure 9.7. If all the geometries of interest are not included, then the process can be repeated by creating profile lines in areas to include. However, these areas should again be found manually.

9.3   COMPARISON

The advantage of the top-down approach lies in the fact that it is very robust to thresholding errors as a wider threshold range is selected. The major disadvantage is that it requires manual correction of the mask. Therefore, this approach is more suited for industrial designers.

The advantage of the bottom-up approach lies in the fact that it provides a lot of control to the user. The major disadvantage is that the user should be able to locate the underlying geometry of interest on the MRI scan. Therefore, this approach is more suited for users with a background in medicine.

9.4   FABRICATION OF PHYSICAL MODEL

After the scan, data was converted into a 3D image. It was saved in STL format and exported for 3D printing using a PolyJet printer (Stratasys). Using default printing parameters the model the material used was biocompatible MED 60. The models were used as an operational physical model to design operative schemes, choose the best operative paths and select suitable aneurysm clips by their high simulation degree and individualised characteristics. The models can also be helpful for surgical planning, especially for the preoperative plan of treating refractory multiple aneurysms and giant aneurysms.

9.5   DISCUSSION

Three-dimensional (3-D) printed anatomic models created from a patient's CT, MRI or 3-D ultrasound imaging datasets are seeing increasing use for procedural planning and hands-on clinical education. Established medical centres along with engineering universities have created their own 3-D printing labs to enable on-demand printing of complex anatomy not only for planning and device sizing, but also to practice dry runs and aid procedural navigation. An emerging trend is the use of new 3-D computer modelling software to enable virtual device implantations for improved patient selection, reduce complications and enable faster development of novel reconstructive surgeries and transcatheter devices.

Also known as medical rapid prototyping, 3D printing has revolutionised the manufacturing segment by producing intricate and complex anatomical parts without human intervention. By producing both soft and hard tissues it is frequently used in the field of reconstructive surgery like oral and maxillofacial, orthopaedics, cardiology and neurosurgery and has become a standard procedure to be adopted for presurgical planning (Marro et al., 2016; Bibb et al., 2014).

Most commonly used in maxillofacial reconstructive surgery, hard tissue management is done pre-surgically on CAD software to analyse the defect and decide the number of osteotomies required. The surgeries are simulated and the defects are reconstructed which are further transformed into physical models. The design of surgical cutting and drilling guides for both maxillofacial and orthopaedic surgery has improved precision by knowing the exact osteotomy site, length and angles. Pre-adaptation of reconstructive plates and mesh plates used for fracture management have eliminated trial and adapt procedures during the surgery and resulted in reduced planning and execution time.

While on the other hand, the soft tissue management has also benefited from the combined applications of CAD/CAM and 3D printing. Being produced in plastic and flexible materials the anatomical components of the brain, heart and liver are accessible to be physically held and observed to create the perspective of the surgical approach. Models used for pre-procedural planning, are printed in multiple materials to simulate the actual anatomy. This includes flexible materials for soft tissues and hard plastics to simulate things like arteries and valves. In case of aneurysms experienced as well as trainee surgeons can practice clipping technique beforehand which gives a feel of the actual plot and transmit confidence in terms of accuracy and eliminates chances of mistakes.

For someone to really understand the anatomy, even experienced surgeons do not always appreciate the complexities by looking at 2D images from ultrasound, CT scans or angiograms. On the other hand, the ability to do multi-material printing of the models can be influential for procedural planning and dry runs. The entire structure could be analysed to see the impact of the angulations and vessel tortuosity. Anticipation of the problem is done with these models which are extremely beneficial for surgical pre-planning which also involves the use of device sizing, and guidance of meticulous procedure for novel devices and techniques (Correy et al., 2005). The selection of clip size is usually unpredictable with the desired diameter by just viewing the imaging data or the type of issues they might run into. The trial for the type of clip and wire for the coiling approach can be changed and used, based on 3D-printed anatomy.

The size and location of the aneurysm vary between patients tremendously. As a result patient selection should be careful to prevent rupture or obstruction. This is where VSP and 3D printing can assist to tackle the fear of what the surgeon would see. Misinterpretation of the size of the clip is also eliminated with the help of models that determine the best development and evaluate the 3D shape, depth and location of an aneurysm anywhere hidden between the networks of the arteries.

Customised implants are frequently used for almost all types of reconstructive surgeries. In the case of brain aneurysms, the surgeon can also design customised clips for a particular aneurysm or even a universal clip that adapts to all aneurysms. This could be a major help in terms of cost and immediate availability in case of emergency surgeries. The design is done virtually along with design engineers and 3D printed in biocompatible titanium (Aggarwal et al., 2018). Models can also be implanted in cadavers to create a real-time scenario for rehearsals for trainee surgeons to practice and expertise in a particular technique (Benet et al., 2015; Kato et al., 2001).

9.6 CONCLUSION

The surgical procedure of the aneurysm is the most complicated in terms of planning and treatment. Any procedure poses a potential risk that requires emergency care. The present chapter introduces a pre-surgical methodology to produce 3D-printed physical models of the aneurysms to be used for pre-surgical planning in order to decide clip size for the closure of an aneurysm and education of young surgeons to help them access the utility for the management of complex cases. Furthermore, it helps surgeons to identify alternatives thereby avoiding any life-threatening risks. The use of imaging and 3D-printed pre-surgical models for unruptured brain aneurysms can generally be recommended to identify alternatives, thereby avoiding any life-threatening risks.

REFERENCES

Aggarwal, A., Singh, M., & Kalra, P. (2018). Proposed solution for dorsal internal carotid artery aneurysms: Suggestion of a novel new clip design. *Neurology India*, 66(3), 804.

Arvier, J. F., Barker, T. M., Yau, Y. Y., D'Urso, P. S., Atkinson, R. L., & McDermant, G. R. (1994). Maxillofacial biomodelling. *British Journal of Oral and Maxillofacial Surgery*, 32(5), 276–283.

Banga, H. K., Belokar, R. M., & Kumar R (2017b). A Novel Approach For Ankle Foot Orthosis Developed By Three Dimensional Technologies, *3rd International Conference on Mechanical Engineering and Automation Science (ICMEAS 2017)*, University of Birmingham, UK, Vol. 8 No. 10, pp. 141–145.

Banga, H. K., Belokar, R. M., Madan, R., & Dhole, S. (2017a). Three dimensional Gait assessments during walking of healthy people and drop foot patients. *Defence Life Science Journal*, 2, 14–20.

Banga, H. K., Kalra, P., Belokar, R. M., & Kumar, R. (2020a). Customized design and additive manufacturing of kids' ankle foot orthosis. *Rapid Prototyping Journal*, 26(10). https://doi.org/10.1108/RPJ-07-2019-0194

Banga, H. K., Kalra, P., Belokar, R. M., & Kumar, R. (2020b). Design and fabrication of prosthetic and orthotic product by 3D printing [Online First]. *IntechOpen*. https://doi.org/10.5772/intechopen.94846. Available from: https://www.intechopen.com/online-first/design-and-fabrication-of-prosthetic-and-orthotic-product-by-3d-printing

Banga, H. K., Kalra, P., Belokar, R. M., & Kumar, R. (2020c). Effect of 3D-printed ankle foot orthosis during walking of foot deformities patients. In: Kumar H., Jain P. (eds) *Recent Advances in Mechanical Engineering*. Lecture Notes in Mechanical Engineering. Springer, Singapore, pp. 275–288.

Banga, H. K., Kalra, P., Belokar, R. M., & Kumar, R. (2020d). Role of finite element analysis in customized design of kid's orthotic product. In: Singh S., Prakash C., Singh R. (eds) *Characterization, Testing, Measurement, and Metrology*, pp. 139–159 CRC Press Taylor & Francis Group, USA.

Banga, H. K., Kalra, P., Belokar, R.M., & Kumar, R. (2020e). Improvement of human gait in foot deformities patients by 3D printed ankle–foot orthosis. In: Singh S., Prakash C., Singh R. (eds) *3D Printing in Biomedical Engineering*. Materials Horizons: From Nature to Nanomaterials. Springer, Singapore.

Banga, H. K., Kumar, P., Kumar, H. (2021). Utilization of additive manufacturing in orthotics and prosthetic devices development. *IOP Conference Series: Materials Science and Engineering*. https://doi.org/10.1088/1757-899X/1033/1/012083

Banga, H. K., Parveen, K., Belokar, R. M., & Kumar, R. (2014). Rapid prototyping applications in medical sciences. *International Journal of Emerging Technologies in Computational and Applied Sciences (IJETCAS)*, 5(8), 416–420.

Banga, H. K., Parveen, K., Belokar, R. M., & Kumar, R. (2018). Fabrication and stress analysis of ankle foot orthosis with additive manufacturing. *Rapid Prototyping Journal Emerald Publishing*, 24(2), 300–312.

Benet, A., Plata-Bello, J., Abla, A. A., Acevedo-Bolton, G., Saloner, D., & Lawton, M. T. (2015). Implantation of 3D-printed patient-specific aneurysm models into cadaveric specimens: A new training paradigm to allow for improvements in cerebrovascular surgery and research. *BioMed Research International*, 939387.

Bibb, R., Eggbeer, D., & Paterson, A. (2014). *Medical Modelling: The Application of Advanced Design and Rapid Prototyping Techniques in Medicine*. Woodhead Publishing.

Casey, S. O., Alberico, R. A., & Ozsvath, R. R. (1997). Operator dependence of cerebral CT angiography in the detection of aneurysms. *American Journal of Neuroradiology*, 18(4), 790–792.

Chong, C. K., Rowe, C. S., Sivancsan, S., Rattray, A., Black, R. A., Shortland, A. P., & How, T. V. (1999). Computer aided design and fabrication of models for in vitro studies of vascular fluid dynamics. *Proceedings of the Institution of Mechanical Engineers, Part H: Journal of Engineering in Medicine*, 213(1), 1–4.

D'Urso, P. S., Atkinson, R. L., Bruce, I. J., Effeney, D. J., Lanigan, M. W., Earwaker, W. J., … & Thompson, R. G. (1998). Stereolithographic (SL) biomodelling in craniofacial surgery. *British Journal of Plastic Surgery*, 51(7), 522–530.

Dillon, E., Van Leeuwen, M., Fernandez, M. A., Eikelboom, B., & Mali, W. (1992). Computed tomographic angiography for carotid imaging. *The Lancet*, 340(8830), 1286.

Edwards, F. H., Wind, G., Thompson, L., Bellamy, R. F., Barry, M. J., & Schaefer, P. S. (1990). Three-dimensional image reconstruction for planning of a complex cardiovascular procedure. *The Annals of Thoracic Surgery*, 49(3), 486–488.

Frego, M., Lumachi, F., Bianchera, G., Pilon, F., Scarpa, M., Ruffolo, C., … & Picchi, G. (2007). Risk factors of endoleak following endovascular repair of abdominal aortic aneurysm. *A Multicentric Retrospective Study. In Vivo*, 21(6), 1099–1102.

Govsa, F., Yagdi, T., Ozer, M. A., Eraslan, C., & Alagoz, A. K. (2017). Building 3D anatomical model of coiling of the internal carotid artery derived from CT angiographic data. *European Archives of Oto-Rhino-Laryngology*, 274(2), 1097–1102.

Hieu, L. C., Zlatov, N., Vander Sloten, J., Bohez, E., Khanh, L., Binh, P. H., … & Toshev, Y. (2005). Medical rapid prototyping applications and methods. *Assembly Automation*.

Kato, K., Ishiguchi, T., Maruyama, K., Naganawa, S., & Ishigaki, T. (2001). Accuracy of plastic replica of aortic aneurysm using 3D-CT data for transluminal stent-grafting: experimental and clinical evaluation. *Journal of Computer Assisted Tomography*, 25(2), 300–304.

Knox, K., Kerber, C. W., Singel, S. A., Bailey, M. J., & Imbesi, S. G. (2005). Stereolithographic vascular replicas from CT scans: Choosing treatment strategies, teaching, and research from live patient scan data. *American Journal of Neuroradiology*, 26(6), 1428–1431.

Markl, M., Schumacher, R., Küffer, J., Bley, T. A., & Hennig, J. (2005). Rapid vessel prototyping: Vascular modeling using 3t magnetic resonance angiography and rapid prototyping technology. *Magnetic Resonance Materials in Physics, Biology and Medicine*, 18(6), 288–292.

Marro, A., Bandukwala, T., & Mak, W. (2016). Three-dimensional printing and medical imaging: A review of the methods and applications. *Current Problems in Diagnostic Radiology*, 45(1), 2–9.

Naftulin, J. S., Kimchi, E. Y., & Cash, S. S. (2015). Streamlined, inexpensive 3D printing of the brain and skull. *PloS One*, 10(8), e0136198.

Ryan, J. R., Chen, T., Nakaji, P., Frakes, D. H., & Gonzalez, L. F. (2015). Ventriculostomy simulation using patient-specific ventricular anatomy, 3D printing, and hydrogel casting. *World Neurosurgery*, 84(5), 1333–1339.

Sodian, R., Weber, S., Markert, M., Rassoulian, D., Kaczmarek, I., Lueth, T. C., … & Daebritz, S. (2007). Stereolithographic models for surgical planning in congenital heart surgery. *The Annals of Thoracic Surgery*, 83(5), 1854–1857.

Sugawara, T., Higashiyama, N., Kaneyama, S., Takabatake, M., Watanabe, N., Uchida, F., … & Mizoi, K. (2013). Multistep pedicle screw insertion procedure with patient-specific lamina fit-and-lock templates for the thoracic spine. *Journal of Neurosurgery: Spine*, 19(2), 185–190.

Swann, S. (1996). Integration of MRI and stereolithography to build medical models: A case study. *Rapid Prototyping Journal*.

Szmidt, J., Galazka, Z., Rowinski, O., Nazarewski, S., Jakimowicz, T., Pietrasik, K., ... & Chudzinski, W. (2007). Late aneurysm rupture after endovascular abdominal aneurysm repair. *Interactive Cardiovascular and Thoracic Surgery*, 6(4), 490–494.

Vannier, M. W., Gutierrez, F. R., Laschinger, J. C., Gronemeyer, S., Canter, C. E., & Knapp, R. H. (1988). Three-dimensional magnetic resonance imaging of congenital heart disease. *Radiographics*, 8(5), 857–871.

Vieco, P. T., Shuman, W. P., Alsofrom, G. F., & Gross, C. E. (1995). Detection of circle of Willis aneurysms in patients with acute subarachnoid hemorrhage: A comparison of CT angiography and digital subtraction angiography. *AJR. American Journal of Roentgenology*, 165(2), 425–430.

Waran, V., Narayanan, V., Karuppiah, R., Pancharatnam, D., Chandran, H., Raman, R., ... & Aziz, T. Z. (2014). Injecting realism in surgical training—initial simulation experience with custom 3D models. *Journal of Surgical Education*, 71(2), 193–197.

Wielopolski, P. A., Haacke, E. M., & Adler, L. P. (1992). Three-dimensional MR imaging of the pulmonary vasculature: preliminary experience. *Radiology*, 183(2), 465–472.

10 Amalgamating Additive Manufacturing and Electrospinning for Fabrication of 3D Scaffolds

Parneet Kaur Deol
G.H.G. Khalsa College of Pharmacy Gurusar Sadhar,
Ludhiana, India

Amoljit Singh Gill
I.K. Gujral Punjab Technical University, Kapurthala, India

Mandeep Singh and Indu Pal Kaur
Panjab University Chandigarh, Chandigarh, India

CONTENTS

10.1 INTRODUCTION

A remarkable shift has been witnessed in the field of tissue engineering with the focus moving from synthetic implants and tissue grafts to the use of three-dimensional (3D), degradable, porous material scaffolds integrated with biological cells or biomolecules to regenerate tissues. Nowadays, great emphasis is made on designing, and then

DOI: 10.1201/9781003301066-10

fabricating an appropriate scaffold structure that provides a novel carrier for cells and drugs (Chaudhary & Garg, 2015; Banga et al., 2020a, 2020b, 2020c, 2020d, 2020e). Features like porous structure, porosity, pore size and pore interconnectivity of the fabricated scaffold, have greatly influenced its biological performance (Yang et al., 2019). Although, appropriate pore size and high porosity are favourable for cell growth as it facilitates the absorption of nutrients and the excretion of metabolic waste. However, it drastically influences the mechanical properties of the scaffold and thus limits its in-vivo performance. Further, variation of mechanical strength during degradation is critical in load-bearing implants, as it is important that load is gradually transferred to the regenerating tissue (Chaudhary & Garg, 2015; Banga et al., 2021; Roseti et al., 2017). A tissue-engineering scaffold must also be biocompatible and bioabsorbable, so that tissue can easily accept and ultimately replace the scaffold. It should possess bioactivity and can interact with the surrounding living tissues or organs. Lastly, and most importantly from a commercial point of view, the 3D scaffold should be easily fabricable in a variety of sizes and shapes (Gu, Choi, Park, Kim, & Kim, 2018).

Various methods have been established for manufacturing 3D scaffolds of natural and synthetic polymers, with their own list of issues and shortcomings. The present chapter will discuss recent advances in combining two separate technologies, namely additive manufacturing and electrospinning for the fabrication of 3D scaffolds for tissue-engineering applications. Emphasis will be made to highlight in detail the issues faced by individual technologies alone and how their amalgamation can benefit scaffold fabrication.

10.2 STATUS OF ADDITIVE MANUFACTURING (AM) IN SCAFFOLD FABRICATION

It was reported that worldwide, on a daily basis, approximately 266.2 to 359.5 million major surgical procedures were performed in 2012 (Chaudhary & Garg, 2015; Banga et al., 2018; Weiser et al., 2016). These procedures generally involve the replacement of damaged tissues/organs or their repair or reconstruction. The present focus of tissue engineering is to provide substitutes for maintaining, improving or restoring the functional tissues in a patient-specific manner (O'Brien, 2011). In recent years, additive manufacturing (AM) or 3D printing has shown promising capabilities for manufacturing scaffolds with different biological and physical requirements (Mota, Puppi, Chiellini, & Chiellini, 2015). This method is different from traditional manufacturing technology because rather than removing material; it is a bottom-up technique that adds materials layer by layer (Javaid & Haleem, 2018; Chaudhary & Garg, 2015; Banga et al., 2017a, 2017b). Complex 3D structures are fabricated via four interconnected steps: generating computer-based 3D models, conversion and preprocessing of data, fabrication or printing, and post-processing (Singh, Singh, & Han, 2016). Initially, a 3D model is generated using precise information about the type and severity of tissue defect and the nature and properties of the biopolymer to be used. The 3D model is sliced horizontally to generate two dimensional (2D) images. The connected printer fabricates each slice by utilising the data of each 2D image in the X-Y plane. The layer-by-layer printing of the slices gives the Z dimension to the structure.

Stable 3D structures with higher Z plane resolution can be fabricated by reducing the thickness of the sliced 2D layers (Gill, Deol, & Kaur, 2019; He et al., 2018).

Presently, various AM techniques are available which are capable of fabricating a variety of intricate structures using different types of biopolymers. Four additive manufacturing techniques namely extrusion-based printing, fluid deposition modelling, inkjet printing and stereolithography, have found immense application in fabricating 3D scaffolds for tissue engineering. Figure 10.1 highlights their brief construction of various AM techniques along with their specific advantages and limitations. The extrusion-based printers use pneumatic or mechanical forces to dispense viscous ink/bio-ink through a syringe or nozzle in a line by line manner according to a computer-based 3D model to print a complex structure (Bishop et al., 2017). It is a slow fabricating process, free from unnecessary stresses in the form of heat or irradiation and thus is capable of fabricating 3D patterns with up to 90 per cent cell viability (Jessop et al., 2017; Mandrycky, Wang, Kim, & Kim, 2016). Further, high cell density bio-ink can be easily handled using this technique (Vijayavenkataraman, Yan, Lu, Wang, & Fuh, 2018; Chaudhary & Garg, 2015; Banga et al., 2017a, 2017b). Inkjet printing is a precise and high-resolution (up to 50 µm) printing technique that utilises actuators based on a piezoelectric, electromagnetic or thermal technique to drop bio-ink continuously on a substrate according to a computer-aided model (Bishop et al., 2017; Jessop et al., 2017). It offers high cell viability (80 to 90 %) but supports low cell densities (Mandrycky et al., 2016). Further, vertical printing abilities with this technology are highly compromised. Stereolithography utilises photopolymerisation as the basis of printing complex structures. In this technique a photo resin is mixed with the polymer to be printed and the printed structure is illuminated with UV light to crosslink it into a hardened structure (Bishop et al., 2017; Chaudhary & Garg, 2015; Jessop et al., 2017). It is very fast, offers good vertical printing ability, has more than 90% cell viability and can handle medium cell density (Kačarević et al., 2018). Fused deposition modelling (FDM) is extrusion-based modelling in which a plastic filament of exact diameter is passed through a heated nozzle, where it is melted and extruded onto a substrate in a definite pattern. Highly interconnected porous structures can be produced using this simple, high speed and low-cost 3D-printing technique (Azad et al., 2020).

To summarise, AM technology can provide highly customised and economical fabrication of scaffolds (Javaid & Haleem, 2018). It has already been used with great success in dentistry where implants with low cost and better strength are manufactured according to patient requirements (Javaid & Haleem, 2019). A remarkable increase in demand for 3D printing in the field of tissue engineering, surgical planning and designing of a therapeutic delivery system is attributed to its high reproducibility, precision and accuracy (Ahangar et al., 2018). Further, the fabricating technique reduces the wastage of material and requires comparatively minimal chemicals (such as cleaning solutions and etching agents), hence making the process environment friendly (Ivanova, Williams, & Campbell, 2013). It also empowers the scholars to fabricate artificial organs to understand the anatomic and pathology variations faced during actual surgery or intervention and plan accordingly. A group of researchers have manufactured a silicon-based artificial heart that can beat like a

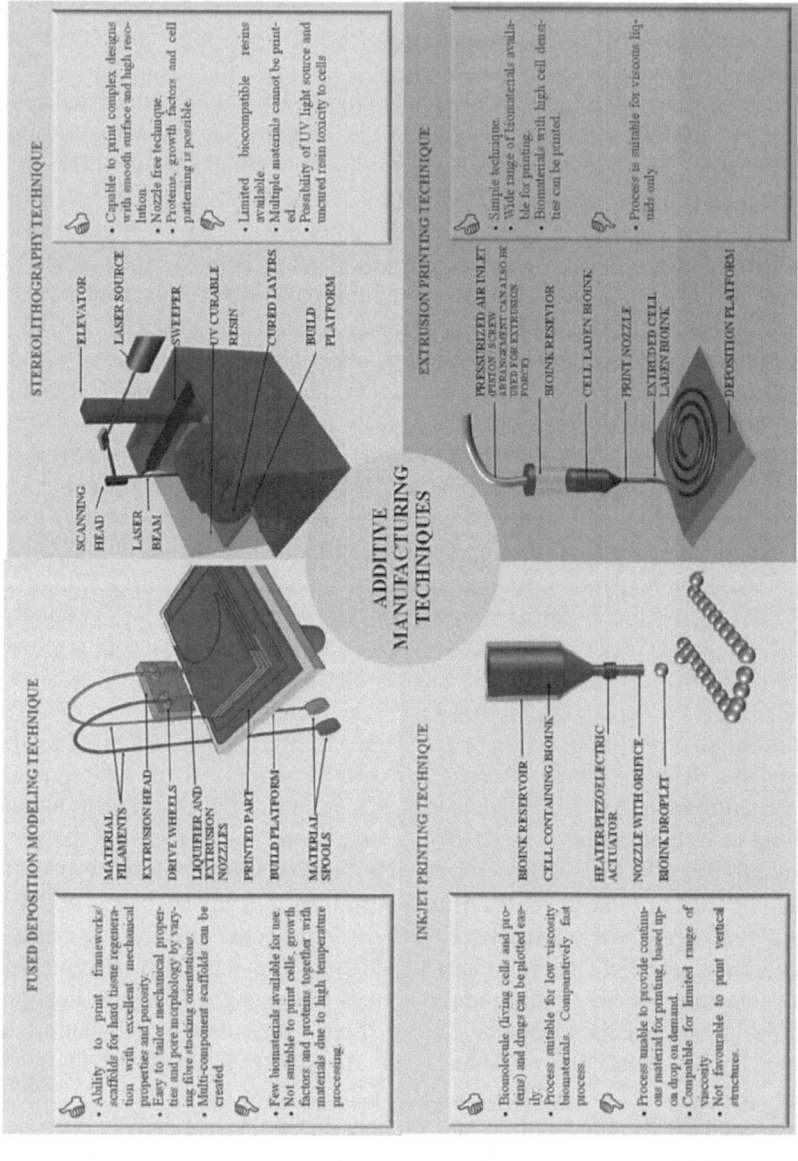

FIGURE 10.1 Different AM techniques commonly used in scaffold fabrication: construction, advantages and limitations.

human heart but has a limited life (Haleem, Javaid, & Saxena, 2018). However, AM technology also has some limitations to its credit. It offers limited building platform size, slow build rates, and has limited compatible biomaterials, and disputed dimensional accuracy (Chia & Wu, 2015). There is also significant labour required for application design, setting process parameters, and necessary post-processing procedures (Tofail et al., 2018).

10.3 STATUS OF ELECTROSPINNING IN SCAFFOLD FABRICATION

Electrospinning or electrostatic spinning is the most common technique for fabricating nano and sub-microfibers. The technique originated back in the seventeenth century when William Gilbert observed that a drop of water on a dry and flat surface was drawn into a conical shape when a rubber amber was held at a particular distance from it (Asmatulu & Khan, 2019). The present form of electrospinning technology with a vast field of application has emerged after the years of invention, refinement and reorientation of the process (Tan, Yang, & Shen, 2017).

The basic electrospinning setup has three components, namely a high voltage source, a spinneret or nozzle and a grounded collector (Hong, Yeo, Yang, & Kim, 2019). The process is capable of processing many different polymers. Most polymers need to be dissolved in some solvent to form a solution for further processing. The polymer solution is then introduced into the capillary tube or syringe having a nozzle connected to high voltage for electrospinning. The process of fibre formation in electrospinning is not only based on the electrostatic interactions between the grounded collector and charged polymer solution but also on the electrostatic repulsion within the charged polymer solution droplet. The electrostatic field between the ground collector and nozzle charges the drop of polymer solution at the nozzle tip. At a certain threshold of charge, the electrostatic repulsion overcomes the surface tension of the solution resulting in a jet eruption from the drop of solution, also referred to as Taylor cone formation (Nagrath, Alhalawani, Rahimnejad Yazdi, & Towler, 2019). Some polymers or their solutions may emit harmful fumes or unpleasant smells, hence the processing needs to be done within the well-ventilated chambers (Bhardwaj & Kundu, 2010).

Various modifications in basic electrospinning techniques have taken place over the years and various researchers have reported different merits and demerits of these techniques. We broadly categorise electrospinning into two major types, solution and melt electrospinning. In solution electrospinning, a polymer solution is extruded into the air through a spinneret under an electric field and fibres (in the range of a few nanometres) are produced as the solvent evaporates from the extruded jets (Gupta & Kothari, 1997; Luo, Stoyanov, Stride, Pelan, & Edirisinghe, 2012). The major concern with solution electrospinning is electrified jet instabilities. The dynamic nature of the electrified jet is attributed to the solvent used in the technique. Its presence not only lowers the surface tensions of polymer solutions but is also responsible for high surface charges on the deposited fibres. If on the one hand, the jet instabilities are responsible for generating nanofibres, on the other hand, it only makes their deposition difficult to control and fails to attain sufficient Z dimensions, thus limiting its application in the fabrication of 3D scaffolds. Researchers have tried to control the collection of nanofibres by altering the design of collectors and have reported significant success (Haifeng Liu et al., 2013; C. Wang et al., 2019; X. Wang, Ding, Sun, Wang, & Yu, 2013). Further, the electrospinning process depends on numerous parameters such as nozzle–collector distance, applied voltage, surrounding humidity and temperature, rate of airflow, ejection speed and solution properties (surface tension, viscosity and electrical conductivity). Hence, the morphology of the nanofibres can be directly controlled by precise control of these parameters (Shi et al., 2015; Tan et al., 2017).

In solution electrospun fibres, the presence of residual solvent may lead to the issue of cell toxicity. Hence, the cells/tissues should not be in direct contact with fibres fabricated by the solution electrospinning process unless all the solvent gets removed (Dalton et al., 2013).

Another type of electrospinning, i.e. melt electrospinning has found immense application in designing 3D scaffolds. The technique is very similar to FDM as in this an extruded polymer melt produces fibres upon cooling (Tourlomousis, Babakhanov, Ding, & Chang, 2015). As melt electrospinning does not use the solvent to generate fibres, it very easily overcomes the limitations of solution electrospinning viz. chaotic fibre placement, inability to attain thickness in electrospun fibres due to high surface charge and toxicity concern due to remaining solvent in electrospun fibres. The only concern with melt electrospinning is that low diameter nanofibres are not easily produced (Lian & Meng, 2017). Although few studies have reported such fibres using melt electrospinning, still majorly the technique is suitable to generate submicron fibres (Muerza-Cascante, Haylock, Hutmacher, & Dalton, 2014) Figure 10.2.

Few other electrospinning techniques like wet and gel electrospinning are also gaining interest in recent years. Wet spinning involves the precipitation of polymer due to a chemical reaction or dilution effect when the polymer solution is extruded into the chemical bath and hence generates polymer fibres upon solidification (Luo et al., 2012). On the other hand, gel spinning involves whirling a polymer in the 'gel' state, followed by air-drying and then cooling in a liquid bath. The technique enables the production of high mechanical strength fibres (Xue, Wu, Dai, & Xia, 2019).

Electrospinning can process a variety of materials including polymers and inorganic compounds into fibres of diameter ranging from several micrometres to tens of nanometers (Shi et al., 2015). Effective and simple procedure, inexpensive setup and ability to control parameters like fibre diameter, orientation and composition make the process highly attractive (Dahlin, Kasper, & Mikos, 2011). Further, the technique is continuous and can generate long electrospun fibres when compared to fibres prepared by other chemical or physical methods (Long et al., 2011). The process is capable of fabricating nanofibres with high design flexibility, high porosity and high surface area (Tan et al., 2017). These electrospun fibres are being used in various applications such as filtration applications, affinity membranes, membranes in biosensors, drug delivery, wound healing, tissue-engineering scaffolds, immobilisation of enzymes, protective clothing, cosmetics, etc. (Bhardwaj & Kundu, 2010). A distinctive benefit of electrospinning is its ability to generate complex hierarchical structures via regulated calcination of inorganic nanofibres. These structures are difficult to manufacture using conventional approaches like CVD, self-assembly,

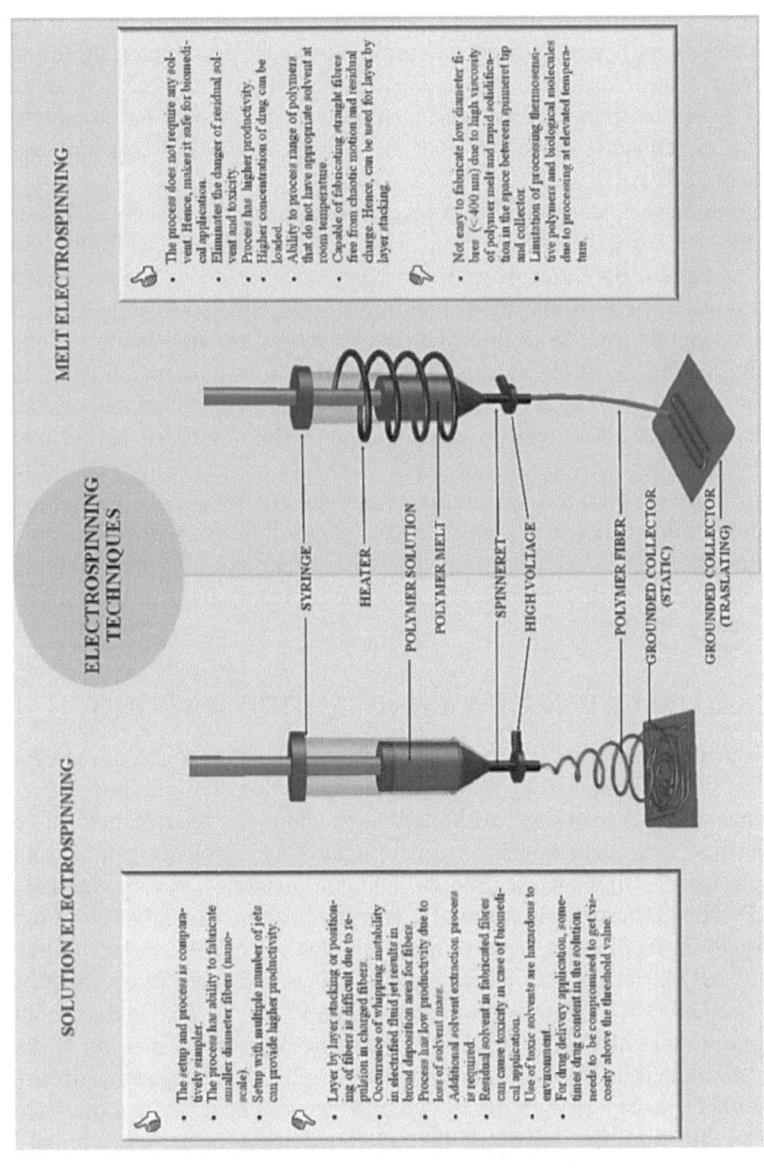

FIGURE 10.2 Electrospinning techniques for scaffolds generation: layout, advantages and limitations.

template-assisted synthesis and other solution-based methods (Shi et al., 2015). The process enables bioactive compounds to achieve high encapsulation efficacy. The process also favours encapsulation of thermosensitive compounds due to its nonthermal nature of processing. This makes its application much greater in food processing and storage as enhancing the stability and functionality and preserving the structure are the main requirements (C. Zhang, Li, Wang, & Zhang, 2020). In medical applications, the electrospun fibres are used for sustained-release drug materials and wound dressings where the requirement is to release the drug continuously without any overdose. The electrospun materials are also used in the field of tissue engineering for repairing or replacing damaged tissues (vascular, nerve and soft bone tissues) (Hao Liu et al., 2020).

There are numerous advantages and successful applications of electrospun nanofibres and the technique. However, some critical limitations such as limited cellular infiltration and small pore size in spun fibres are also reported. The use of organic solvents in solution electrospinning further limits its application (Dahlin et al., 2011). Many efforts are being made to improve cellular migration and the design through multilayering, inclusion of Heprasil and combination with polymers having distinct degradation behaviour (Ekaputra, Prestwich, Cool, & Hutmacher, 2008). If controlled calcination can assist electrospun inorganic nanofibres to obtain complex structures, it also limits its applications as it markedly increases fibre friability (Shi et al., 2015). Further, even though simple equipment and procedure are required for electrospun nanofibre generation, its industrial translatability is still a serious issue (Hao Liu et al., 2020). Also, there is a need to evaluate the UV, thermal and time-dependent stabilities of these materials as no significant study has been reported (C. Zhang et al., 2020).

10.4 AMALGAMATION OF AM AND ELECTROSPINNING

AM and electrospinning are two separate techniques that have found immense application in scaffold fabrication for tissue engineering. Both techniques have their share of advantages and shortcomings. Although AM techniques provide precise control over the scaffold architecture which is manufactured using biocompatible and bioabsorbable materials, at the same time the filament resolution is very small (Dalton et al., 2013). The highest resolution of 3D printing is approximately 300 mm which is large enough for facilitating the attachment of most cells on the surface of the scaffold (Kwan, 2013). Further, the fabricated scaffold surfaces are too smooth and do not support cell adhesion (Nguyen, Rahman, & San Wong, 2012). On the other hand, electrospinning faces the issue of chaotic filament deposition, making it difficult to create a reproducible 3D scaffold (Dalton et al., 2013). Charge accumulation on deposited fibres restricts the number of layers which can be deposited on one above the other and thus limit the maximum thickness which can be achieved in the fabricated scaffold to not more than 3–4 mm (Vaquette & Cooper-White, 2012). Solution electrospun fibre meshes have limited porosity (Dalton et al., 2013). Cells are not able to infiltrate such tightly packed meshes but grow on their top thus limiting their applications in tissue engineering. Although many researchers have worked in this area using structured collectors to electrospun porous scaffolds (Neves et al., 2007;

Vaquette & Cooper-White, 2011; Y. Wang et al., 2009; D. Zhang & Chang, 2007), the technique is not very reliable to ensure accurate placement of fibres.

Thus, the strong need to precisely control the pore distribution within the scaffolds and to ensure its precise reproducibility has resulted in combining these two processing methods in recent times. With the increased desire of the tissue-engineering scientist to repair and replace the tissues and organs of high complexity, this amalgamation was considered the only way out as it offers the researchers options to develop more elaborate structures incorporating micro- and nano-scale elements together. On screening the literature reports in this area, it is evident that the research in the generation of 3D scaffolds using electrospun nano/microfibers can be broadly grouped into two categories: (a) electrospinning used in combination with AM technique, and (b) melt electrospinning as AM technique. In the following sections, we will discuss both these options in detail.

10.4.1 ELECTROSPINNING USED IN COMBINATION WITH AM TECHNIQUE

For the first time in 2008, three research labs independently reported the fabrication of a bimodal scaffold, combining both micro- (via. AM) and nano- (via electrospinning) scale elements (Moroni, de Wijn, & van Blitterswijk, 2008; Park, Kim, Kim, Yang, & Park, 2008). They fabricated scaffolds by alternating depositions from the fused deposition modelling (FDM) process and electrospinning. The resulting scaffold had large pores for easy cell invasion and electrospun fibres provide a suitable structure for cell adhesion. Later, Centola et al. (2010) reported the fabrication of tubular structure for vascular grafts using the same principle (Centola et al., 2010). Vaquette et al. (2012) developed a biphasic scaffold composed of a solution electrospun membrane and an FDM scaffold with application in ectopic periodontal regeneration. The electrospun layer acted as a supportive membrane which enabled the adhesion of seeded periodontal ligament cells or mesenchymal stem cells, while the FDM scaffold ensured biomedical stability and provided space for bone regeneration (Vaquette et al., 2012). Later the same group loaded the FDM scaffold with bone morphogenic protein-7 loaded hydrogel and evaluated its effect on the stimulation of bone growth. The results were very encouraging and the biphasic scaffold permitted a high level of bone formation without any traces of mineralisation in the periodontal compartment (Dalton et al., 2013). Yu et al. (2016) reported the fabrication of a composite 3D scaffold by infusing discontinuous polycaprolactone/gelatine electrospun nanofibres into the mesh of a 3D-printed polycaprolactone scaffold. The developed 3D composite scaffold had higher mechanical strength than a scaffold made of only electrospun fibres, and good biocompatibility and better cell migration and proliferation compared to the only 3D-printed scaffold (Yu et al., 2016). Chen et al. (2019) combined electrospinning, 3D printing, freeze-drying, and crosslinking to fabricate 3D-printed scaffolds with precisely controlled shapes and large pores, in addition to fibrous surface morphologies similar to that of a native extracellular matrix. In the study, initially they developed gelatin/poly (lactic-co-glycolic acid) electrospun fibres. The fibres were then dehydrated to maintain fibre structure during future processing and later homogenised to give small stands which avoid clogging the nozzle of the 3D printer. The homogenised and dried fibre powder was then blended with small amounts of hyaluronic acid and polyethylene oxide solutions to form ink that could be smoothly extruded from the needle of a 3D printer to form continuous strands. Finally, the developed scaffold was freeze-dried and crosslinked to improve its mechanical strength. Features such as water-induced shape memory and good elasticity were exhibited by the novel scaffolds which mimic the extracellular matrix structures. Moreover, the developed scaffold had shown potential to use in cartilage regeneration as it satisfactorily combined with chondrocytes (Chen et al., 2019) (Table 10.1).

10.4.2 MELT ELECTROSPINNING AS AM APPROACH

It was 2006 when the 'near-field' electrospinning technology was introduced for direct writing using electrospinning. The setup facilitates the single-layer deposition of fibres on the collector stage using its controlled movement and keeping the collector distance very short (Sun, Chang, Li, & Lin, 2006). In general, electrospinning, more specifically solution electrospinning, faces two major issues which hasten the prospects of using it as AM technique. Firstly, the electrified jet of solution often shows 'whipping' instability and results in a wide deposition area. Secondly, the deposited fibres repel the next layer of fibre and thus limit the achievable maximum thickness. These problems can be attributed to the use of charged solvent in this electrospinning technique (Dalton et al., 2013). In recent years, another electrospinning technique called melt electrospinning has emerged as a newer AM technique using which complex and porous scaffolds with high levels of reproducibility can be fabricated (Dalton, 2017). The absence of solvent in melt electrospinning results in the generation of straight fibres free from chaotic motion and residual charge and is very effective in view of environmental considerations and productivity (Haleem et al., 2018). This successfully addresses both the limitations of solution electrospinning and the electrified molten jet can be used for direct-writing purposes with accurate stacking. However, the process has the limitation of fabricating nanofibres with narrow thickness distribution and attaining a diameter of less than 400 nm, which is easier to attain by the solvent electrospinning process. Three research labs in 2010 individually reported the generation of 3D bimodal scaffolds by combining micro (via melt electrospinning) and nano (via solvent electrospinning) fibres obtained from electrospinning alone without involving any AM technique (Chung et al., 2010; Gentsch, Boysen, Lankenau, & Börner, 2010; S. J. Kim et al., 2010; Soliman et al., 2010). The generated scaffold offered the advantage of better cell penetration and adhesion.

The most related AM technique to the melt electrospinning is FDM. Melt electrospinning can result in the fabrication of highly porous scaffolds when compared to FDM fabricated ones. Major differences between the two techniques can be attributed to the production of lower diameter filaments in melt electrospinning under the electric field. Further, the nozzle-to-collector distance is much lower for FDM, and a z-stage controlling the height of deposition is required. On the other hand, for melt electrospinning, sufficient spinneret to collector distance permits accurate control of scaffold properties (Dalton, 2017). Various materials that are compatible and processed with melt electrospinning are polyurethane (PU), poly(e-caprolactone) (PCL),

TABLE 10.1

Literature Reporting Fabrication of 3D Scaffolds Using Electrospinning Alone or in Combination with AM Technique

S. No.	Technique Used	Polymers Used	Important Findings	References
A.	*Electrospinning used in combination with AM technique*			
1.	Direct polymer melt deposition (DPMD)/ Solution electrospinning	• In DPMD: PCL polymer was melted at 150°C. • In solution electrospinning, 10% concentration solution of PCL/ collagen (6/4 weight ratio) blend and PCL in HFIP were used.	• Developed bimodal or hybrid scaffold. • Layer-by-layer approach was followed to generate a 3D hybrid structure having alternate layers of microfibers (via DPMD process) and nanofibre (via solution electrospinning). • In the electrospinning process, a syringe pump with a 22-gauge needle was used to electrospin fibres onto a grounded collector placed at a distance of 10 cm. PCL/collagen and PCL nanofibres having diameters of 325 ± 128 and 431 ± 148 nm respectively were fabricated with an applied voltage of 18 kV.	Park et al. (2008)
2.	3D rapid prototyping system/ Solution electrospinning	• In 3D rapid prototyping: PCL melted polymer was used. • In solution electrospinning; PCL polymer in methylene chloride (80 wt.%)/ dimethylformamide solvent system (20 wt.%) was used.	• Developed bimodal or hybrid scaffold. • In 3D rapid prototyping, a dispensing needle of 250 µm tip diameter was used for plotting layer by layer. • In solution electrospinning, a setup consisting of syringe pump along with a 20 mL glass syringe was used for controlling the flow rate of polymer solution. • Scaffolds of approximate size 10 × 10 × 5 mm were fabricated. • The diameter and thickness of the deposited spun fibres were 700–2000 nm and 10–25 µm and respectively.	G. Kim, Son, Park, & Kim (2008)

(Continued)

TABLE 10.1 (CONTINUED)

Literature Reporting Fabrication of 3D Scaffolds Using Electrospinning Alone or in Combination with AM Technique

S. No.	Technique Used	Polymers Used	Important Findings	References
3.	Fused deposition modelling/ Solution electrospinning	In FDM: PCL polymer was melted at 80°C. In solution electrospinning: The polymer solution of PLLA (13% w/w) was made using dichloromethane solvent. The polymer solution was then added with unfractionated heparin along with methanol as a cosolvent.	• Developed bimodal or hybrid scaffold. • In the electrospinning process, a 28-gauge needle with an applied voltage of 15 kV was used to electrospin fibres onto a grounded collector placed at a distance of 15 cm. • The combination of FDM and electrospinning enhanced the mechanical properties of the fabricated structure without affecting the optimal fibre arrangement for tissue formation and cell attachment.	Centola et al. (2010)
4.	FDM scaffold/ Solution electrospinning	In FDM: β-tricalcium phosphate (β-TCP, 20% wt) in PCL was used. In solution electrospinning: A mixture of chloroform and dimethylformamide (9/1) was used to dissolve PCL.	• Developed bimodal or hybrid scaffold containing a flexible electrospun membrane for the periodontal compartment and an FDM component for the bone compartment. • In solution electrospinning, the solution of polymer was loaded into a 10 mL syringe and electrospun fibres are collected on collector placed 20 cm apart using a voltage of 10 kV.	Vaquette et al. (2012)
5.	Three-dimensional (3D) printing/ Solution electrospinning	In solution electrospinning: the polymers PCL and gelatin (mass ratio w/w- 2:8) were dissolved in HFIP (w/v- 12%). In 3D printing: PCL solid particles melted at 80°C.	• Developed bimodal or hybrid scaffold. • Cut pieces (2×2 mm²) of the collected electrospun PCL/gelatin nanofibre films were submerged into tert-butanol solution using high-speed dispersion homogeniser. • Further, in the 3D-printing approach melted PCL solid particles used to prepare scaffold which was printed through the layers stacking and controlled with a computer.	Yu et al. (2016)

(Continued)

6.	3D printing/ Freeze-drying/ Solution electrospinning	• In solution electrospinning: Solvent 1,1,1,3,3,3-hexafluoro-2-propanol was used to dissolve Gelatin and PLGA polymers for fabricating electrospun nanofibres. • In 3D printing: Electrospun fibre-based inks were developed using HA and PEO in deionised water.	• In the solution electrospinning process a high voltage of 16 kV was applied to generate gelatin/PLGA fibre membranes. Spinneret-collector distance was kept as 15 cm. High temperature (180°C) was used to dehydrate the developed fibres. • Pieces of nanofibres were dispersed in HA and PEO with deionised water to develop fibre-based ink. • In the 3D-printing process, a 3D plotting system was used to extrude electrospun fibre-based ink through nozzles. The moving speed of the plotting head was 0.5 mms^{-1}, and the dosing speed was 0.0018 mms^{-1}. Fabricated scaffolds were freeze-dried.	Chen et al. (2019)
B.	***Melt electrospinning as AM approach***			
1.	Melt electrospinning/ Solution electrospinning	• In melt electrospinning: PLGA was melted at 210°C. • In solution electrospinning: PLGA polymer was used to prepare solution (1–10 wt%) in HFIP.	• In melt electrospinning method, PLGA microfibers collection was done from a distance of 8 cm on target drum from syringe tip (18 G) with applied voltage of 17.5 kV. Whereas, in solution electrospinning method, nanofibres were collected on a target drum placed 8.5 cm from the syringe tip (21G) at a voltage of 17.5 kV. • Both the PLGA solution and PLGA melt were electrospun at the same time in opposite directions onto a rotating collector for fabricating nano/microfibre composite scaffolds. • It was found that prepared PLGA nano/microfibre scaffolds were functionally active in terms of cell attachment for both NHEF and NHEK.	S. J. Kim, Jang, Park, & Min (2010)

(Continued)

TABLE 10.1 (CONTINUED)
Literature Reporting Fabrication of 3D Scaffolds Using Electrospinning Alone or in Combination with AM Technique

S. No.	Technique Used	Polymers Used	Important Findings	References
2.	Melt electrospinning/ Solution electrospinning	In melt electrospinning: PLCL copolymer was melted at 155°C and the PLCL copolymer contained L-lactide and ε-caprolactone monomers in the molar ratio of 50:50. In solution electrospinning: Acetone (15%) and HFIP (9%) i.e., two solvents were used for dissolving PLCL copolymer.	• In melt electrospinning, a predetermined winding angle was set by providing a transverse motion to the wind-up unit while collecting the melt-spun monofilament fibres. • In solution electrospinning, the distance between the collector and needle tip was 15 cm with applied voltage of 10–14 kV. • As a result, double-layered tubular scaffolds were formed containing both melt-spun macrofibres (<200 μm in diameter) and electrospun submicron fibres (>400 nm in diameter).	Chung, Ingle, Montero, Kim, & King (2010)
3.	Melt electrospinning writing	PCL polymer melted at 65–82°C.	• In melt electrospinning, the motion of collector was programmed using software and the dispensing head remains at the fixed position. • The low pressure promoted the formation of small fibres (3–10 μm in diameters) whereas, larger fibres (10–20 μm in diameters) were manufactured at higher pressure as it induced more flow of molten polymer.	Wunner et al. (2017)
4.	Melt electrospinning writing	PCL polymer melted at 65–82°C.	• A scaffold was printed with an eagle pattern. • To achieve fibres with the smallest diameter, a combination of low collection distance, low flow rate, high applied voltage and high printing speed were used. • The resulting fibres diameter ranged from 3.59 ± 0.62 μm to 22.9 ± 0.53 μm.	Jin et al. (2020)

HFIP: hexafluoroisopropanol; PCL: polycaprolactone; PLCL: poly(l-lactide-co-ε-caprolactone); PCL: polycaprolactone; PLGA: poly (lactic-co-glycolic acid); PLLA: poly-L-lactide; NHEF: normal human epidermal fibroblasts; NHEK: normal human epidermal keratinocytes poly(ethylene terephthalate) (PET), polyamide 12 (PA12), poly(lactic-co-glycolic acid) (PLGA), polylactic acid (PLA), polypropylene (PP) and polyethylene (PE) (Jin et al., 2020; S. J. Kim et al., 2010; Koenig, Beukenberg, Langensiepen, & Seide, 2019; Koenig et al., 2020).

10.5 CONCLUSION AND FUTURE PERSPECTIVE

In the present era of personalised and consumer-friendly products, tissue-engineering research has shifted its focus from synthetic implants and tissue grafts to 3D porous scaffolds which can mimic the natural tissue environment at nanoscale. These scaffolds have been used to deliver drugs and to support cell implantation and growth at the site of application. In recent times, the amalgamation of novel technologies like AM and electrospinning has provided a unique opportunity for researchers to develop low-cost, high-resolution, 3D scaffolds for better clinical translation. The research in the area is still in its infancy and exciting avenues are still unexplored awaiting recognition.

ACKNOWLEDGEMENT

The authors are grateful to DST SERB for the research project sanctioned to Professor Indu Pal Kaur under the CRG Scheme.

ANNEXURE FOR ABBREVIATIONS

AM   Additive manufacturing
CVD   Chemical vapour deposition
DPMD   Direct polymer melt deposition
FDM   Fused deposition modelling
HFIP   1,1,1,3,3,3-hexafluoro-2-propanol
HA   Hydroxyapatite
NHEF   Normal human epidermal fibroblasts
NHEK   Normal human epidermal keratinocytes
PCL   Polycaprolactone (PCL)
PEO   Polyethylene oxide
PLCL   Poly(l-lactide-co-ε-caprolactone)
PLGA   Poly (lactic-co-glycolic acid)
PLLA   Poly-L-lactide
UV   Ultraviolet

REFERENCES

Ahangar, P., Akoury, E., Ramirez Garcia Luna, A. S., Nour, A., Weber, M. H., & Rosenzweig, D. A.-O. (2018). Nanoporous 3D-printed scaffolds for local doxorubicin delivery in bone metastases secondary to prostate cancer. *Materials (Basel)*, 11, 1485.

Asmatulu, R., & Khan, W. S. (2019). Chapter 2 – Historical background of the electrospinning process. In R. Asmatulu & W. S. Khan (Eds.), *Synthesis and Applications of Electrospun Nanofibers* (pp. 17–39): Elsevier.

Azad, M. A., Olawuni, D., Kimbell, G., Badruddoza, A. Z. M., Hossain, M. S., & Sultana, T. (2020). Polymers for extrusion-based tissing of pharmaceuticals: A holistic materials-process perspective. *Pharmaceutics*, *12*(2). doi:10.3390/pharmaceutics12020124

Banga, H.K., Belokar, R.M., Kumar, R., (2017a). A Novel Approach For Ankle Foot Orthosis Developed By Three Dimensional Technologies, *3rd International Conference on Mechanical Engineering and Automation Science (ICMEAS 2017)*, University of Birmingham, UK, Vol. 8 No. 10, pp. 141–145.

Banga, H.K., Belokar, R.M., Madan, R., Dhole, S. (2017b). Three dimensional Gait assessments during walking of healthy people and drop foot patients. *Defence Life Science Journal*, 2, 14–20.

Banga, H.K., Parveen, K., Belokar, R.M., Kumar R, (2018). Fabrication and stress analysis of ankle foot orthosis with additive manufacturing. *Rapid Prototyping Journal Emerald Publishing*, 24(2), 300–312.

Banga, H.K., Parveen, K., Belokar, R.M. and Kumar, R. (2020a). Customized design and additive manufacturing of kids' ankle foot orthosis. *Rapid Prototyping Journal*, 26, 10. doi:10.1108/RPJ-07-2019-0194

Banga, H.K., Parveen, K., Belokar, R.M. and Kumar, R. (2020b). Design and fabrication of prosthetic and orthotic product by 3D printing [Online First], *IntechOpen*. doi:10.5772/intechopen.94846. Available from: https://www.intechopen.com/online-first/design-and-fabrication-of-prosthetic-and-orthotic-product-by-3d-printing

Banga, H.K., Parveen, K., Belokar, R.M., Kumar, R. (2020c). Effect of 3D-printed ankle foot orthosis during walking of foot deformities patients. In: Kumar H., Jain P. (eds) *Recent Advances in Mechanical Engineering*. Lecture Notes in Mechanical Engineering. Springer, Singapore, pp. 275–288.

Banga, H.K., Parveen, K., Belokar R.M., Kumar R. (2020d). Role of finite element analysis in customized design of kids' orthotic product'. In: Singh S., Prakash C., Singh R. (eds) *Characterization, Testing, Measurement, and Metrology*, pp. 139–159. CRC Press Taylor & Francis Grpoup, USA.

Banga H.K., Parveen, K., Belokar R.M., Kumar R. (2020e). Improvement of human gait in foot deformities patients by 3D printed ankle–foot orthosis. In: Singh S., Prakash C., Singh R. (eds) *3D Printing in Biomedical Engineering*. Materials Horizons: From Nature to Nanomaterials. Springer, Singapore.

Banga, H.K., Parveen, K., Kumar, H. (2021). Utilization of additive manufacturing in orthotics and prosthetic devices development. *IOP Conference Series: Materials Science and Engineering*. doi:10.1088/1757-899X/1033/1/012083

Bhardwaj, N., & Kundu, S. C. (2010). Electrospinning: A fascinating fiber fabrication technique. *Biotechnology Advances*, 28(3), 325–347. doi:10.1016/j.biotechadv.2010.01.004

Bishop, E., Mostafa, S., Pakvasa, M., Luu, H., Lee, M., Wolf, J.,... Reid, R. (2017). 3-D bioprinting technologies in tissue engineering and regenerative medicine: Current and future trends. *Genes & Diseases*, 4, 185–195. doi:10.1016/j.gendis.2017.10.002

Centola, M., Rainer, A., Spadaccio, C., De Porcellinis, S., Genovese, J. A., & Trombetta, M. (2010). Combining electrospinning and fused deposition modeling for the fabrication of a hybrid vascular graft. *Biofabrication*, 2(1), 014102. doi:10.1088/1758-5082/2/1/014102

Chaudhary, C., & Garg, T. (2015). Scaffolds: A novel carrier and potential wound healer. *Critical Reviews in Therapeutic Drug Carrier Systems*, 32, 277–321. doi:10.1615/CritRevTher DrugCarrierSyst.2015011246

Chen, W., Xu, Y., Liu, Y., Wang, Z., Li, Y., Jiang, G.,... Zhou, G. (2019). Three-dimensional printed electrospun fiber-based scaffold for cartilage regeneration. *Materials & Design*, *179*, 107886. doi:10.1016/j.matdes.2019.107886

Chia, H. N., & Wu, B. M. (2015). Recent advances in 3D printing of biomaterials. *Journal of Biological Engineering*, *9*(1), 4. doi:10.1186/s13036-015-0001-4

Chung, S., Ingle, N. P., Montero, G. A., Kim, S. H., & King, M. W. (2010). Bioresorbable elastomeric vascular tissue engineering scaffolds via melt spinning and electrospinning. *Acta Biomater, 6*(6), 1958–1967. doi:10.1016/j.actbio.2009.12.007

Dahlin, R. L., Kasper, F. K., & Mikos, A. G. (2011). Polymeric nanofibers in tissue engineering. *Tissue Engineering. Part B, Reviews, 17*(5), 349–364. doi:10.1089/ten.TEB.2011.0238

Dalton, P. D. (2017). Melt electrowriting with additive manufacturing principles. *Current Opinion in Biomedical Engineering, 2,* 49–57. doi:10.1016/j.cobme.2017.05.007

Dalton, P. D., Vaquette, C., Farrugia, B. L., Dargaville, T. R., Brown, T. D., & Hutmacher, D. W. (2013). Electrospinning and additive manufacturing: Converging technologies. *Biomaterials Science, 1*(2), 171–185. doi:10.1039/C2BM00039C

Ekaputra, A., Prestwich, G., Cool, S., & Hutmacher, D. (2008). Combining electrospun scaffolds with electrosprayed hydrogels leads to three-dimensional cellularization of hybrid constructs. *Biomacromolecules, 9,* 2097–2103. doi:10.1021/bm800565u

Gentsch, R., Boysen, B., Lankenau, A., & Börner, H. G. (2010). Single-step electrospinning of bimodal fiber meshes for ease of cellular infiltration. *Macromol Rapid Communication, 31*(1), 59–64. doi:10.1002/marc.200900431

Gill, A., Deol, P., & Kaur, I. P. (2019). An update on use of alginate in additive biofabrication techniques. *Current Pharmaceutical Design, 25,* 1249–1264. doi:10.2174/1381612825 666190423155835

Gu, B. K., Choi, D. J., Park, S. J., Kim, Y. J., & Kim, C. H. (2018). 3D bioprinting technologies for tissue engineering applications. *Advances in Experimental Medicine and Biology, 1078,* 15–28. doi:10.1007/978-981-13-0950-2_2

Gupta, V. B., & Kothari, V. K. (1997). *Manufactured Fibre Technology.* London: Chapman & Hall.

Haleem, A., Javaid, M., & Saxena, A. (2018). Additive manufacturing applications in cardiology: A review. *The Egyptian Heart Journal, 70*(4), 433–441. doi:10.1016/j.ehj.2018.09.008

He, P., Zhao, J., Zhang, J., Li, B., Gou, Z., Gou, M., & Li, X. (2018). Bioprinting of skin constructs for wound healing. *Burns & Trauma, 6,* 5–5. doi:10.1186/s41038-017-0104-x

Hong, J., Yeo, M., Yang, G. H., & Kim, G. (2019). Cell-electrospinning and its application for tissue engineering. *International Journal of Molecular Sciences, 20*(24), 6208. doi:10.3390/ijms20246208

Ivanova, O., Williams, C., & Campbell, T. (2013). Additive manufacturing (AM) and nanotechnology: Promises and challenges. *Rapid Prototyping Journal, 19,* 353. doi:10.1108/rpj-12-2011-0127

Javaid, M., & Haleem, A. (2018). Additive manufacturing applications in orthopaedics: A review. *Journal of Clinical Orthopaedics & Trauma, 9*(3), 202–206. doi:10.1016/j.jcot.2018.04.008

Javaid, M., & Haleem, A. (2019). Current status and applications of additive manufacturing in dentistry: A literature-based review. *Journal of Oral Biology and Craniofacial Research, 9*(3), 179–185. doi:10.1016/j.jobcr.2019.04.004

Jessop, Z. M., Al-Sabah, A., Gardiner, M. D., Combellack, E., Hawkins, K., & Whitaker, I. S. (2017). 3D bioprinting for reconstructive surgery: Principles, applications and challenges. *Journal of Plastic, Reconstructive & Aesthetic Surgery, 70*(9), 1155–1170. doi:10.1016/j.bjps.2017.06.001

Jin, Y., Gao, Q., Xie, C., Li, G., Du, J., Fu, J., & He, Y. (2020). Fabrication of heterogeneous scaffolds using melt electrospinning writing: Design and optimization. *Materials & Design, 185,* 108274. doi:10.1016/j.matdes.2019.108274

Kačarević Ž. P., Rider, P. M., Alkildani, S., Retnasingh, S., Smeets, R., Jung, O.,… Barbeck, M. (2018). An introduction to 3D bioprinting: Possibilities, challenges and future aspects. *Materials (Basel), 11*(11). doi:10.3390/ma11112199

Kim, G., Son, J.-G., Park, S., & Kim, W. (2008). Hybrid process for fabricating 3D hierarchical scaffolds combining rapid prototyping and electrospinning. *Macromolecular Rapid Communications, 29,* 1577–1581. doi:10.1002/marc.200800277

Kim, S. J., Jang, D. H., Park, W. H., & Min, B.-M. (2010). Fabrication and characterization of 3-dimensional PLGA nanofiber/microfiber composite scaffolds. *Polymer*, *51*(6), 1320–1327. doi:10.1016/j.polymer.2010.01.025

Koenig, K., Beukenberg, K., Langensiepen, F., & Seide, G. (2019). A new prototype melt-electrospinning device for the production of biobased thermoplastic sub-microfibers and nanofibers. *Biomaterials Research*, *23*(1), 10. doi:10.1186/s40824-019-0159-9

Koenig, K., Hermanns, S., Ellerkmann, J., Saralidze, K., Langensiepen, F., & Seide, G. (2020). The effect of additives and process parameters on the pilot-scale manufacturing of polylactic acid sub-microfibers by melt electrospinning. *Textile Research Journal*, *90*(17–18), 1948–1961. doi:10.1177/0040517520904019

Kwan, J. (2013). *Design of Electronics for a High-Resolution, Multi-Material, and Modular 3D Printer*.

Lian, H., & Meng, Z. (2017). Melt electrospinning vs. solution electrospinning: A comparative study of drug-loaded poly (ε-caprolactone) fibres. *Materials for Biological Applications. Materials Science and Engineering: C*, *74*, 117–123. doi:10.1016/j.msec.2017.02.024

Liu, H., Ding, X., Zhou, G., Li, P., Wei, X., & Fan, Y. (2013). Electrospinning of nanofibers for tissue engineering applications. *Journal of Nanomaterials*, *2013*, 495708. doi:10.1155/2013/495708

Liu, H., Gough, C., Deng, Q., Gu, Z., Wang, F., & Hu, X. (2020). Recent advances in electrospun sustainable composites for biomedical, environmental, energy, and packaging applications. *International Journal of Molecular Sciences*, *21*, 4019. doi:10.3390/ijms21114019

Long, Y.-Z., Li, M.-M., Gu, C., Wan, M., Duvail, J.-L., Liu, Z., & Fan, Z. (2011). Recent advances in synthesis, physical properties and applications of conducting polymer nanotubes and nanofibers. *Progress in Polymer Science*, *36*(10), 1415–1442. doi:10.1016/j.progpolymsci.2011.04.001

Luo, C. J., Stoyanov, S. D., Stride, E., Pelan, E., & Edirisinghe, M. (2012). Electrospinning versus fibre production methods: From specifics to technological convergence. *Chemical Society Reviews*, *41*(13), 4708–4735. doi:10.1039/c2cs35083a

Mandrycky, C., Wang, Z., Kim, K., & Kim, D.-H. (2016). 3D bioprinting for engineering complex tissues. *Biotechnol Advance*, *34*(4), 422–434. doi:10.1016/j.biotechadv.2015.12.011

Moroni, L., de Wijn, J. R., & van Blitterswijk, C. A. (2008). Integrating novel technologies to fabricate smart scaffolds. *Journal of Biomaterials Science, Polymer Edition*, *19*(5), 543–572. doi:10.1163/156856208784089571

Mota, C., Puppi, D., Chiellini, F., & Chiellini, E. (2015). Additive manufacturing techniques for the production of tissue engineering constructs. *Journal of Tissue Engineering and Regenerative Medicine*, *9*(3), 174–190. doi:10.1002/term.1635

Muerza-Cascante, M., Haylock, D., Hutmacher, D., & Dalton, P. (2014). Melt electrospinning and its technologization in tissue engineering. *Tissue Engineering. Part B, Reviews*, *21*. doi:10.1089/ten.TEB.2014.0347

Nagrath, M., Alhalawani, A., Rahimnejad Yazdi, A., & Towler, M. R. (2019). Bioactive glass fiber fabrication via a combination of sol-gel process with electro-spinning technique. *Materials Science and Engineering: C*, *101*, 521–538. doi:10.1016/j.msec.2019.04.003

Neves, N. M., Campos, R., Pedro, A., Cunha, J., Macedo, F., & Reis, R. L. (2007). Patterning of polymer nanofiber meshes by electrospinning for biomedical applications. *International journal of nanomedicine*, *2*(3), 433–448. Retrieved from https://pubmed.ncbi.nlm.nih.gov/18019842

Nguyen, M. D., Rahman, M., & San Wong, Y. (2012). Simultaneous micro-EDM and micro-ECM in low-resistivity deionized water. *International Journal of Machine Tools and Manufacture*, *54*, 55–65.

O'Brien, F. J. (2011). Biomaterials & scaffolds for tissue engineering. *Materials Today*, *14*(3), 88–95. doi:10.1016/S1369-7021(11)70058-X

Park, S. H., Kim, T. G., Kim, H. C., Yang, D.-Y., & Park, T. G. (2008). Development of dual scale scaffolds via direct polymer melt deposition and electrospinning for applications in tissue regeneration. *Acta Biomater, 4*(5), 1198–1207. doi:10.1016/j.actbio.2008.03.019

Roseti, L., Parisi, V., Petretta, M., Cavallo, C., Desando, G., Bartolotti, I., & Grigolo, B. (2017). Scaffolds for bone tissue engineering: State of the art and new perspectives. *Materials for Biological Applications. Materials Science and Engineering: C, 78,* 1246–1262. doi:10.1016/j.msec.2017.05.017

Shi, X., Zhou, W., Ma, D., Ma, Q., Bridges, D., Ma, Y., & Hu, A. (2015). Electrospinning of nanofibers and their applications for energy devices. *Journal of Nanomaterials, 2015,* 140716. doi:10.1155/2015/140716

Singh, D., Singh, D., & Han, S. S. (2016). 3D printing of scaffold for cells delivery: advances in skin tissue engineering. *Polymers, 8*(1), 19. doi:10.3390/polym8010019

Soliman, S., Pagliari, S., Rinaldi, A., Forte, G., Fiaccavento, R., Pagliari, F.,... Traversa, E. (2010). Multiscale three-dimensional scaffolds for soft tissue engineering via multimodal electrospinning. *Acta Biomaterialia, 6*(4), 1227–1237. doi:10.1016/j.actbio.2009. 10.051

Sun, D., Chang, C., Li, S., & Lin, L. (2006). Near-field electrospinning. *Nano Letters, 6*(4), 839–842. doi:10.1021/nl0602701

Tan, R., Yang, X., & Shen, Y. (2017). Robot-aided electrospinning toward intelligent biomedical engineering. *Robotics and Biomimetics, 4*(1), 17. doi:10.1186/s40638-017-0075-1

Tofail, S. A. M., Koumoulos, E. P., Bandyopadhyay, A., Bose, S., O'Donoghue, L., & Charitidis, C. (2018). Additive manufacturing: Scientific and technological challenges, market uptake and opportunities. *Materials Today, 21*(1), 22–37. doi:10.1016/j. mattod.2017.07.001

Tourlomousis, F., Babakhanov, A., Ding, H., & Chang, R. (2015). *A Novel Melt Electrospinning System for Studying Cell Substrate Interactions* (Vol. 2).

Vaquette, C., & Cooper-White, J. (2012). The use of an electrostatic lens to enhance the efficiency of the electrospinning process. *Cell and Tissue Research, 347*(3), 815–826. doi:10.1007/s00441-011-1318-z

Vaquette, C., & Cooper-White, J. J. (2011). Increasing electrospun scaffold pore size with tailored collectors for improved cell penetration. *Acta Biomater, 7*(6), 2544–2557. doi:10.1016/j.actbio.2011.02.036

Vaquette, C., Fan, W., Xiao, Y., Hamlet, S., Hutmacher, D. W., & Ivanovski, S. (2012). A biphasic scaffold design combined with cell sheet technology for simultaneous regeneration of alveolar bone/periodontal ligament complex. *Biomaterials, 33*(22), 5560–5573. doi:10.1016/j.biomaterials.2012.04.038

Vijayavenkataraman, S., Yan, W.-C., Lu, W. F., Wang, C.-H., & Fuh, J. Y. H. (2018). 3D bioprinting of tissues and organs for regenerative medicine. *Advanced Drug Delivery Reviews, 132,* 296–332. doi:10.1016/j.addr.2018.07.004

Wang, C., Wang, J., Zeng, L., Qiao, Z., Liu, X., Liu, H.,... Ding, J. (2019). Fabrication of electrospun polymer nanofibers with diverse morphologies. *Molecules, 24*(5). doi:10.3390/molecules24050834

Wang, X., Ding, B., Sun, G., Wang, M., & Yu, J. (2013). Electro-spinning/netting: A strategy for the fabrication of three-dimensional polymer nano-fiber/nets. *Progress in Materials Science, 58*(8), 1173–1243. doi:10.1016/j.pmatsci.2013.05.001

Wang, Y., Wang, G., Chen, L., Li, H., Yin, T., Wang, B.,... Yu, Q. (2009). Electrospun nanofiber meshes with tailored architectures and patterns as potential tissue-engineering scaffolds. *Biofabrication, 1*(1), 015001. doi:10.1088/1758-5082/1/1/015001

Weiser, T. G., Haynes, A. B., Molina, G., Lipsitz, S. R., Esquivel, M. M., Uribe-Leitz, T.,... Gawande, A. A. (2016). Size and distribution of the global volume of surgery in 2012. *Bulletin of the World Health Organization, 94*(3), 201–209F. doi:10.2471/BLT.15.159293

Wunner, F. M., Bas, O., Saidy, N. T., Dalton, P. D., Pardo, E. M. D.-J., & Hutmacher, D. W. (2017). Melt electrospinning writing of three-dimensional Poly(ε-caprolactone) scaffolds with controllable morphologies for tissue engineering applications. *Journal of visualized experiments* : *JoVE*(130), 56289. doi:10.3791/56289

Xue, J., Wu, T., Dai, Y., & Xia, Y. (2019). Electrospinning and electrospun nanofibers: Methods, materials, and applications. *Chemical Reviews*, *119*(8), 5298–5415. doi:10.1021/acs.chemrev.8b00593

Yang, Y., Wang, G., Liang, H., Gao, C., Peng, S., Shen, L., & Shuai, C. (2019). Additive manufacturing of bone scaffolds. *International Journal of Bioprinting*, *5*(1), 2019. doi:10.18063/ijb.v5i1.148

Yu, Y., Hua, S., Yang, M., Fu, Z., Teng, S., Niu, K.,... Yi, C. (2016). Fabrication and characterization of electrospinning/3D printing bone tissue engineering scaffold. *RSC Advances*, *6*(112), 110557–110565. doi:10.1039/C6RA17718B

Zhang, C., Li, Y., Wang, P., & Zhang, H. (2020). Electrospinning of nanofibers: Potentials and perspectives for active food packaging. *Comprehensive Reviews in Food Science and Food Safety*, *19*. doi:10.1111/1541-4337.12536

Zhang, D., & Chang, J. (2007). Patterning of electrospun fibers using electroconductive templates. *Advanced Materials*, *19*, 3664–3667. doi:10.1002/adma.200700896

11 Usage of Additive Manufacturing in Customised Bone Tissue-Engineering Scaffold

Shipra Gupta and Vaibhav Sahni
Post Graduate Institute of Medical Education & Research
(PGIMER), Chandigarh, India

CONTENTS

DOI: 10.1201/9781003301066-11

11.1   INTRODUCTION TO BONE BIOFABRICATION: HISTORY, ROLE AND CHALLENGES

It was on 8 August 1984 that Charles W. 'Chuck' Hull applied for a US patent number (US4575330 A). The details stated that the patent filed was for an 'Apparatus for production of three-dimensional objects by stereolithography' (Hull, 1986). This was essentially the first 3D printer in the world. Additive Manufacturing (AM) purportedly had several advantages over subtractive manufacturing such as those of precision, speed and the potential to produce customised tailor-made constructs. As time progressed the applications of AM increased and the related cost of purchase and use declined to a point wherein 3D printers can be bought off Amazon for as little as 500 pounds sterling. This has invited hobbyists and amateur inventors to utilise the process for their own ends. Chuck Hull himself conceded that he did not foresee the medical applications of his invention and was informed by medical counterparts of its utility (Ponsford & Glass, 2014).

Before 3D printing made its way into mainstream medicine, it was heralded by a series of trials carried out at Boston Children's Hospital. These trials involved the manufacture of urinary bladders for seven patients utilising collagen and synthetic polymer scaffolds which were layered with patient-derived cells and allowed to grow into functional organs. Although the trials were a success, it was realised that a 'built by hand' construction methodology was not feasible and the process needed to be automated which led to the team beginning its experiments with 3D printing.

At around the same time, the philosophy of utilising 'scaffolds' was being utilised in other fields of medicine such as orthopaedics. The ability to exactly mimic biological tissue to suit patient-specific needs was deemed invaluable. Three-dimensional printing in medicine, over the years, has undergone an evolution beyond simply building scaffolds. A significant majority of work has been done in order to facilitate orthopaedic procedures; however, recent years have seen a very real and commercial foray into other branches of medicine as well with reports in the news about 3D-printed bone being utilised in the reconstruction of jaws, hips and even skulls in their entirety. Other advances relating to this work involve using live cells to print anatomical structures which can be applied as replacements for actual human organs and tissues (Figure 11.1). It was in 2013, that Organovo, a US-based company, developed the first 3D-printed completely cellular liver tissue in the world. It would be reasonable to state that the availability of 3D-printed transplantable organs are a question of when, not if (Bhat, 2020; Leukers et al., 2005a, 2005b; Whitaker, 2014).

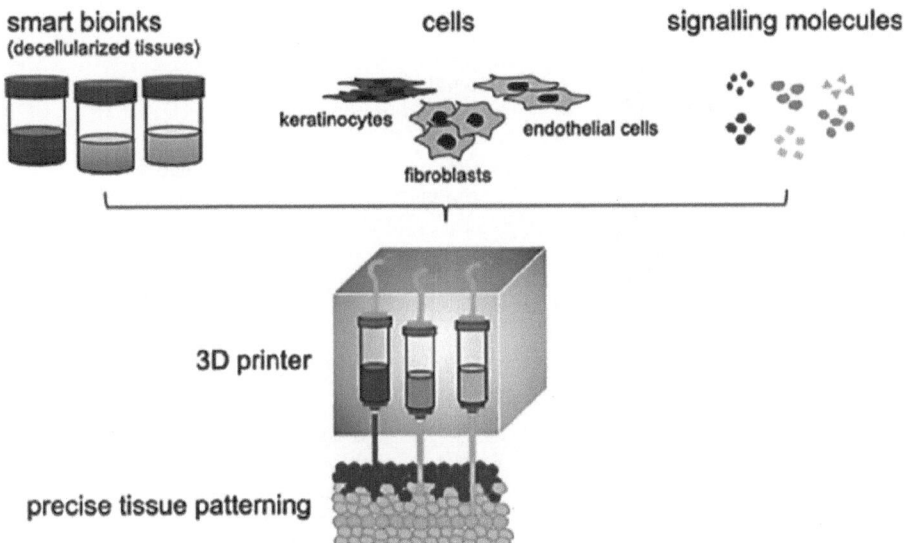

smart bioinks
(decellularized tissues)

cells

signalling molecules

keratinocytes

endothelial cells

fibroblasts

3D printer

precise tissue patterning

FIGURE 11.1 3D-printing approach for fabrication of tissues. A combination of smart bio-inks, ideally derived from decellularised tissues for the preservation of the tissue-specific matrix components together with the signalling molecules (epidermal growth factor – EGF, fibroblast growth factor-2 – FGF2, tumour growth factor beta – TGFβ, platelet-derived growth factor – PDGF, vascular endothelial growth factor – VEGF) can be precisely patterned via extrusion, laser-assisted, and inkjet 3D or stereolithography bioprinting to mimic the complex tissue architecture. Reproduced with permission (Nesic et al., 2020); Copyright 2020, Elsevier Ltd.

11.2 BONE STRUCTURE AND PHYSIOLOGY

11.2.1 BONE

The organic matrix, inorganic matrix and cells are what make up the bone. Amongst these, the cellular component can be divided into that which constitutes the bone marrow, namely, haematopoietic and non-haematopoietic stem cells which are blood forming and non-blood forming respectively. The next cell lineage is that of osteo-blasts or bone-forming cells of which some line cortical inner surfaces and trabecular bone present between these cortices. Others make up the cambium or inner layer of the periosteum. Osteoblasts upon maturation become encased in a mineralised matrix to form osteocytes. Osteoclasts, or bone-resorbing cells on being activated, initiate bone turnover or remodelling (Bayliss, Mahoney & Monk, 2012) (Figure 11.2).

The organic matrix is mainly composed of collagen type I. Incidentally, this comprises 98.5 per cent of the acellular component of the organic matrix, with hydroxy-apatite forming the major part of the inorganic matrix. Since the organic and inorganic matrices are present together, the bone matrix essentially consists of type 1 collagen along with hydroxyapatite crystals. That said, there are several important non-colla-gen proteins present in bone such as BMP (Bone Morphogenic Protein), sialoprotein, insulin-like growth factor (IGF-1 & 2) and osteopontin (Carda, Silvestrini, de Ferraris, Peydro & Bonucci, 2005). From an evolutionary perspective, the bone and

Features of main bone cells

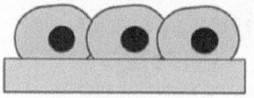

Osteoblast
- Derived from mesenchymal progenitors
- Produce collagen and other matrix proteins

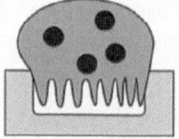

Osteoclast
- Derived from haematopoietic progenitors
- Resorb bone

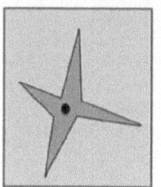

Osteocytes and lining cells
- Mature osteoblasts
- Line bone surface or become embedded in bone matrix
- Homoeostatic function (e.g. mechanostat)

FIGURE 11.2   Features of main bone cells. Reproduced with permission (Bayliss et al., 2012); Copyright 2012, Elsevier Ltd.

by that virtue the skeleton are responsible for conferring integrity of internal structure, providing a stem cell reserve and sites for muscle attachment. It also functions as the prime regulator of serum calcium levels in order to mediate muscle contraction and hence aid in locomotion and perfusion of organs.

11.2.2 Bone Remodelling

The bone-cell interaction model can best be utilised to explain bone biochemistry. Osteoblasts secrete osteoprotegerin (OPG), which acts in an inhibitory capacity upon osteoclasts and ultimately prevents resorption of bone. Gradually, the osteoblast matures to become entrapped in the mineralised matrix to form an osteocyte and in the process loses its OPG secreting capacity, thereby becoming vulnerable to osteoclast-mediated resorption. It is for this reason that injured, dead or old bones undergo resorption.

Macrophages present in the bone marrow are responsible for giving rise to osteoclasts from their mononuclear precursor cell lineage (Figure 11.3). Upon formation, they undergo rapid maturation upon receiving stimulation from interleukin-1 & 6 along with macrophage colony-stimulating factor. After completion of the maturation process, these osteoclasts enter the circulation in a resting i.e. non-resorbing state owing to the inhibitory effects exerted by calcitonin. The signal to override this inhibitory effect is provided systemically by parathormone and by RANKL (receptor activator nuclear Rankl kappa-beta ligand) locally. Not only is RANKL secreted by cancers to form pathological bone cavities, it is also a feature of normal osteoblast

Stages in the development of osteoclasts from monocyte/macrophage cell lineage and contributing factors

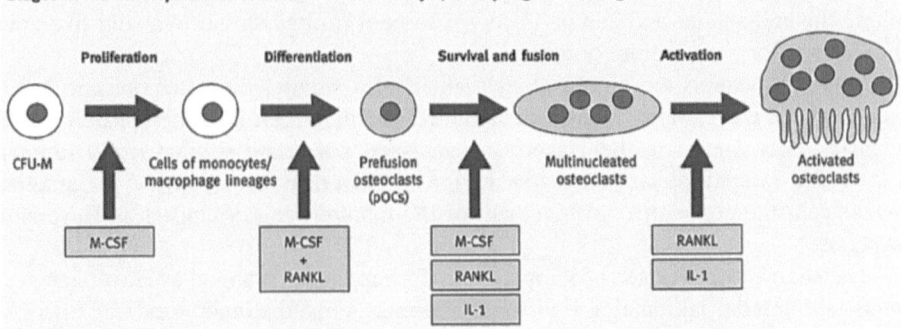

FIGURE 11.3   Stages in the development of osteoclasts from monocytes/macrophage cell lineage and contributing factors. Reproduced with permission (Bayliss et al., 2012); Copyright 2012, Elsevier Ltd.

secretion to upregulate bone resorption. RANKL undergoes binding to osteoclast membrane RANK receptors to facilitate resorption. To maintain a check on this process in terms of physiology, normal osteoblasts also secrete OPG which plays the role of a false ligand that acts as a competitor with RANKL to bind with the RANK receptor on the osteoclast membrane (Feng, 2005; Kostenuik, 2005; Wada, Nakashima, Hiroshi & Penninger, 2006; Xing, Schwarz & Boyce, 2005).

Normal bone resorption brought about by osteoclasts is responsible for initiating the bone remodelling process. The osteoclast upon activation subsequently adheres to the surface of the bone and progressively undergoes the development of a ruffled border as it apposes the bone surface which it eventually seals to form Howship's lacunae. It is at this site that hydrochloric acid and collagenases are secreted to break down the matrices, both organic and inorganic. A cutting cone is defined when a number of osteoblasts act in unison in order to carve out a large area of old bone. Since IGF-1 & 2 and BMP are not acid-soluble, they remain active as cytokines upon their release during bone resorption. These factors then bind to local and circulating stem cells in order to stimulate them into forming osteoblasts. The osteoblasts so formed secrete osteoid (Bayliss et al., 2012).

Bone metabolic unit (BMU) is a term used to denote a cutting cone with a trail of osteoclasts. With a life span of 14 days, osteoclasts need to be constantly replenished in order to sustain a cutting cone that lasts 150–180 days (termed sigma). These values translate to explain how bone may replace itself in the capacity of 0.5 per cent per day. Two BMUs forming bone, upon coming into contact with each other undergo coalescence to become integrated, which appears as a cementing/resting or reversal line histologically. Osteopontin and sialoprotein form this 'cementing' substance (Bayliss et al., 2012; Feng, 2005; Xing et al., 2005).

11.2.3   BONE STRUCTURE

The identifying features of mature bone are the Haversian systems. These are interconnecting osteocytes arranged in a concentric ring-like fashion around a Haversian canal through which lymphatics, arterioles and venules pass. The osteoblasts line up along the endosteum and can be observed to be forming osteoid in a ring-like configuration along the mature bone.

Volkmann canals are similar canals albeit of a smaller diameter present at 90° angles to the Haversian system which connects them to their neighbours. Being concentric in arrangement, the Haversian canals do not relate geometrically to each other. The interstitial lamella is the region of mature bone organised as lamellae which join the concentric arrangement of the mature bone organised as Haversian systems.

The shaft of long bones is comprised of cortical bone arranged as Haversian systems with interstitial lamella. Endosteal osteoblasts line the inner cortex and periosteal osteoblasts, the outer cortex.

The mid-shaft bone marrow is primarily composed of cellular components. The proximal and distal regions of vertebrae, long bones, cranium, facial skeleton and pelvis in adults are composed of interconnected trabecular bone. As ageing progresses, the bone marrow stem cells are replaced by a fibro-fatty component (Wada et al., 2006).

11.2.4 BONE REGENERATION AND HEALING

There are three distinct stages in bone healing that overlap each other – namely, a. early inflammatory stage, b. repair stage, and c. late remodelling stage. The inflammatory stage involves the development of a haematoma at the injury site within the first few hours or days. Monocytes, macrophages, polymorphonuclear cells, lymphocytes and fibroblasts form the infiltrate which enters the site of injury upon prostaglandin mediation. This process leads to the development of a granulation tissue, angiogenesis and mesenchymal cell migration. The nourishment at this stage of healing is provided by muscle and exposed cancellous bone. As the repair stage begins, fibroblasts initiate stroma formation which in turn provides support to vascular ingrowth. With the progression of vascular ingrowth, collagen matrix begins to become established with the laying down of osteoid which in turn undergoes mineralisation. These events eventuate into soft callus formation at the repair site (Bayliss et al., 2012).

This soft callus ultimately ossifies, forming a bony bridge between the fracture fragments. The remodelling stage involves the completion of the bone healing process. This phase lasts from months to years with adequate strength being achieved typically between 3 and 6 months. Bone healing involving grafting exhibits the phenomenon of 'creeping substitution' which is the incorporation of a bone graft by an incremental and gradual resorption of old necrosed bone with the simultaneous replacement being performed with viable new bone formation. The first 1–2 weeks are the most critical for bone healing which involves inflammation and re-vascularisation. It is imperative for mesenchymal cells to have access to the bone graft via vasculature in order for them to differentiate into osteoblasts and osteoclasts and promote bone graft incorporation and subsequent remodelling (Burchardt & Enneking, 1978; Daftari et al., 1994; DePalma et al., 1972; Prolo, 1990).

Systemic factors such as diabetes, malnutrition, cigarette smoking, osteoporosis and rheumatoid arthritis. Particularly during the first week of healing, cytotoxic drugs, steroid medications and non-steroidal anti-inflammatory drugs can cause harm. Subjecting the healing site to radiation within the first 2–3 weeks can impair cell proliferation and further induce vasculitis (Prolo, 1990). Local mechanical forces during the remodelling stage also influence bone grafts. Wolff (1892) first propounded the structural bone adaptation concept. He stated that bone being subjected to tensile or compressive stress undergoes remodelling. So essentially, bone forms and resorbs as a function of the stress to which it is subjected (Wolff, 1986).

11.3   ESSENTIAL ELEMENTS OF BONE BIOFABRICATION TRIAD

Biofabrication is a highly versatile and futuristic technology that aims to replace, restore or regenerate diseased and damaged human tissues with fully functional engineered tissue constructs. The tissue-engineering triad comprises a scaffold which is usually a solid structural support construct with an inherent network of pores that are interconnected and a matrix, cells and regulatory signals, most times in the form of appropriate growth factors.

Each of these elements must play its part in order to achieve the end goal of bone biofabrication. Scaffolds need to be porous in order to allow internal pathways for cell adhesion, proliferation, differentiation, attachment and migration. At the same time, they need to ensure that nutrient and oxygen transfer to the encapsulated cells is not hampered in any manner. Their mechanical characteristics need to match those of bone in order to provide adequate support. The transplanted cells in the tissue-engineering triad need to be available in abundance, be easily harvested and be able to bear the brunt of the printing process and the extreme condition changes associated with it. They must remain viable to the count of 90 per cent of the total number of printed cells for the construct to function and successfully integrate with the native bone tissue. It is desirable that they actively initiate new bone formation by facilitating osteogenic differentiation and regulating the behaviour of other cells. In the complex cascade initiated at the time of tissue injury, various growth factors, proteins and other cytokines play a significant role in stimulating various biological functions like chemotaxis, angiogenesis, proliferation and differentiation. They hence form an integral part of the triad, working in tandem with the scaffold and cells to regulate wound healing, repair and immune response.

11.4   SCAFFOLDS

Scaffolds form an indispensable component of osseous tissue engineering. They are, in essence, three-dimensional constructs that are biocompatible and simulate the properties of the extracellular matrix (ECM). Properties such as cell activity, mechanical strength and production of proteins in addition to those pertaining to stimulation of osteogenesis and provision of a template for attachment of cellular components are what make scaffolds an integral part of the bone tissue-engineering process (Salgado, Coutinho & Reis, 2004; Seitz, Rieder, Irsen, Leukers & Tille, 2005).

The chemistry of these scaffolds apart, the porosity in terms of its size and volume is also a critical determinant of scaffold performance. After positioning of a scaffold, the ingrowth of bone is initiated at their periphery from an early stage following a negative mineralisation gradient towards the more central parts (Jones et al., 2007). For this growth to continue, porosities must be interconnected as these pores provide an opportunity for nutrients and other molecules of import to be transported to the central region of the scaffold thereby facilitating vascularisation, ingrowth of cells and waste removal (Jones et al., 2007; Salgado et al., 2004). As can be logically presumed, a higher porosity would increase the per unit volume surface area of scaffolds which would allow one to optimise the kinetics of biodegradation. Biodegradation assumes importance in ensuring stable repair and scaffold replacement with novel bone in the absence of any remnants by means of chemical dissolution or cellular level interactions. Bone formation is conducive with a pore dimension between 100–150 microns with a further enhancement along with vascularisation taking place at a pore size of 300 microns or more (Jones et al., 2007; Otsuki et al., 2006). Effective formation of ECM is also influenced by the pore dimension with reports stating that PDLLA scaffolds possessing pore size between 325–420 microns provided for a collagen type 1 network of a well-organised structure. At the same time, it has been reported that a pore dimension of 275 microns did not allow for the proliferation and differentiation of human osteoblasts for the purpose of ECM formation (Stoppato et al., 2013).

Pore volume is also responsible for the permeability of nutrients into the scaffold and also influences its eventual mechanical structure. All other pore dimensions being constant, polycaprolactone (PCL) permeability was increased with an increase in pore volume resulting in optimisation of vascularisation, regeneration and mechanical properties in vivo. The scaffold should possess primary mechanical properties which should match the tissue it aims to mimic. The kinetics of strength degradation is influenced to a large extent by the size, geometry and strut orientation of pores (Banerjee, Tarafder, Davies, Bandyopadhyay & Bose, 2010; Das, Bose & Bandyopadhyay, 2007; Sultana & Wang, 2008; Tarafder, Banerjee, Bandyopadhyay & Bose, 2010). The cell-material interactions are determined by scaffold surface properties such as those of charge, topography and overall chemistry.

Manufacture of porous bone scaffolds can be accomplished by utilising a variety of methods such as solvent casting, gas foaming, freeze-drying, salt leaching, foam-gel and thermal induction of phase separation (Sultana & Wang, 2008). Most of these methods, however, fail to provide tailor-made scaffold solutions with a lack of control over pore dimensions. Where such exacting requirements are necessitated, methods such as additive manufacturing (AM) in the form of 3D printing (3DP), rapid prototyping (RP) and solid free-form fabrication (SFF) can be utilised directly along with CAD files to derive scaffolds (Bose, Suguira & Bandyopadhyay, 1999). Most of the commercially available AM approaches involve the construction of 3D approaches in a layer-by-layer fashion (Figure 11.4). AM techniques can therefore be classified as one of the following types: a. extrusion, b. laser-assisted sintering, c. polymerisation and d. direct writing-based (Darsell, Bose, Hosick & Bandyopadhyay, 2003; Doraiswamy et al., 2007; Q. Fu, Saiz & Tomsia, 2011; C. X. Lam, Teoh & Hutmacher, 2007; Lee et al., 2009; Ronca, Ambrosio & Grijpma, 2013; Serra, Planell & Navarro, 2013; Sobral, Caridade, Sousa, Mano & Reis, 2011; Tsang & Bhatia, 2004; Williams et al., 2005).

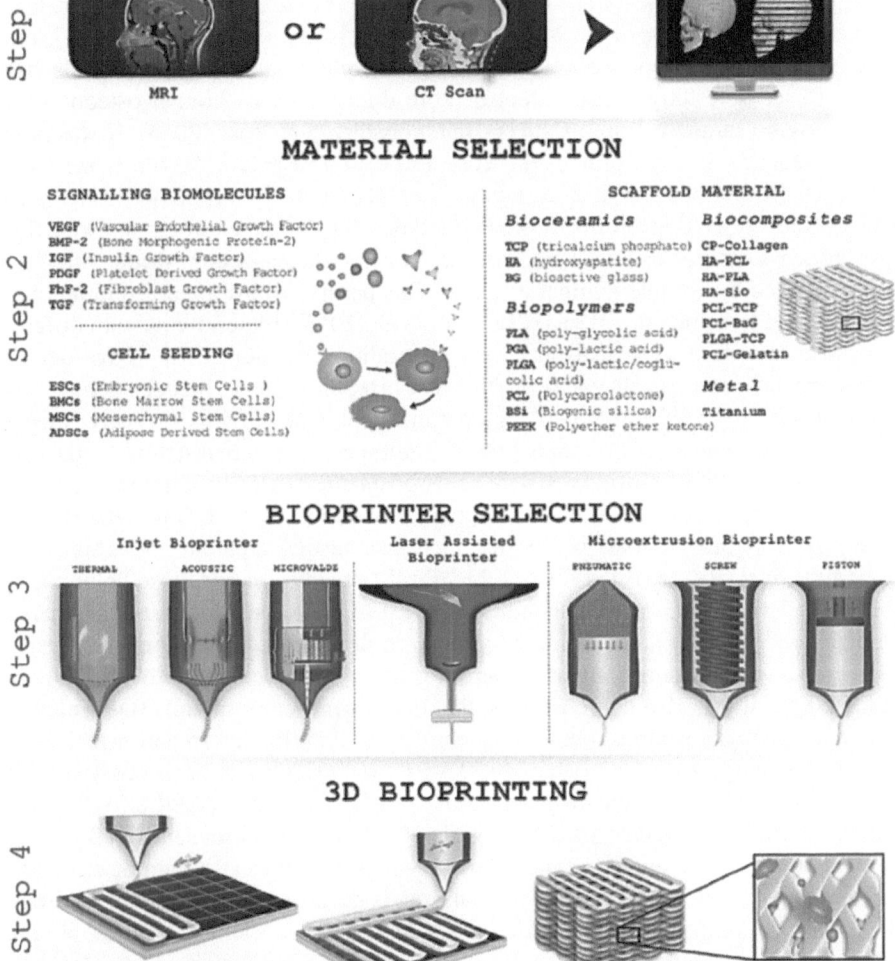

FIGURE 11.4 Process of 3D bioprinting. Reproduced with permission (Maroulakos, Kamperos, Tayebi, Halazonetis & Ren, 2019); Copyright 2019, Elsevier Ltd.

11.4.1 3D-Printed Bone Scaffolds

One of the candidates for applications pertaining to bone replacement are starch-based binders. These are biocompatible and allow for the production of constructs that have mechanical strength comparable to that of trabecular bone. 3D-printed scaffolds made from polyethylene (PE) with porosity dimensions in the range of 22.3–49.7 per cent have demonstrated maximum tensile strengths of 4 MPa and are devoid of any toxic influences upon human osteoblasts (C. X. F. Lam, Mo, Teoh & Hutmacher, 2002; J Suwanprateeb, Thammarakcharoen, Wongsuvan & Chokevivat, 2012).

Calcium phosphate ceramics are commonly utilised in tissue engineering of bone. This is owed to their properties of osteoconduction, biocompatibility as well as comparability to physiological bone composition (Becker et al., 2012). There is evidence in the literature of 3D-printed hydroxyapatite blocks demonstrating vascularisation and homogenous osteoconductivity. Tricalcium phosphate (TCP) scaffolds have been utilised for studying the effect of pore dimensions on human osteoblasts of foetal origin (Tarafder, Balla, Davies, Bandyopadhyay & Bose, 2013). It was noted that a reduction in pore dimension from 1,000 to 750 and/or 500 microns led to increased proliferated cell density. Upon analysing the histomorphometric characteristics of doped TCP scaffolds, it was concluded that these scaffolds allowed for a greater proportion of osteoid type bone at the early stages of deposition which was later followed by complete mineralisation. This points toward the translational benefits of rapid bone healing in vivo (Tarafder et al., 2013). Experiments with different pore dimensions of TCP scaffolds with the addition of SiO_2 – ZnO have demonstrated an increase in cell viability. Not just osteoblasts, but osteoclasts have also been utilised in ratifying the biocompatibility of CaP ceramics. There was an observed differentiation of monocytes to multinuclear osteoclast type cells upon microscopy following tartrate resistant acid phosphatase (TRAP) staining and formation of lacunae (Detsch et al., 2011; Fielding, Bandyopadhyay & Bose, 2012).

Hydroxyapatite scaffolds possessing increased surface area did not exhibit cytotoxicity and in fact, provided for suitable fibroblast adhesion for those belonging to the MC3T3-E1 lineage. A study conducted on a goat model concluded that 3D-printed cements of brushite and monetite with controlled pore dimensions resulted in increased levels of osteoconduction thereby ratifying its biocompatibility (Habibovic et al., 2008). It was also demonstrated, that in a rodent femur model, 3D-printed tricalcium phosphate samples possessing porosity at both the micro and macro levels exhibited osteogenesis. However, MC3T3-E1 cytotoxicity has been observed with bone cement compositions involving beta TCP/TTCP and $TTCP/CaSo_4.2H_2O$. A variety of binders have been utilised to date. 20–40 per cent citric acid and 30–40 per cent lactic acid have exhibited the shortest hardening times (Khalyfa et al., 2007). Lower ranges of these binders with varying concentrations of sodium hydrogen phosphate coupled with phosphoric and sulphuric acids can be used to produce increased hardening times.

11.4.2 Mechanical Properties

Porous scaffolds are haunted by less than adequate mechanical strength by virtue of their pore volume. The same problem lies with 3D-printed CaP scaffolds which is responsible for confining their application to situations involving none or low levels of load bearing. In such situations, modifications made at the post-processing stage and those in the composition of materials can be utilised to make the mechanical properties of these materials more amenable to use. Microwave sintering causes shrinkage and increase in density which eventually results in elevated compressive strength of the resulting construct. A reduction in the pore volume or size can be correlated with a concomitant elevation of the scaffold strength. Contrary to these observations, sintering of a TTCP/CaSO$_4$.2H$_2$O scaffold resulted in decreased strength as a consequence of water release (Khalyfa et al., 2007). An effective densification approach has been described which involves utilising microwave sintering as opposed to conventional heating resulting in enhanced mechanical properties of TCP scaffolds (Vorndran et al., 2008). Alongside this, bioactive liquid phase sintering has also been described to enhance the strength of constructs (Jintamai Suwanprateeb, Sanngam, Suvannapruk & Panyathanmaporn, 2009).

Monomer/polymer infiltration has also been described in literature as an approach that aims to enhance the strength of ceramic scaffolds, all the while leaving its biological properties unimpaired (Khalyfa et al., 2007).

11.4.3 BIOPRINTING OF SCAFFOLDS

AM has also been utilised to study live cells and tissue-incorporated scaffold fabrication. Liver tissue has been demonstrated to be constructed utilising such methodologies in vitro. The process of 3D fibre deposition involves the preparation of a viscous paste of polymer laden with cells which is printed utilising a syringe dispenser. Chondrocytes or multipotent stromal cells with embedded alginate hydrogel were subsequently printed using this methodology and were demonstrated to possess adequate cell viability. Further, the incorporation of these chondrocytes and multipotent stromal cells, both in vitro and in vivo led to the formation of a distinct brand of ECM.

In addition to this, an attempt to increase porosity by means of increasing strand distance was successfully demonstrated while maintaining a low elastic modulus. On the contrary, a change in strand orientation from 90 to 45 degrees resulted in an increase in the elastic modulus (Fedorovich et al., 2012). Laser-assisted bioprinting to produce human osteoprogenitor cells alone or in conjunction with hydroxyapatite has also been demonstrated to maintain functionality and osteoblast lineage phenotype as ratified by the expression of alkaline phosphatase.

11.4.4 BIO-INKS

Direct ink writing (DIW) and inkjet bioprinting are the preferred 3DP technologies for the printing of live cells (Gudapati, Dey & Ozbolat, 2016; Ozbolat, Peng & Ozbolat, 2016). DIW involves the extrusion of hydrogel/cell suspensions or highly viscous solutions in order to derive 3D structures. These structures may be obtained either with or without a carrier (Jakus, Rutz & Shah, 2016). Inkjet bioprinting involves the deposition of low viscosity cellular suspensions or colloidal solutions in the form of droplets at increased shear rates. Naturally, the bio-ink forms an important part of the bioprinting process. It should be able to sustain live cells, be biocompatible and should remain mechanically stable after printing has been accomplished. Hydrogels are the commonest materials utilised for bioprinting. This is chiefly attributable to their chemical structure being amenable to modifications, ability to sustain live cells, biodegradation and mechanical properties which can be adjusted and the satisfactory resolution it provides upon printing.

Grouping of bio-ink materials can be done into two important categories pertaining to 3DP for the development of tissues and/or organ constructs. The first approach is cell-scaffold-based in which the bio-ink involves live cells and a biomaterial that are used for printing. In this approach, the scaffold undergoes degradation and the encapsulated live cells grow to occupy the spaces so created to form biostructures. The second approach is a scaffold-free one, which involves the printing of living cells directly, resembling physiologic embryonic growth (Kaushik et al., 2016). These groups of live cells undergo transformation into neo-tissues which are then deposited in a particular larger arrangement (Hospodiuk, Dey, Sosnoski & Ozbolat, 2017).

Polymers obtained from natural resources are termed natural biomaterials in biomedical fields. These materials have distinct advantages over their synthetic counterparts such as those of ECM mimicking, biocompatibility, self-assembly and biodegradation. This is not to say that synthetic polymers have no favourable properties of their own. These materials possess the advantages of mechanical stability control, pH, ability to photo-cross-link and tunable temperature response amongst others. Recent times have observed the emergence of multi-material bio-inks which aim to provide improved cell survival and stability of structure. Polymeric hydrogels form the most preferred class of bio-inks utilised for 3DP as a result of their ability to mimic host ECM and allow adhesion of cell load and subsequent matrix integration. Some recently reported natural hydrogel bio-inks have been composed of biomaterials such as alginate, collagen, chitosan, agarose, fibrin, hyaluronic acid, gelatin and Matrigel. Their synthetic counterparts have involved the utilisation of materials such as methacrylated gelatin, pluronic F-127 and poly(ethylene glycol). Multimaterial bio-inks have been synthesised by utilising components such as sodium alginate, hydroxyapatite, gellan gum, gelatin methacrylate, alginate/polyvinyl acetate and polylactic acid (Adepu et al., 2017).

11.5   STEM CELLS

Bone is a dynamic tissue. Scaffolds used in 3D printing of bone have the inherent limitation of being synthetic in origin. The placing of a synthetic material in a biological environment, expecting it to possess biological functionality like enhancing cell survival, proliferation and differentiation, is unrealistic. To overcome this particular limitation, researchers all over the world have been experimenting with stem cells as the second essential element of tissue engineering. These third-generation scaffolds are primed to be osteoinductive on account of the inclusion of stem cells in addition to the incorporation of growth factors like BMPs and VEGF.

Stem cells are cells with the unique ability to differentiate into different cell types. On the division of a stem cell, the daughter cell can remain either as a stem cell or go on to differentiate into a specialised cell like a brain cell or muscle cell. They were first reported in bone marrow. They can be embryonic (ESCs) which are pluripotent; mesenchymal stem cells (MSCs)/adult stem cells which are multipotent or induced pluripotent stem cells (iPSCs). An ideal stem cell is expected to agree with the Good Manufacturing Practice Guidelines; be available in large amounts; be isolated painlessly and have the property of multiple differentiation (Trohatou & Roubelakis, 2017).

11.5.1   EMBRYONIC STEM CELLS (ESCs)

Derived from blastocysts of human lineage, these cells can develop into those of all three embryonic germ layers. Studies have reported that though they possess desirable properties like favourable viability of cells and osteogenic differentiation, certain demerits exist (W. Chen et al., 2018; S. Kim et al., 2008; X. Liu et al., 2014; Tang, Chen, Weir, Thein-Han & Xu, 2012). As isolating them has ethical issues associated on account of embryo destruction during the isolation process, limited research data is available in literature. Other limitations to their use comprise immune reactions and the potential for unexpected differentiation and teratoma formation (Cunningham, Ulbright, Pera & Looijenga, 2012; Iaquinta et al., 2019).

11.5.2   INDUCED PLURIPOTENT STEM CELLS (iPSCs)

To avoid the problem of embryo destruction, iPSCs were developed using lentiviruses. They express the same marker genes as ESCs but are devoid of their drawbacks of immune rejection (B. Fu, Tian, & Wei, 2014; Perez et al., 2018; Takahashi & Yamanaka, 2006). When cultured with collagen, chitosan and hydroxylapatite, they have been found to induce osteogenesis (Xie et al., 2016). Scaffolds containing iPSCs isolated from gingival fibroblasts have also been studied in bone biofabrication (Ji et al., 2016).

11.5.3   MESENCHYMAL STEM CELLS (MSCs)

These are adult stem cells that can go on to differentiate into adipocytes, osteoblasts, chondroblasts, myocytes, endothelial cells, smooth muscle cells, ligament cells, hepatocytes etc. They also have the inherent property of self-renewal, multi-differentiation and have remarkable anti-inflammatory and immuno modulatory properties.

They can be obtained from a number of body tissues, the various sources being (J. Liu et al., 2015a; Pisciotta et al., 2015; Chongyang Shen, Yang, Xu & Zhao, 2019; Ullah, Subbarao & Rho, 2015):

1. Adipose tissues (ADSCs)
2. Bone marrow (BM-MSCs)
3. Amniotic fluid (AF-MSCs)
4. Umbilical cord MSCs (UC-MSCs)
5. Placental-derived MSCs (PD-MSCs) like amniotic membrane MSCs (AM-MSCs), chorionic membrane MSCs (CM-MSCs), deciduas MSCs (DC-MSCs)
6. Dental pulp tissues (DPSCs)
7. MSCs derived from human primary teeth (SHED)
8. Tooth germ progenitor cells (TGPCs)
9. Dental follicle progenitor cells (DFPCs)
10. Periodontal ligament (PDLSCs)
11. Alveolar bone-derived MSCs (AB-MSCs)
12. Stem cells derived from apical papilla (SCAP)
13. Gingival MSCs (G-MSCs)

Amniotic membrane MSCs, umbilical cord MSCs and dental pulp tissues (DPSCs) have the maximum osteogenic differentiation potential (Jensen et al., 2016; Chongyang Shen et al., 2019). Unwanted cell differentiation, immune rejection, limited availability, issues in maintaining cell viability and ethical concerns are a few of the limitations associated with MSCs. Their mode of delivery to the site of bone defect and the absence of standardised SOPs associated with their ex vivo expansion are challenges for researchers to further work upon.

Multiple stem cells of different lineages and potency have been studied in tissue engineering. The bone marrow, adipose tissue by liposuction, blood apheresis, or creation from skin biopsy as well as peripheral blood mononuclear cells form possible routes of harvest (Figure 11.5). An ideal stem cell needs to have the ability to expand adequately for bioprinting in addition to retaining its ability to function biologically. Balanced momentum and sufficient proliferation into the scaffold are also desirable qualities when selecting the cell lines. Stem cells can be either seeded onto 3D-printed preformed acellular scaffolds via chemical binding or be bioprinted onto the scaffolds simultaneously during the 3D-printing process (Boland, Xu, Damon & Cui, 2006; Keriquel et al., 2010; Langer & Vacanti, 1993). The simultaneous process, though being superior due to the precise distribution of cells into the scaffold, is not without its inherent disadvantages of low mechanical strength in addition to the chances of cells getting damaged during the printing process due to temperature or pressure incurred. Ink jet printers designed specially to respond to computer-aided design templates working on the layer-by-layer deposition principle of bioprinting are one such device (Jakab et al., 2008). Micro-extrusion bioprinters can print bio-inks containing hydroxyapatite-incorporating particles, thereby improving the 3D geometry (Tasnim et al., 2018). In vivo bioprinting has also been made possible by the development of biological laser printing (BioLP) and bioplotters (Barron, Ringeisen, Kim, Spargo, & Chrisey, 2004; Dinca et al., 2008; Ringeisen, Othon, Barron, Young, & Spargo, 2006) Recently a newer technology comprising of scaffold-free spheroid- based bioprinting has also been developed. The entire process of 3D bioprinting revolves around two main components, the biopaper and the bio-ink. Biopaper refers to the substrate on which printing is done, and bio-ink is the material, usually hydrogel-based, which resembles the extracellular matrix and has cells dispersed throughout it. The bioprinter deposits bio-ink onto the biopaper, creating predefined cell patterns. Bio-ink has stem cells and bioactive molecules like BMP, FGF, IGF-1 and VEGF incorporated within ECM in order to enhance neovascularisation and osteogenesis. Microfluidic/valve-based extrusion bioprinting methods have opened up unique possibilities to predictably influence cell viability and proliferation in bone biofabrication.

11.5.4 APPLICATIONS

Bone marrow stromal cells have been extensively studied as a source of cells in studies attempting to regenerate bone. Adipose tissue-derived stem cells are another member of the group which has been preferred over BM-MSCs in certain situations due to their ease of availability and ability to survive in low oxygen environments. Oral cavity MSCs are gaining popularity too. Mohammed et al. (2019) in their in

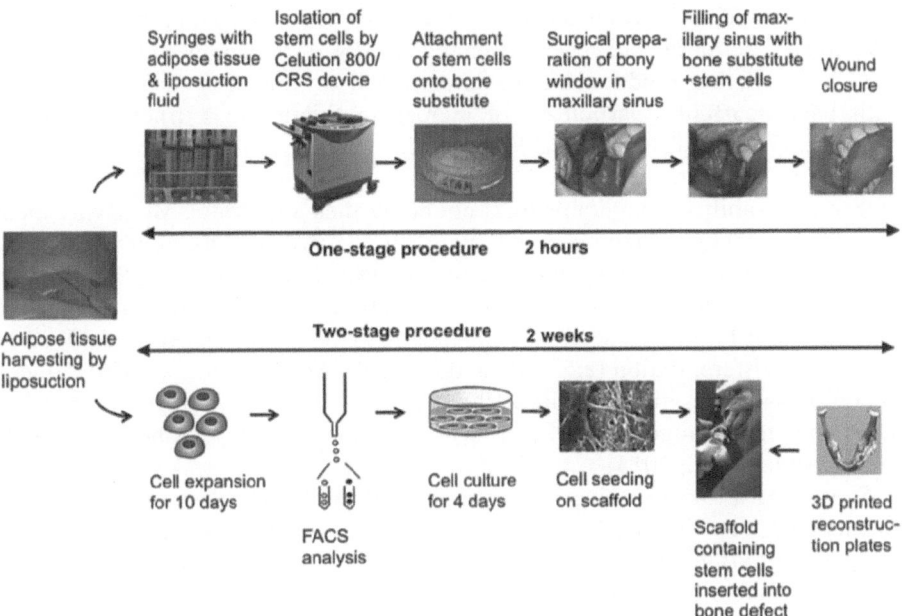

FIGURE 11.5 Image display of 1-stage and 2-stage procedures using bone substitutes in combination with 2-week expanded (2-stage procedure) or freshly isolated adipose stem cells (1-stage procedure) for treatment of large oral and maxillofacial bone defects. Top, One-stage procedure. 1) Adipose tissue is harvested by liposuction. 2) The adipose tissue and liposuction fluid are collected in syringes. 3) The filled syringes are transferred into a Celution 800/CRS system (Cytori Therapeutics, Inc, San Diego, CA). This device washes, digests and centrifugates the adipose tissue to obtain the fresh vascular fraction containing the adipose stem cells. After isolation of the stromal vascular fraction, cells can be briefly stimulated with growth factors before seeding the stimulated cells onto a 3D-printed scaffold material. 4) The freshly isolated adipose stem cells are seeded onto the scaffold. Unattached cells are washed off, and the scaffold is combined with stem cells. 5) During the short attachment period of the cells (30 minutes), the patient is prepared for the surgical procedure (ie, maxillary sinus floor elevation). 6) The tissue-engineered construct containing the scaffold and adipose stem cells is inserted immediately into the patient, and the space created in the maxillary sinus is filled with the 3D-printed construct combined with adipose stem cells. 7) The wound is closed. Bottom, Two-stage procedure. 1) Cells are cultured and expanded on tissue culture plastic for 10 days. 2) Adipose stem cells are collected by FACS analysis. 3) Adipose stem cells are cultured again for a few days. 4) Cells are seeded on the scaffolds. 5) The tissue-engineered construct containing the scaffold and adipose stem cells is inserted immediately into the patient, and the space created is filled. 6) In the 2-stage procedure, 3D stereolithographic medical skull models are fabricated using the patient's preoperative computed tomographic non-compressed Digital Imaging and Communications in Medicine voxel-based dataset. The medical skull models allow visualisation and assessment of the planned resection defects and are used to pre-bend commercially available reconstruction plates and titanium meshes for later use in the reconstructions. The 2-stage procedure has often been performed in conjunction with 3D-printed reconstruction plates. Reproduced with permission (Farré-Guasch et al., 2015); Copyright 2015, Elsevier Ltd.

vivo study on AF-MSCs and BM-MSCs found AF-MSCs loaded on gel-foam scaffolds to be superior in bone regeneration to BM-MSCs (Mohammed et al., 2019).

MSCs once delivered to the bone defect via direct injection or in combination with bone scaffolds, participate in increasing the tissue stiffness and burst strength. They possess remarkable bone regenerating abilities due to their differentiation into osteoblasts. Cell seeded calcium phosphate scaffolds have bone regeneration ability comparable to, if not better than autografts. Modifying them in order to generate osteogenic and angiogenic growth factors to promote bone regeneration has also been investigated (Nauth, Miclau III, Li & Schemitsch, 2010). D'Agostino et al. (2016) attempted to observe how human ADSCs loaded onto HA/type I collagen scaffold influence the expression of genes involved in osteogenic differentiation (e.g., SP7 and ALP) (D'Agostino et al., 2016). Sándor et al. (2014) successfully repaired 10 out of 13 cranio-maxillofacial hard-tissue defects using autologous ADSCs seeded onto bioactive glass or beta TCP scaffolds (Sándor et al., 2014).

Saos-eGFP are novel engineered human osteoblast-like cells that express enhanced Green Fluorescent Protein. They can be added along with ADSCs onto HA/collagen-derived scaffolds to attempt bone regeneration (Manfrini et al., 2015).

Usage of more than one cell type in order to utilise the abilities of two different cell sets is another field of research in stem cell therapy. There have been studies where researchers have co-cultured osteoblasts with umbilical vein endothelial cells in an attempt to increase the cell population and enzyme activity (Y. Liu, Chan & Teoh, 2015b; Unger, Dohle & Kirkpatrick, 2015). Both umbilical vein endothelial cells and human foetal BM-MSCs have the ability of neovascularisation in the presence of seeded osteogenic cells and increase ectopic bone formation in vivo (Koob et al., 2011; Y. Liu et al., 2013).

Cell sheets developed by seeding MSCs onto temperature-responsive culture dishes in an attempt to retain cell-cell interactions have also gained recognition in 3D bioprinting. These alone or alongside 3D-printed scaffolds have been utilised for targetting accelerated bone formation, Kim et al. in 2016 reported enhanced in vitro bone formation (Y. Kim et al., 2016).

Stem cells have also been utilised in the generation of decellularised extracellular matrix (ECM) in an attempt to improve cellular responses of a synthetic scaffold, or to function directly as a bioscaffold for tissue engineering (Bhrany et al., 2006; Flynn, Prestwich, Semple & Woodhouse, 2008; Y. S. Kim, Majid, Melchiorri & Mikos, 2019). ECM when ornamented onto 3D-printed scaffolds, mimics the bony microenvironment, thereby acting as a reservoir of physiologically active biosignals, upregulating the osteoblastic differentiation of seeded stem cells and/or osteoblastic genes. Researchers have successfully evaluated the distinct advantages of Cell-laid bone-like ECM while cultured on titanium fibre mesh (Datta et al., 2006; Pham et al., 2008); beta -TCP scaffolds (Kang, Kim, Bishop, Khademhosseini & Yang, 2012; Kang, Kim, Khademhosseini & Yang, 2011); as well as a composite of polycaprolactone (PCL), poly(lactic-co-glycolic acid), and beta-TCP (Pati et al., 2015). Pati et al. (2015) in their study on ECM- ornamented 3 D printed scaffolds seeded with human nasal inferior turbinate tissue-derived mesenchymal stromal cells (hTMSCs) found four genes (RUNX2, ALP, osteopontin, osteocalcin) involved in osteogenesis to be upregulated, with higher deposition of calcium as compared to bare scaffolds (Pati et al., 2015).

11.6   GROWTH FACTORS

A number of signals, both physical and biochemical are required as a part of engineering bone tissue in order to bring about the formation of new bone and its subsequent host tissue integration (Samorezov & Alsberg, 2015).

Growth factors (GFs) comprise a class of signalling molecules that can be utilised for bone tissue engineering. The direct application of GFs, though attractive in terms of its therapeutic potential, has failed to achieve much success commercially. BMP-2 and BMP-7 are Food and Drug Administration (FDA) approved GFs which can be applied in place of autografting in cases of long bone fractures, spinal fusion and bone fractures that have failed to unite (Nauth, Ristevski, Li & Schemitsch, 2011). Numerous systems, namely, osmotic pumps, scaffold degradation, bolus injection and surface-adsorbed protein release have been utilised for the administration of GFs (Porter, Ruckh & Popat, 2009). Methods which involve rapid diffusion of molecules of interest or their enzymatic deactivation are unsuitable for application as it is imperative to tailor the timed release of these molecules or drugs to run parallel with the process of tissue repair. Such a tuned delivery would also ensure the delivery of molecules of interest to the intended sites. A number of GF delivery systems only incorporate a single delivery mechanism which is in contrast to the actual bone healing process which is simultaneously multifactorial. It would, therefore, seem logical to utilise multiple GF delivery modalities to achieve suitable bone repair (R. R. Chen & Mooney, 2003; Rambhia & Ma, 2015).

The bone repair process involves both an osteogenic and an angiogenic component wherein vascularisation is essential to maintain the vitality of the structure, making the simultaneous use of GFs which promote both these processes desirable (Kolambkar et al., 2011). There is evidence in literature to support the sequential provision of BMP-2 and vascular endothelial growth factor (VEGF) to have an effect on bone regeneration which is synergistic in nature (Shah et al., 2011). It would be important to note that merely providing two GFs would not achieve the desired result, the two factors would have to be tuned in terms of both their dose and kinetics within the same delivery system to have the desired outcome (Tayalia & Mooney, 2009).

It is essential to understand and correlate the natural physiology of bone in order to mimic or engineer the same. The extracellular matrix (ECM), initially thought of as a scaffold that could provide structural support to the bone tissue has now been established to be the bed of chemical activity which promotes processes such as those of cellular proliferation and migration by virtue of the various binding sites it expresses (Y.-H. Kim & Tabata, 2015; Patel et al., 2008; Reed & Wu, 2014; Vonau, Bostrom, Aspenberg & Sams, 2001; Young et al., 2009; Yu, Khalil, Dang, Alsberg & Murphy, 2014). A representation of this can be made by the fact that VEGF, BMP-2 and platelet-derived growth factor (PDGF) can utilise binding sites to bind with heparin sulphate (Badylak, Freytes & Gilbert, 2009; Brown & Badylak, 2014; Macri, Silverstein & Clark, 2007; Schultz & Wysocki, 2009). While fibronectin, tenascin, fibrinogen and vitronectin offer GF binding sites to promote the process of bone regeneration. Glycosaminoglycans (GAGs) can also provide binding sites for GFs and cytokines. Both these interactions are responsible for promoting bone regeneration. However, the high physiological levels of GFs required to effect bone healing in the absence of an appropriate delivery vehicle for these can pose safety and economical conundrums. A possible way out could be to devise delivery systems to be regulated by the ECM itself which can provide a situation-specific delivery mechanism in vivo (Martino, Briquez, Maruyama & Hubbell, 2015; Martino & Hubbell, 2010; Upton et al., 2008).

11.6.1 BIOMOLECULES IN BONE HEALING

In the first, i.e. inflammatory stage of bone healing, there occurs an influx of inflammatory cells such as lymphocytes, monocytes, neutrophils, macrophages and platelets. Under mediation by prostaglandins, there occurs fibroblast invasion which is followed by the expression of a number of biomolecules at the site of injury. The result of this cascade is the formation of granulation tissue, vascular infiltration and mesenchymal stem cell (MSC) migration. Transforming growth factor beta (TGF beta), BMP-2, BMP-7, BMP-4, fibroblast growth factor (FGF) -1, -2, interleukin (IL)-2, -6, PDGF and osteonectin are expressed at this stage.

The next phase involves the appropriation of cartilaginous tissue brought about by MSC differentiation into chondrocytes. The callus so formed requires fresh stromal tissue to be laid down in order to sustain itself. This stromal growth is effected by fibroblasts which in turn provide adequate support for vascular invasion. BMP-2, BMP-7, BMP-4, TGFb, FGF-1 and -2, IL-6, IL-1, VEGF, fibronectin, angiopoietin -1 and -2 along with collagens (type 2, 3, 4, 5, 6, 9 and 10) are involved.

As the stroma is laid down, vascular invasion occurs along with osteoid formation and subsequent mineralisation. Additional involvement of macrophage colony-stimulating factor (M-CSF) and RANKL is observed at this stage. The final stage of bone healing is marked by conversion of woven bone and cartilage to trabecular bone which subsequently undergoes remodelling. IL-6 and -1, RANKL and M-CSF are involved at the bone remodelling stage. It is important to have knowledge of biomolecules involved at each stage of bone regeneration in order to devise delivery mechanisms to effect the same. GFs expressed by one cell lineage (e.g. osteoblasts) can critically influence the behaviour of others (e.g. osteoclasts). A prime example here would be that of VEGF which is expressed by osteoblasts and influences osteoclast function (Abou-Khalil et al., 2014; Detsch & Boccaccini, 2015; Lauzon, Bergeron, Marcos & Faucheux, 2012; Sfeir, Ho, Doll, Azari & Hollinger, 2005; Tanaka, Nakayamada & Okada, 2005).

11.6.2 DELIVERY SYSTEMS

Biomolecules require control of both a spatial and temporal nature for their effective utilisation (Minh Khanh Nguyen & Alsberg, 2014). A common strategy to achieve this is to physically entrap bioactive molecules in biomaterials. Several purported delivery vehicles such as hydrogels, liposomes, microparticulate polymer and bone cements have been utilised for this purpose. The rate of diffusion and degradation of scaffold material form the basis of fast release of GFs. Conversely, the structurally determined affinity of the biomolecule for the scaffold material can be utilised to achieve their sustained release. Factors such as functional group charge and hydrophilic/phobic nature influence the kinetics of biomolecule release. Physical entrapment aside, physisorption and adsorption form alternative biomolecule delivery mechanisms. BMP delivery can be brought about by its impregnation into absorbable collagen material (Piskin, 1992; Riedl & Valentin-Opran, 1999).

Covalent binding of the biomolecule to the scaffold material is another alternative delivery system. An internal stimulus-dependent delivery system would seem to be an appropriate assembly to provide release control. A delivery system should allow for appropriate dose and time-dependent biomolecule release, improve cell attachment subsequent to recruitment along with initiating angiogenesis and cell migration.

The system should have adequate mechanical strength and be suitably biodegradable and biocompatible at the same time. It should be reproducible, malleable and should provide for all this while being cost-effective. Both natural and synthetic polymers can be utilised for bone GF delivery. Natural polymers possess properties such as biodegradability, biocompatibility and biomimetic chemical properties which qualify them as possible delivery system candidates. Silk, collagen, fibrin, alginate, chitosan, starch and hyaluronic acid are a few examples (Ivanova, Bazaka & Crawford, 2014). However, problems such as inter-batch variations, sterilisation method susceptibility and immunogenicity cast a shadow over their usage. Synthetic polymers can be utilised to overcome such limitations (S.-H. Lee & Shin, 2007). Polymers such as polylactic-co-glycolic acid (PLGA) and polylactic acid (PLA), with their suitable physiochemistry, mechanical properties and tailorable processability can be utilised. Even synthetic polymers which have exhibited undesirable properties such as increased levels of immunogenicity, poor clearance and degradation of bulk, can be redesigned to suit specific applications. This is generally achieved by either combining them with other polymers or adding varied functional groups to their structure (van de Watering, Molkenboer-Kuenen, Boerman, van den Beucken & Jansen, 2012).

Three-dimensional scaffolds utilising PLA, PLGA and polyglycolic acid (PGA) have been established in literature as delivery vehicles for TGF beta, BMP-2 and BMP-7. BMPs can also be delivered via vehicles such as those of an inorganic construct namely, calcium phosphate ceramics (CPCs), beta-tricalcium phosphate (bTCP) and hydroxyapatite (HA). Numerous options aside, no singularly established delivery vehicle can cater to all GFs of import in biological systems (Odelius, Plikk & Albertsson, 2008).

11.6.3 Sterilisation

Graft sterilisation is a surprisingly overlooked issue in the literature, despite its irrefutable importance in medicine. Routine biomedical sterilisation methodologies may not be suitable for all systems. An example to cite here can be that of PCL sensitivity at temperatures exceeding 60 degrees Celsius thereby ruling out autoclavation and sterilisation by means of hot air ovens (Odelius et al., 2008). Ethylene oxide can be a possible option for materials sensitive to heat and moisture because of its activity at low temperatures (cold sterilisation). However, it has its own problems in terms of incomplete removal of toxic ethylene oxide residues at the completion of the sterilisation process. This can be circumvented by degassing the material at 50 degrees Celsius in a vacuum for at least 48 hours but then again this makes it unsuitable for use in polymers with low melting temperatures such as PCL.

Gamma (ionising) irradiation is a time-tested cold sterilisation methodology for foods and drugs. It finds use in the sterilisation of materials that are sensitive to heat. Radiation dosage must be tuned so as not to compromise the polymer structure and drug activity. Analytic methods to determine structural changes can be employed after the conclusion of the sterilisation cycle as a means of assessing unintentional alterations (Baume, Boughton, Coleman & Ruys, 2016).

Apart from gamma radiation, there has been a focus on e-beam sterilisation and its effect on pharmaceuticals and biomaterials. It can be safely stated that radiation sterilisation methods have several advantages over thermal methods (dry or moist) in terms of being suitable and tunable for a variety of materials that can be subject to structural analysis post-sterilisation (Silindir & Özer, 2009).

11.7   APPLICATIONS IN LIFE SCIENCES

11.7.1   APPLICATIONS IN MEDICAL SCIENCES

3D printing as applied to medical sciences has a role to play in almost every aspect of healthcare, ranging from bioprinted tissues and organs, manufacturing of custom-fit prostheses, implants and simulated models to gain insight into the mimicked anatomy, to its potential applications in formulation of personalised 3D-printed drugs and implantable drug delivery devices. Although the prospects are exciting, the technology has a long way to go before it becomes the mainstay of how clinicians treat.

Additive manufacturing 3D technology finds numerous applications in orthopaedics for making surgical instruments, anatomical and simulation models for mock surgeries, splints, implants, orthosis and custom-fit prostheses. They aid by enhancing the surgeon's accessibility, his tactile and visual understanding, reducing the operating time and giving the patient a perfectly fitted implant (Bagaria & Chaudhary, 2017; Lal & Patralekh, 2018). Complex shapes in nylon, metals and polymers can be reproduced to meet the structural and functional requirements. The material properties can be changed to make the prosthesis or implant lightweight. Artificial bone created by layer to layer fabrication has elastic properties and strength relatively similar to natural bone. Zou et al. from their study on the precision and reliability of 3D-printed models regarding anatomical parameters like the height of bone made using stereolithography techniques concluded that 3D-printed models are reliable and precise when used for the treatment of complex orthopaedic deformities (Zou et al., 2018).

The ease by which it can be given desired shape and size makes it attractive to clinicians and patients alike (Javaid & Haleem, 2018). 3D-printing technology has been successfully used to reconstruct the articular surface and osseous component in a patient with severe open distal humerus fracture (Luenam et al., 2018). Implants are routinely being printed for pelvis, spine, jaw, skull and hip bones following medical imaging via computed tomography (CT), X-rays and magnetic resonance imaging (MRI).

Kim et al. made use of 3D-printed clavicular models to help the surgeon plan and rehearse his fracture reduction treatment and select a pre-contoured locking plate in seven cases of unilateral comminuted clavicular fractures (H. N. Kim, Liu & Noh, 2015). Good elbow function in cases of distal humerus fracture treated using 3D-printed plates has also been demonstrated (J. W. Kim et al., 2018). It has also found application in the treatment of proximal humerus fractures and in cases of cubitus varus deformities (Luenam et al., 2018). PLA is considered the material of choice in elbow fractures. Calcaneal fractures can be effectively reduced with minimum invasion by 3D printing the fractured calcanei and mirror image of its contralateral side (Wu et al., 2017). Be it fractures of the tibia, talar neck, tibial plateau, distal femur, pelvis, radius or any other bone of the upper and lower limbs, 3D printing can be used to understand the complex anatomies and fracture patterns, prepare templates for the selection of anatomical plates and aid the surgeon in planning screw trajectories for reduction and fixation (Chung et al., 2014).

Customised sockets for rehabilitation after leg amputation are considered durable and mechanically strong. In neurosurgery, after the removal of skull bone in an attempt to give space for the brain to swell, 3D-printed cranial bones are preferred because of their ease of construction and perfect fit. 3D-printed external fixators obviate the need for extensive invasive procedures for fracture reduction (Qiao et al., 2015).

3D-printed bone chips made from PLA/HA/silk composites have been advocated by Yeon et al. to be relatively non-invasive and possible internal fixation devices (Yeon et al., 2018).

3D printing is also gaining popularity in infant and neonate care, both as surgical guides as well as supporting systems for body parts. Oncological resections have been made easy with the precise simulated models generated by 3D printers. From 3D-printed heart simulation models to 3D-printed air splints for tracheobronchomalacia, this technology has revolutionised paediatric care. In a 9-month-old child, a 3D-printed sternum was utilised at the surgical planning stage, which was further treated by a 3D-printed titanium implant. In bone regeneration, 3D printing for devices functions as custom-fit orthoses, that is, as external assisting devices protecting body segments post-trauma and supporting weak joints. Cranial caps (Craniocap®) and cranial bands (SnugKap®) are medical non-invasive cranial orthoses made by FDM technology, that have been utilised to aid in the correction of cranial defects in Plagiocephaly patients. They also aid in redirecting the growth of the cranium in these patients (Geoffroy, Gardan, Goodnough & Mattie, 2018; Sukanya, Panigrahy & Rath, 2021). 3D-printed club feet comprising rigid foot bones in a gel matrix have also been tried for the pre-analysis stage of corrective surgery for the procedure. As it is desirable for the implants to grow as the child grows, 3D printing with smart bioresponsive materials, which can alter their behaviour according to stimulus, are the need of the hour.

11.7.2 APPLICATIONS IN DENTISTRY

The concept of digital workflow has revolutionised dentistry. Be it diagnosis, treatment or education, 3D printing has found numerous applications. Almost all branches of dentistry are benefitting from this innovative technology, be it for socket preservation, guided endodontics, clear aligners, surgical guides, fabrication of complete and partial prosthesis, guided implant placement, simulation education models for teaching purposes, alveolar ridge preservation, periodontal repair and regeneration, peri-implant maintenance, facial prosthesis, surgical instruments, customised splints or 3D-printed brackets, etc. (Kohli Tarika, 2019).

As far as reconstruction of bone is concerned, additive manufacturing primarily plays a major role in oral and maxillofacial reconstruction and in periodontal regeneration and repair, and is still in its inception stage. Additive manufacturing technology has made it possible to come up with customised scaffolds and implants by virtue of the biocompatible materials developed to date (Hixon, Melvin, Lin, Hall & Sell, 2017; Tsai et al., 2017; Wurm et al., 2017). These materials are expected to integrate with the host bone and vascular supply, bear loads, adequately stabilise blood clots and have the ability to remodel.

3D printing has been used for constructing tissue scaffolds in bone grafting procedures such as socket preservation, guided bone regeneration and sinus augmentation (Lei, Yu, Ke, Sun & Chen, 2019; Rasperini et al., 2015; Sumida et al., 2015). Such bioresorbable scaffolds have been found to preserve alveolar bone better in extraction sockets, than those without scaffolds, especially those using 3D-printed hydroxyapatite (Goh, Teh, Tan, Zhang & Teoh, 2015; Kijartorn, Thammarakcharoen, Suwanprateeb & Buranawat, 2017; Park et al., 2018). Guided tissue regeneration (GTR) using a scaffold made from a CT scan of the bone defect has been tried by a few researchers (Oberoi et al., 2018; Pilipchuk et al., 2016). Natural polymers like gelatin can be combined with mechanically stronger materials to help the scaffolds function as both a graft and a membrane. Collagen/bioceramic mix closely resembles ECM of bone and can present an adequate degradation profile. These scaffolds are able to closely mimic the lost bony architecture and duplicate the internal porous structure. Less chair side time, availability of material and near to no risk of infection transfer make them materials of choice (Gul, Arif & Ghafoor, 2019). Allogenic grafts prepared using this technology are also advantageous as they lack ethical and donor site morbidity issues. The addition of calcium phosphate powder to calcium sulphate-based 3D powders has been found to enhance the bone augmentation potential of the scaffold. The incorporation of growth factors further stimulates osteogenic differentiation. In periodontal regeneration, 3D-printed triphasic scaffolds allowing spatiotemporal delivery of a number of proteins have been developed for better control over tissue infiltration and regeneration of periodontal fibres, and cementum in addition to alveolar bone (C. H. Lee et al., 2014). Cell sheets enclosed in electrospun PCL membrane, thermally incorporated with a FDM-developed TCP-PCL bone compartment have also shown promise when tested in animal models (Akizuki et al., 2005).

In the field of maxillofacial reconstructive surgery, the role of bone tissue engineering is even more critical as the complex architecture of craniofacial bones

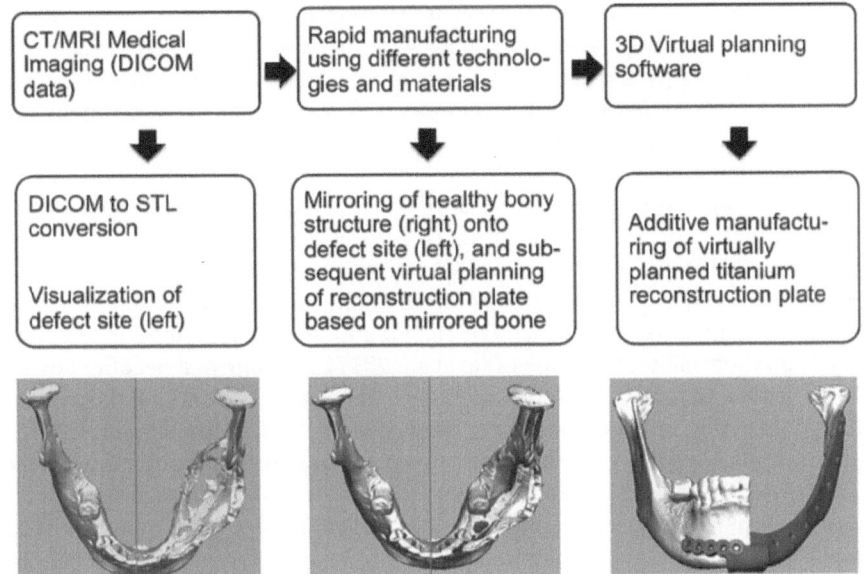

FIGURE 11.6 Schematic representation of a bony reconstruction showing the three basic steps of the 3D-printing system. (1) Acquisition of high definition 3D imaging data with CT. (2) Image processing, including segmentation steps and surface modelling. (3) Manufacturing with a 3D printer. 3D, 3-dimensional; CT, computed tomography; DICOM, Digital Imaging and Communications in Medicine; MRI, magnetic resonance imaging; STL, stereo lithography. Reproduced with permission (Farré-Guasch et al., 2015); Copyright 2015, Elsevier Ltd.

including the temporomandibular joint (TMJ), temple, mandible, nose, zygomatic arch, orbital bone etc. needs to be replicated (Brie et al., 2013; Salah, Tayebi, Moharamzadeh & Naini, 2020) (Figure 11.6). The bone being anisotropic poses unique challenges for preparing these patient-specific reconstructions. In addition, each of these individual bones has typical characteristics of its own which the clinician must keep in mind. For example, in the TMJ the density of the bone matrix increases from the inferior to the superior condylar region in the vertical cancellous bone lamina. Grayson et al. have successfully in their reconstruction of TMJ simulated these anatomical challenges, thereby generating an anatomically shaped scaffold seeded with human MSCs (Grayson et al., 2010). Formation of lamellar bone and osteoids with fully viable cells in a bone matrix resembling the natural bone in both architecture and density indicated the potential of the biomimetic scaffold-bioreactor system to come up with patient-specific bone grafts.

Scaffolds made using the CAD/CAM system and bioprinted with single component or multicomponent bio-inks have been found to be predictable and effective in the construction of defects due to craniofacial injuries, congenital abnormalities or tumour excision (Liao et al., 2019; Congcong Shen et al., 2014). One of the more studied scaffold materials is polycaprolactone (PCL), which is extensively used due to its inherent resemblance to ECM. Scaffolds can be built using this material to closely mimic the anisotropic nature of condyle. TCP scaffolds made using an inkjet printer and implanted in patients with maxillofacial defects have been found to reduce surgery time and favourably unite with the surrounding bone (Saijo et al., 2009). The technology allows the developer to adjust the porosity, design and texture of these scaffolds as per desired requirements. The addition of bioceramics helps combat the slow degradation profile. Scaffolds with added hydroxyapatite have more bone regenerating ability than scaffolds with bioactive glass. Monolithic monetite and biphasic calcium phosphate have also gained popularity in sinus augmentation techniques and as potential bone grafts (Inzana et al., 2014; Tamimi et al., 2009; Torres et al., 2011).

As with any other 3D-printed scaffold, the addition of stem cells and growth factors increases the osteogenic potential, enabling these 'smart' scaffolds to enhance the cell adhesion and proliferation (Tsai et al., 2017). For maximal benefit, they need to be programmed to be activated in a timely and phased manner, with the cytokines coming into action at the earliest, upregulating the cell migration and proliferation, followed by the release of osteogenic factors for guiding bone formation (Figure 11.2). BMP-2, FGF, IGF-1 and PDGF have all been studied in this regard. Cells from platelet-rich plasma, bone marrow, dental pulp and adipose tissue have been harvested for seeding into scaffolds and have shown promising results (Boo et al., 2002; Caplan, 2005; Gimble, Katz & Bunnell, 2007; Marx, 2004; Mendonça & Juiz-Lopez, 2010; Monaco, Bionaz, Hollister & Wheeler, 2011; Yamada et al., 2004). iPSCs have some inherent limitations like low yield and slow evolution in culture, which must be overcome before they are actively used for maxillofacial reconstructions.

In implant dentistry, in addition to 3D printing being used for the manufacture of surgical guides for the guided placement of dental implants, additive technologies are used for the construction of bioactive implants, with silver added onto the implant surface by AM techniques to benefit from the antimicrobial efficacy of silver. The porous silver scaffolds have been found to be mechanically similar to cancellous bone in terms of their ultimate strength, yield strength, Young's modulus and elastic limit. These were reported to reduce Staphylococcus aureus numbers by 90 per cent within 4 hours and by 99 per cent within a 14-hour duration (Arjunan et al., 2020). Also under research are hybrid scaffolds which are filled with bone graft particles and have implant fixtures in them to save cost and time of an otherwise multistep surgical procedure (Jeong et al., 2020).

Fibre-guided scaffolds for GTR have been successful when tested in rat models, but discrepancies amongst humans and animals in terms of host response and time taken for complete healing pre-empt their duplication in routine therapy. However, literature is lacking in terms of randomised control trials and follow-up studies with further validation being required before they are labelled as the mainstay of dental reconstruction modalities and the results of preclinical trials are translated into clinical reality.

11.8 FUTURE DIRECTIONS

Constant innovation to parallel the complexities of bone physiology is required in order to provide the most desirable of outcomes. Numerous advances have been made towards achieving suitable scaffold materials for this purpose. It has already been mentioned how scaffold materials possessing the properties of both osteogenesis and angiogenesis would aid in mimicking and reproducing normal bone physiology. Tailored biodegradable scaffold materials with controlled ranges of porosity are possible in today's day and age. A possible drawback of porous scaffolds is their structural weakness and the relatively uniform distribution of porosity throughout their structure. This is in contrast with what is observed in human bone specimens wherein the core is more porous than the relatively denser shell. Complexity of design and manufacturing is required in order to achieve similar results and at the same time ensure structural robustness and interconnectivity within the scaffold (Bose, Roy & Bandyopadhyay, 2012; Mironov, Reis & Derby, 2006).

Strong materials with desirable bioresorption times also need to be developed in order to provide effective solutions. Generally, composite scaffolds comprising polymers and ceramics are utilised to address these situations. A challenge with these constructs is that the resorption time of the two elements does not match, with the polymeric components tending to degrade faster than the ceramic in the scaffold. A possible solution may be offered in the form of utilising an amorphous variant of calcium phosphate which characteristically degrades more rapidly than its crystalline form. Alternatively, polymers with slower degradation times may also be utilised. A fine-tuned orchestrated response is desired from the entire endeavour of bone printing as this is what goes on in the human bone as well. Any attempt to mimic this would have to achieve levels of complexity to rival what it aims to imitate in the first place. Sustained and sequential activity of biomolecules is as important as incorporating the right elements into the construct. The pore size of scaffolds may aid in influencing the efficiency and delivery rate of the intended bioactive molecules. Scaffold micropores can potentially be tuned to the extent that the burst release of entrapped biomolecules is prevented by capillary action. This would ensure that it is the degradation of the scaffold itself which determines the release of biomolecules in a time-dependent manner. This incidentally formed a requirement that is anticipated and very much essential for third-generation scaffolds. The timed and sequential release of biomolecules can optimise the levels of growth factor requirements in vivo, thereby effectively enhancing tissue integration (Marga et al., 2012; Skardal, Zhang & Prestwich, 2010).

It is not just the sustainability of biomolecule release, but the longevity of cell lineage survival that would need to be addressed. It is only when the intended cells survive for sufficient periods that they will be effective in fulfilling their purpose. Most reports in literature peg the viability of cell function to range from days to a few weeks, while the actual demand is for these to function for considerably longer periods. Rapid scaffolding has been handicapped for a long time as a result of material development inadequacies with high temperatures, ultraviolet light and chemical cross-linking rendering undesirable outcomes upon most constructs. To avoid these undesirable curing processes, cell pastes and cellularised matrix gels were developed only to discover that a significant majority of these prints were devoid of primary mechanical integrity and were susceptible to a multitude of external influences which led to their dissolution, melting or warpage. A high cell concentration can also be held responsible for inhibiting certain hydrogel-based cross-links. A reasonable approach would be to aim for maintaining cell cultures at levels that are relevant biologically and producing biopolymer constructs capable of tackling the mechanical and chemical demands of the construct. Biomedical implant and micro-fluidic vasculature composite scaffold applications are severely limited in the attempt to achieve the right amount of compromise between ensuring mechanical strength and utilising processing that is biocompatible. Codeposition, or simultaneous printing of biomolecules along with their structural components, with or without non-deleterious post-processing, can be a possible solution to this problem. Based on literature, it can be stated that bioprinting in vivo is now a possibility as well with potential applications in medicine viz a viz robotics and computer-assisted interventions. A significant issue in medicine is the rehabilitation of large bone defects and/or discontinuities, a step in this direction would be to attempt an optimisation of vascularised scaffolds with a mechanical structure. Another prospect of promise is the development of multiple-layer scaffolds to address the issue of osteochondral tissue regeneration or repair. With no effective solution at present, it poses quite the conundrum in orthopaedics (Marques et al., 2019; Roseti et al., 2017).

A variety of therapeutics based on RNA have been developed to facilitate bone regeneration. These include microRNA (miRNA), messenger RNA (mRNA), long coding RNA (lncRNA) and small interfering RNA (siRNA) (Elangovan et al., 2015; Eskildsen et al., 2011; Hao et al., 2019; Lin et al., 2019; H. Liu et al., 2019; Minh K Nguyen et al., 2018; Takayama et al., 2009). These act by enhancing bone defect repair by virtue of being embedded in the scaffolds. miRNA is responsible for the upregulation of genes related to osteogenesis and the downregulation of post-translational level adverse genes. siRNA can be tailor-made to silence a gene of choice, perhaps one which causes inhibition of bone formation through a specific endogenous pathway. lncRNA is expressed through indirect gene regulation by binding competing endogenous RNA (ceRNA) with miRNA during the process of osteogenesis. RNA centric treatment methodologies have only recently incited interest in their applications as treatment methodologies (Winkler, Sass, Duda & Schmidt-Bleek, 2018).

Amongst others, lipid nanoparticles and polymer nanoparticles have been described as the chief vectors for the carriage of these RNA particles with collagen and hydrogels forming the commonest materials for use in the construction of scaffolds to accomplish in vivo RNA delivery at bone sites. However, bone healing is a complex process and RNA methodologies aiming to address its needs have to be further fine-tuned to fit the system they aim to mimic. The influence of the physical environment and chemical factors is well established in the process of bone healing by the utilisation of scaffolds. Such parameters have not been explored in RNA-based therapies yet. Several findings in vitro do not find sustenance when translated in vivo (Wang, Tran, Shen & Grainger, 2012). Finally, however effective these modalities may purportedly be, a low-cost RNA-based solution for bone healing challenges is yet to be developed and remains another significant challenge to plague the translational benefits of these novel therapeutic approaches.

ANNEXURE FOR ABBREVIATIONS

3D	Three-dimensional
3DP3	Three-dimensional printing
AB MSCs	Alveolar bone-derived mesenchymal stem cells
ADSCs	Adipose tissue-derived stem cells
AF-MSCs	Amniotic fluid mesenchymal stem cells
ALP	Alkaline phosphatase
AM	Additive manufacture/ Additive manufacturing
AM-MSCs	Amniotic membrane mesenchymal stem cells
BioLP	Biological laser printing
BM-MSCs	Bone marrow mesenchymal stem cells
BMP	Bone morphogenic protein
BMU	Bone metabolic unit
bTCP/TTCP	Beta-tricalcium phosphate/ Tetracalcium phosphate
CAD	Computer-aided design
CAM	Computer-aided manufacture
CaP	Calcium phosphate
ceRNA	Competing endogenous RNA
CFU	Colony-forming unit
CM-MSCs	Chorionic membrane mesenchymal stem cells
CPCs	Calcium phosphate ceramics
CT	Computed tomography
DC-MSCs	Deciduous mesenchymal stem cells
DFPCs	Dental follicle progenitor cells
DICOM	Digital imaging and communications in medicine
DIW	Direct ink writing
DPSCs	Dental pulp stem cells
ECM	Extracellular matrix
EGF	Epidermal growth factor
ESCs	Embryonic stem cells
FACS	Fluorescence-activated cell sorting
FDA	Food and Drug Administration
FDM	Fused deposition modelling
FGF2	Fibroblast growth factor-2
GAGs	Glycosaminoglycans
GF	Growth factors
G-MSCs	Gingival mesenchymal stem cells
GTR	Guided tissue regeneration
HA	Hydroxyapatite
hT-MSCs	Human thymus-derived mesenchymal stem cells
IGF	Insulin-like growth factor
IL	Interleukin
iPSCs	Induced pluripotent stem cells
lncRNA	Long coding RNA
M-CSF	Macrophage colony-stimulating factor

miRNA	Micro RNA
MPa	Megapascal
MRI	Magnetic resonance imaging
mRNA	Messenger RNA
MSCs	Mesenchymal stem cells
OPG	Osteoprotegerin
PCL	Polycaprolactone
PDGF	Platelet-derived growth factor
PDLLA	Poly-d,l-lactic acid
PDLSCs	Periodontal ligament stem cells
PD-MSCs	Placental-derived mesenchymal stem cells
PE	Polyethylene
PGA	Polyglycolic acid
PLA	Polylactic acid
PLGA	Polylactic-co-glycolic acid
RANK	Receptor activator nuclear kappa-B
RANKL	Receptor activator nuclear kappa-B ligand
RNA	Ribonucleic acid
RP	Rapid prototyping
RUNX2	Runt-related transcription factor 2
Saos-eGFP	Sarcoma osteogenic enhanced green fluorescent protein
SCAP	Stem cells derived from apical papilla
SFF	Solid free-form fabrication
SHED	Stem cells from exfoliated deciduous teeth
SiO$_2$	Silicon dioxide
siRNA	Small interfering RNA
SOP	Standard operating procedure
STL	Stereolithography
TCP	Tricalcium phosphate
TGFβ	Tumour growth factor beta/ Transforming growth factor beta
TGPCs	Tooth germ progenitor cells
TMJ	Temporomandibular ljoint
TRAP	Tartrate-resistant acid phosphatase
TTCP/CaSo$_4$.2H$_2$O	Tetracalcium phosphate/Calcium sulphate dihydrate
UC-MSCs	Umbilical cord mesenchymal stem cells
VEGF	Vascular endothelial growth factor
ZnO	Zinc oxide

REFERENCES

Abou-Khalil, R., Yang, F., Mortreux, M., Lieu, S., Yu, Y. Y., Wurmser, M., … Marcucio, R. S. (2014). Delayed bone regeneration is linked to chronic inflammation in murine muscular dystrophy. *Journal of Bone and Mineral Research*, 29(2), 304–315.

Adepu, S., Dhiman, N., Laha, A., Sharma, C. S., Ramakrishna, S., & Khandelwal, M. (2017). Three-dimensional bioprinting for bone tissue regeneration. *Current Opinion in Biomedical Engineering*, 2, 22–28.

Akizuki, T., Oda, S., Komaki, M., Tsuchioka, H., Kawakatsu, N., Kikuchi, A., ... Ishikawa, I. (2005). Application of periodontal ligament cell sheet for periodontal regeneration: A pilot study in beagle dogs. *Journal of Periodontal Research, 40*(3), 245–251.

Arjunan, A., Robinson, J., Al Ani, E., Heaselgrave, W., Baroutaji, A., & Wang, C. (2020). Mechanical performance of additively manufactured pure silver antibacterial bone scaffolds. *Journal of the Mechanical Behavior of Biomedical Materials, 112*, 104090.

Badylak, S. F., Freytes, D. O., & Gilbert, T. W. (2009). Extracellular matrix as a biological scaffold material: Structure and function. *Acta Biomaterialia, 5*(1), 1–13.

Bagaria, V., & Chaudhary, K. (2017). A paradigm shift in surgical planning and simulation using 3Dgraphy: Experience of first 50 surgeries done using 3D-printed biomodels. *Injury, 48*(11), 2501–2508.

Banerjee, S. S., Tarafder, S., Davies, N. M., Bandyopadhyay, A., & Bose, S. (2010). Understanding the influence of MgO and SrO binary doping on the mechanical and biological properties of β-TCP ceramics. *Acta Biomaterialia, 6*(10), 4167–4174.

Barron, J. A., Ringeisen, B. R., Kim, H., Spargo, B. J., & Chrisey, D. B. (2004). Application of laser printing to mammalian cells. *Thin Solid Films, 453*, 383–387.

Baume, A., Boughton, P., Coleman, N., & Ruys, A. (2016). Sterilization of tissue scaffolds. In *Characterisation and Design of Tissue Scaffolds* (pp. 225–244): Elsevier.

Bayliss, L., Mahoney, D. J., & Monk, P. (2012). Normal bone physiology, remodelling and its hormonal regulation. *Surgery (Oxford), 30*(2), 47–53.

Becker, S. T., Bolte, H., Schünemann, K., Seitz, H., Bara, J., Beck-Broichsitter, B., ... Warnke, P. H. (2012). Endocultivation: The influence of delayed vs. simultaneous application of BMP-2 onto individually formed hydroxyapatite matrices for heterotopic bone induction. *International Journal of Oral and Maxillofacial Surgery, 41*(9), 1153–1160.

Bhat, S. (2020). 3D printing equipment in medicine. In *3D Printing in Medicine and Surgery* (pp. 223–261): Elsevier.

Bhrany, A. D., Beckstead, B. L., Lang, T. C., Farwell, D. G., Giachelli, C. M., & Ratner, B. D. (2006). Development of an esophagus acellular matrix tissue scaffold. *Tissue Engineering, 12*(2), 319–330.

Boland, T., Xu, T., Damon, B., & Cui, X. (2006). Application of inkjet printing to tissue engineering. *Biotechnology Journal: Healthcare Nutrition Technology, 1*(9), 910–917.

Boo, J. S., Yamada, Y., Okazaki, Y., Hibino, Y., Okada, K., Hata, K.-I., ... Ueda, M. (2002). Tissue-engineered bone using mesenchymal stem cells and a biodegradable scaffold. *Journal of Craniofacial Surgery, 13*(2), 231–239.

Bose, S., Roy, M., & Bandyopadhyay, A. (2012). Recent advances in bone tissue engineering scaffolds. *Trends in Biotechnology, 30*(10), 546–554.

Bose, S., Suguira, S., & Bandyopadhyay, A. (1999). Processing of controlled porosity ceramic structures via fused deposition. *Scripta Materialia, 41*(9), 1009–1014.

Brie, J., Chartier, T., Chaput, C., Delage, C., Pradeau, B., Caire, F., ... Moreau, J.-J. (2013). A new custom made bioceramic implant for the repair of large and complex craniofacial bone defects. *Journal of Cranio-Maxillofacial Surgery, 41*(5), 403–407.

Brown, B. N., & Badylak, S. F. (2014). Extracellular matrix as an inductive scaffold for functional tissue reconstruction. *Translational Research, 163*(4), 268–285.

Burchardt, H., & Enneking, W. (1978). Transplantation of bone. *Surgical Clinics of North America, 58*(2), 403–427.

Caplan, A. I. (2005). Mesenchymal stem cells: cell-based reconstructive therapy in orthopedics. *Tissue engineering, 11*(7-8), 1198–1211.

Carda, C., Silvestrini, G., de Ferraris, M. G., Peydro, A., & Bonucci, E. (2005). Osteoprotegerin (OPG) and RANKL expression and distribution in developing human craniomandibular joint. *Tissue and Cell, 37*(3), 247–255.

Chen, R. R., & Mooney, D. J. (2003). Polymeric growth factor delivery strategies for tissue engineering. *Pharmaceutical Research, 20*(8), 1103–1112.

Chen, W., Liu, X., Chen, Q., Bao, C., Zhao, L., Zhu, Z., & Xu, H. H. (2018). Angiogenic and osteogenic regeneration in rats via calcium phosphate scaffold and endothelial cell co-culture with human bone marrow mesenchymal stem cells (MSCs), human umbilical cord MSCs, human induced pluripotent stem cell-derived MSCs and human embryonic stem cell-derived MSCs. *Journal of Tissue Engineering and Regenerative Medicine*, *12*(1), 191–203.

Chung, K. J., Hong, D. Y., Kim, Y. T., Yang, I., Park, Y. W., & Kim, H. N. (2014). Preshaping plates for minimally invasive fixation of calcaneal fractures using a real-size 3D-printed model as a preoperative and intraoperative tool. *Foot & Ankle International*, *35*(11), 1231–1236.

Cunningham, J. J., Ulbright, T. M., Pera, M. F., & Looijenga, L. H. (2012). Lessons from human teratomas to guide development of safe stem cell therapies. *Nature Biotechnology*, *30*(9), 849–857.

Daftari, T. K., Whitesides Jr, T. E., Heller, J. G., Goodrich, A. C., McCarey, B. E., & Hutton, W. C. (1994). Nicotine on the revascularization of bone graft. An experimental study in rabbits. *Spine*, *19*(8), 904–911.

D'Agostino, A., Trevisiol, L., Favero, V., Gunson, M. J., Pedica, F., Nocini, P. F., & Arnett, G. W. (2016). Hydroxyapatite/collagen composite is a reliable material for malar augmentation. *Journal of Oral and Maxillofacial Surgery*, *74*(6), e1231–1238. e1215.

Darsell, J., Bose, S., Hosick, H. L., & Bandyopadhyay, A. (2003). From CT scan to ceramic bone graft. *Journal of the American Ceramic Society*, *86*(7), 1076–1080.

Das, K., Bose, S., & Bandyopadhyay, A. (2007). Surface modifications and cell–materials interactions with anodized Ti. *Acta Biomaterialia*, *3*(4), 573–585.

Datta, N., Pham, Q. P., Sharma, U., Sikavitsas, V. I., Jansen, J. A., & Mikos, A. G. (2006). In vitro generated extracellular matrix and fluid shear stress synergistically enhance 3D osteoblastic differentiation. *Proceedings of the National Academy of Sciences*, *103*(8), 2488–2493.

DePalma, A. F., Rothman, R. H., Lewinnek, G. E., Canale, S. T. (1972). Anterior interbody fusion for severe cervical disc degeneration. *Surgery, Gynecology and Obstetrics*, *134*, 755–758.

Detsch, R., & Boccaccini, A. R. (2015). The role of osteoclasts in bone tissue engineering. *Journal of Tissue Engineering and Regenerative Medicine*, *9*(10), 1133–1149.

Detsch, R., Schaefer, S., Deisinger, U., Ziegler, G., Seitz, H., & Leukers, B. (2011). In vitro-osteoclastic activity studies on surfaces of 3D printed calcium phosphate scaffolds. *Journal of Biomaterials Applications*, *26*(3), 359–380.

Dinca, V., Ranella, A., Farsari, M., Kafetzopoulos, D., Dinescu, M., Popescu, A., & Fotakis, C. (2008). Quantification of the activity of biomolecules in microarrays obtained by direct laser transfer. *Biomedical Microdevices*, *10*(5), 719–725.

Doraiswamy, A., Narayan, R., Harris, M., Qadri, S., Modi, R., & Chrisey, D. (2007). Laser microfabrication of hydroxyapatite-osteoblast-like cell composites. *Journal of Biomedical Materials Research Part A*, *80*(3), 635–643.

Elangovan, S., Khorsand, B., Do, A.-V., Hong, L., Dewerth, A., Kormann, M., ... Salem, A. K. (2015). Chemically modified RNA activated matrices enhance bone regeneration. *Journal of Controlled Release*, *218*, 22–28.

Eskildsen, T., Taipaleenmäki, H., Stenvang, J., Abdallah, B. M., Ditzel, N., Nossent, A. Y., ... Kassem, M. (2011). MicroRNA-138 regulates osteogenic differentiation of human stromal (mesenchymal) stem cells in vivo. *Proceedings of the National Academy of Sciences*, *108*(15), 6139–6144.

Farré-Guasch, E., Wolff, J., Helder, M. N., Schulten, E. A., Forouzanfar, T., & Klein-Nulend, J. (2015). Application of additive manufacturing in oral and maxillofacial surgery. *Journal of Oral and Maxillofacial Surgery*, *73*(12), 2408–2418.

Fedorovich, N. E., Schuurman, W., Wijnberg, H. M., Prins, H.-J., Van Weeren, P. R., Malda, J., ... Dhert, W. J. (2012). Biofabrication of osteochondral tissue equivalents by printing topologically defined, cell-laden hydrogel scaffolds. *Tissue Engineering Part C: Methods*, *18*(1), 33–44.

Feng, X. (2005). RANKing intracellular signaling in osteoclasts. *IUBMB Life*, *57*(6), 389–395.

Fielding, G. A., Bandyopadhyay, A., & Bose, S. (2012). Effects of silica and zinc oxide doping on mechanical and biological properties of 3D printed tricalcium phosphate tissue engineering scaffolds. *Dental Materials*, *28*(2), 113–122.

Flynn, L. E., Prestwich, G. D., Semple, J. L., & Woodhouse, K. A. (2008). Proliferation and differentiation of adipose-derived stem cells on naturally derived scaffolds. *Biomaterials*, *29*(12), 1862–1871.

Fu, B., Tian, Z., & Wei, H. (2014). TH17 cells in human recurrent pregnancy loss and preeclampsia. *Cellular & Molecular Immunology*, *11*(6), 564–570.

Fu, Q., Saiz, E., & Tomsia, A. P. (2011). Direct ink writing of highly porous and strong glass scaffolds for load-bearing bone defects repair and regeneration. *Acta Biomaterialia*, *7*(10), 3547–3554.

Geoffroy, M., Gardan, J., Goodnough, J., & Mattie, J. (2018). Cranial remodeling orthosis for infantile plagiocephaly created through a 3D scan, topological optimization, and 3D printing process. *JPO: Journal of Prosthetics and Orthotics*, *30*(4), 247–258.

Gimble, J. M., Katz, A. J., & Bunnell, B. A. (2007). Adipose-derived stem cells for regenerative medicine. *Circulation Research*, *100*(9), 1249–1260.

Goh, B. T., Teh, L. Y., Tan, D. B. P., Zhang, Z., & Teoh, S. H. (2015). Novel 3 D polycaprolactone scaffold for ridge preservation–a pilot randomised controlled clinical trial. *Clinical Oral Implants Research*, *26*(3), 271–277.

Grayson, W. L., Fröhlich, M., Yeager, K., Bhumiratana, S., Chan, M. E., Cannizzaro, C., … Vunjak-Novakovic, G. (2010). Engineering anatomically shaped human bone grafts. *Proceedings of the National Academy of Sciences*, *107*(8), 3299–3304.

Gudapati, H., Dey, M., & Ozbolat, I. (2016). A comprehensive review on droplet-based bioprinting: Past, present and future. *Biomaterials*, *102*, 20–42.

Gul, M., Arif, A., & Ghafoor, R. (2019). Role of three-dimensional printing in periodontal regeneration and repair: Literature review. *Journal of Indian Society of Periodontology*, *23*(6), 504.

Habibovic, P., Gbureck, U., Doillon, C. J., Bassett, D. C., van Blitterswijk, C. A., & Barralet, J. E. (2008). Osteoconduction and osteoinduction of low-temperature 3D printed bioceramic implants. *Biomaterials*, *29*(7), 944–953.

Hao, F., Lee, R. J., Zhong, L., Dong, S., Yang, C., Teng, L., … Teng, L. (2019). Hybrid micelles containing methotrexate-conjugated polymer and co-loaded with microRNA-124 for rheumatoid arthritis therapy. *Theranostics*, *9*(18), 5282.

Hixon, K. R., Melvin, A. M., Lin, A. Y., Hall, A. F., & Sell, S. A. (2017). Cryogel scaffolds from patient-specific 3D-printed molds for personalized tissue-engineered bone regeneration in pediatric cleft-craniofacial defects. *Journal of Biomaterials Applications*, *32*(5), 598–611.

Hospodiuk, M., Dey, M., Sosnoski, D., & Ozbolat, I. T. (2017). The bioink: A comprehensive review on bioprintable materials. *Biotechnology Advances*, *35*(2), 217–239.

Hull, C. (1986). US Patent No. 4,575,330.

Iaquinta, M. R., Mazzoni, E., Bononi, I., Rotondo, J. C., Mazziotta, C., Montesi, M., … Martini, F. (2019). Adult stem cells for bone regeneration and repair. *Frontiers in Cell and Developmental Biology*, *7*, 268. doi:10.3389/fcell.2019.00268

Inzana, J. A., Olvera, D., Fuller, S. M., Kelly, J. P., Graeve, O. A., Schwarz, E. M., … Awad, H. A. (2014). 3D printing of composite calcium phosphate and collagen scaffolds for bone regeneration. *Biomaterials*, *35*(13), 4026–4034.

Ivanova, E. P., Bazaka, K., & Crawford, R. J. (2014). *New Functional Biomaterials for Medicine and Healthcare* (Vol. 67): Woodhead Publishing, New Delhi, India.

Jakab, K., Norotte, C., Damon, B., Marga, F., Neagu, A., Besch-Williford, C. L., … Mironov, V. (2008). Tissue engineering by self-assembly of cells printed into topologically defined structures. *Tissue Engineering Part A*, *14*(3), 413–421.

Jakus, A. E., Rutz, A. L., & Shah, R. N. (2016). Advancing the field of 3D biomaterial printing. *Biomedical Materials*, *11*(1), 014102.

Javaid, M., & Haleem, A. (2018). Additive manufacturing applications in orthopaedics: A review. *Journal of Clinical Orthopaedics and Trauma*, *9*(3), 202–206.

Jensen, J., Tvedesøe, C., Rölfing, J. H. D., Foldager, C. B., Lysdahl, H., Kraft, D. C. E., … Bünger, C. E. (2016). Dental pulp-derived stromal cells exhibit a higher osteogenic potency than bone marrow-derived stromal cells in vitro and in a porcine critical-size bone defect model. *Sicot-J*, *2*.

Jeong, H.-J., Gwak, S.-J., Seo, K. D., Lee, S., Yun, J.-H., Cho, Y.-S., & Lee, S.-J. (2020). Fabrication of three-dimensional composite scaffold for simultaneous alveolar bone regeneration in dental implant installation. *International Journal of Molecular Sciences*, *21*(5), 1863.

Ji, J., Tong, X., Huang, X., Zhang, J., Qin, H., & Hu, Q. (2016). Patient-derived human induced pluripotent stem cells from gingival fibroblasts composited with defined nanohydroxy-apatite/chitosan/gelatin porous scaffolds as potential bone graft substitutes. *Stem Cells Translational Medicine*, *5*(1), 95–105.

Jones, A. C., Arns, C. H., Sheppard, A. P., Hutmacher, D. W., Milthorpe, B. K., & Knackstedt, M. A. (2007). Assessment of bone ingrowth into porous biomaterials using MICRO-CT. *Biomaterials*, *28*(15), 2491–2504.

Kang, Y., Kim, S., Bishop, J., Khademhosseini, A., & Yang, Y. (2012). The osteogenic differ-entiation of human bone marrow MSCs on HUVEC-derived ECM and β-TCP scaffold. *Biomaterials*, *33*(29), 6998–7007.

Kang, Y., Kim, S., Khademhosseini, A., & Yang, Y. (2011). Creation of bony microenviron-ment with CaP and cell-derived ECM to enhance human bone-marrow MSC behavior and delivery of BMP-2. *Biomaterials*, *32*(26), 6119–6130.

Kaushik, S. N., Kim, B., Walma, A. M. C., Choi, S. C., Wu, H., Mao, J. J., … Cheon, K. (2016). Biomimetic microenvironments for regenerative endodontics. *Biomaterials Research*, *20*(1), 14.

Keriquel, V., Guillemot, F., Arnault, I., Guillotin, B., Miraux, S., Amédée, J., … Catros, S. (2010). In vivo bioprinting for computer-and robotic-assisted medical intervention: pre-liminary study in mice. *Biofabrication*, *2*(1), 014101.

Khalyfa, A., Vogt, S., Weisser, J., Grimm, G., Rechtenbach, A., Meyer, W., & Schnabelrauch, M. (2007). Development of a new calcium phosphate powder-binder system for the 3D printing of patient specific implants. *Journal of Materials Science: Materials in Medicine*, *18*(5), 909–916.

Kijartorn, P., Thammarakcharoen, F., Suwanprateeb, J., & Buranawat, B. (2017). *The use of three dimensional printed hydroxyapatite granules in alveolar ridge preservation*. Paper presented at the *Key Engineering Materials*.

Kim, H. N., Liu, X. N., & Noh, K. C. (2015). Use of a real-size 3D-printed model as a preop-erative and intraoperative tool for minimally invasive plating of comminuted midshaft clavicle fractures. *Journal of Orthopaedic Surgery and Research*, *10*(1), 1–6.

Kim, J. W., Lee, Y., Seo, J., Park, J. H., Seo, Y. M., Kim, S. S., & Shon, H. C. (2018). Clinical experience with three-dimensional printing techniques in orthopedic trauma. *Journal of Orthopaedic Science*, *23*(2), 383–388.

Kim, S., Kim, S.-S., Lee, S.-H., Ahn, S. E., Gwak, S.-J., Song, J.-H., … Chung, H.-M. (2008). In vivo bone formation from human embryonic stem cell-derived osteogenic cells in poly (d, l-lactic-co-glycolic acid)/hydroxyapatite composite scaffolds. *Biomaterials*, *29*(8), 1043–1053.

Kim, Y., Lee, S. H., Kang, B. J., Kim, W. H., Yun, H. S., & Kweon, O. K. (2016). Comparison of osteogenesis between adipose-derived mesenchymal stem cells and their sheets on poly--caprolactone/-tricalcium phosphate composite scaffolds in canine bone defects. *Stem Cells International*, *2016*.

Kim, Y.-H., & Tabata, Y. (2015). Dual-controlled release system of drugs for bone regenera-tion. *Advanced Drug Delivery Reviews*, *94*, 28–40.

Kim, Y. S., Majid, M., Melchiorri, A. J., & Mikos, A. G. (2019). Applications of decellular-ized extracellular matrix in bone and cartilage tissue engineering. *Bioengineering & Translational Medicine*, *4*(1), 83–95.

Kohli Tarika, M. (2019). 3D printing in dentistry–An overview. *Acta Scientific Dental Sciences*, *3*, 35–41.

Kolambkar, Y. M., Boerckel, J. D., Dupont, K. M., Bajin, M., Huebsch, N., Mooney, D. J., … Guldberg, R. E. (2011). Spatiotemporal delivery of bone morphogenetic protein enhances functional repair of segmental bone defects. *Bone*, *49*(3), 485–492.

Koob, S., Torio-Padron, N., Stark, G. B., Hannig, C., Stankovic, Z., & Finkenzeller, G. (2011). Bone formation and neovascularization mediated by mesenchymal stem cells and endothelial cells in critical-sized calvarial defects. *Tissue Engineering Part A*, *17*(3–4), 311–321.

Kostenuik, P. J. (2005). Osteoprotegerin and RANKL regulate bone resorption, density, geom-etry and strength. *Current Opinion in Pharmacology*, *5*(6), 618–625.

Lal, H., & Patralekh, M. K. (2018). 3D printing and its applications in orthopaedic trauma: A technological marvel. *Journal of Clinical Orthopaedics and Trauma*, *9*(3), 260–268.

Lam, C. X., Teoh, S. H., & Hutmacher, D. W. (2007). Comparison of the degradation of polycaprolactone and polycaprolactone–(β-tricalcium phosphate) scaffolds in alkaline medium. *Polymer International*, *56*(6), 718–728.

Lam, C. X. F., Mo, X., Teoh, S.-H., & Hutmacher, D. (2002). Scaffold development using 3D printing with a starch-based polymer. *Materials Science and Engineering: C*, *20*(1-2), 49–56.

Langer, R., & Vacanti, J. P. (1993). Tissue engineering. *Science (New York, NY)*, *260*(5110), 920–926.

Lauzon, M.-A., Bergeron, É., Marcos, B., & Faucheux, N. (2012). Bone repair: New develop-ments in growth factor delivery systems and their mathematical modeling. *Journal of Controlled Release*, *162*(3), 502–520.

Lee, C. H., Hajibandeh, J., Suzuki, T., Fan, A., Shang, P., & Mao, J. J. (2014). Three-dimensional printed multiphase scaffolds for regeneration of periodontium complex. *Tissue Engineering Part A*, *20*(7–8), 1342–1351.

Lee, S. H., Zhou, W.Y., Wang, M., Cheung, W.L., & Ip, W.Y. (2009). Selective laser sintering of poly (1-lactide) porous scaffolds for bone tissue engineering. *Journal of Biomimetics, Biomaterials and Biomedical Engineering*, *1*, 81–89.

Lee, S.-H., & Shin, H. (2007). Matrices and scaffolds for delivery of bioactive molecules in bone and cartilage tissue engineering. *Advanced Drug Delivery Reviews*, *59*(4–5), 339–359.

Lei, L., Yu, Y., Ke, T., Sun, W., & Chen, L. (2019). The application of three-dimensional print-ing model and platelet-rich fibrin technology in guided tissue regeneration surgery for severe bone defects. *Journal of Oral Implantology*, *45*(1), 35–43.

Leukers, B., Gülkan, H., Irsen, S., Milz, S., Tille, C., Seitz, H., & Schieker, M. (2005b). Biocompatibility of ceramic scaffolds for bone replacement made by 3D print-ing. *Materialwissenschaft und Werkstofftechnik: Entwicklung, Fertigung, Prüfung, Eigenschaften und Anwendungen technischer Werkstoffe*, *36*(12), 781–787.

Leukers, B., Gülkan, H., Irsen, S. H., Milz, S., Tille, C., Schieker, M., & Seitz, H. (2005a). Hydroxyapatite scaffolds for bone tissue engineering made by 3D printing. *Journal of Materials Science: Materials in Medicine*, *16*(12), 1121–1124.

Liao, W., Xu, L., Wangrao, K., Du, Y., Xiong, Q., & Yao, Y. (2019). Three-dimensional print-ing with biomaterials in craniofacial and dental tissue engineering. *PeerJ*, *7*, e7271.

Lin, C. Y., Crowley, S. T., Uchida, S., Komaki, Y., Kataoka, K., & Itaka, K. (2019). Treatment of intervertebral disk disease by the administration of mrna encoding a cartilage-ana-bolic transcription factor. *Molecular Therapy Nucleic Acids*, *16*, 162–171. doi:10.1016/j.omtn.2019.02.012

Liu, H., Dong, Y., Feng, X., Li, L., Jiao, Y., Bai, S., … Zhao, Y. (2019). miR-34a promotes bone regeneration in irradiated bone defects by enhancing osteoblastic differentiation of mesenchymal stromal cells in rats. *Stem Cell Research & Therapy*, *10*(1), 1–14.

Liu, J., Yu, F., Sun, Y., Jiang, B., Zhang, W., Yang, J., … Liu, S. (2015a). Concise reviews: Characteristics and potential applications of human dental tissue-derived mesenchymal stem cells. *Stem cells*, *33*(3), 627–638.

Liu, X., Wang, P., Chen, W., Weir, M. D., Bao, C., & Xu, H. H. (2014). Human embryonic stem cells and macroporous calcium phosphate construct for bone regeneration in cranial defects in rats. *Acta Biomaterialia*, *10*(10), 4484–4493.

Liu, Y., Chan, J. K., & Teoh, S. H. (2015b). Review of vascularised bone tissue-engineering strategies with a focus on co-culture systems. *Journal of Tissue Engineering and Regenerative Medicine*, *9*(2), 85–105.

Liu, Y., Teoh, S.-H., Chong, M. S., Yeow, C.-H., Kamm, R. D., Choolani, M., & Chan, J. K. (2013). Contrasting effects of vasculogenic induction upon biaxial bioreactor stimulation of mesenchymal stem cells and endothelial progenitor cells cocultures in three-dimensional scaffolds under in vitro and in vivo paradigms for vascularized bone tissue engineering. *Tissue Engineering Part A*, *19*(7–8), 893–904.

Luenam, S., Kosiyatrakul, A., Hansudewechakul, C., Phakdeewisetkul, K., Lohwongwatana, B., & Puncreobutr, C. (2018). The patient-specific implant created with 3D printing technology in treatment of the irreparable radial head in chronic persistent elbow instability. *Case Reports in Orthopedics*, 9272075.

Macri, L., Silverstein, D., & Clark, R. A. (2007). Growth factor binding to the pericellular matrix and its importance in tissue engineering. *Advanced Drug Delivery Reviews*, *59*(13), 1366–1381.

Manfrini, M., Mazzoni, E., Barbanti-Brodano, G., Nocini, P., D'agostino, A., Trombelli, L., & Tognon, M. (2015). Osteoconductivity of complex biomaterials assayed by fluorescent-engineered osteoblast-like cells. *Cell Biochemistry and Biophysics*, *71*(3), 1509–1515.

Marga, F., Jakab, K., Khatiwala, C., Shepherd, B., Dorfman, S., Hubbard, B., … Forgacs, G. (2012). Toward engineering functional organ modules by additive manufacturing. *Biofabrication*, *4*(2), 022001.

Maroulakos, M., Kamperos, G., Tayebi, L., Halazonetis, D., & Ren, Y. (2019). Applications of 3D printing on craniofacial bone repair: A systematic review. *Journal of Dentistry*, *80*, 1–14.

Marques, C., Diogo, G., Pina, S., Oliveira, J. M., Silva, T., & Reis, R. (2019). Collagen-based bioinks for hard tissue engineering applications: A comprehensive review. *Journal of Materials Science: Materials in Medicine*, *30*(3), 1–12.

Martino, M. M., Briquez, P. S., Maruyama, K., & Hubbell, J. A. (2015). Extracellular matrix-inspired growth factor delivery systems for bone regeneration. *Advanced Drug Delivery Reviews*, *94*, 41–52.

Martino, M. M., & Hubbell, J. A. (2010). The 12th–14th type III repeats of fibronectin function as a highly promiscuous growth factor-binding domain. *The FASEB Journal*, *24*(12), 4711–4721.

Marx, R. E. (2004). Platelet-rich plasma: Evidence to support its use. *Journal of Oral and Maxillofacial Surgery*, *62*(4), 489–496.

Mendonça, J. J., & Juiz-Lopez, P. (2010). Regenerative facial reconstruction of terminal stage osteoradionecrosis and other advanced craniofacial diseases with adult cultured stem and progenitor cells. *Plastic and Reconstructive Surgery*, *126*(5), 1699–1709.

Mironov, V., Reis, N., & Derby, B. (2006). Bioprinting: A beginning. *Tissue Engineering*, *12*(4), 631–634.

Mohammed, E. E., El-Zawahry, M., Farrag, A. R. H., Aziz, N. N. A., Sharaf-ElDin, W., Abu-Shahba, N., … Mossaad, M. M. (2019). Osteogenic differentiation potential of human bone marrow and amniotic fluid-derived mesenchymal stem cells in vitro & in vivo. *Open Access Macedonian Journal of Medical Sciences*, *7*(4), 507.

Monaco, E., Bionaz, M., Hollister, S., & Wheeler, M. (2011). Strategies for regeneration of the bone using porcine adult adipose-derived mesenchymal stem cells. *Theriogenology*, 75(8), 1381–1399.

Nauth, A., Miclau III, T., Li, R., & Schemitsch, E. H. (2010). Gene therapy for fracture healing. *Journal of Orthopaedic Trauma*, 24, S17–S24.

Nauth, A., Ristevski, B., Li, R., & Schemitsch, E. H. (2011). Growth factors and bone regeneration: How much bone can we expect? *Injury*, 42(6), 574–579.

Nesic, D., Durual, S., Marger, L., Mekki, M., Sailer, I., & Scherrer, S. S. (2020). Could 3D printing be the future for oral soft tissue regeneration? *Bioprinting*, 20, e00100.

Nguyen, M. K., & Alsberg, E. (2014). Bioactive factor delivery strategies from engineered polymer hydrogels for therapeutic medicine. *Progress in Polymer Science*, 39(7), 1235–1265.

Nguyen, M. K., Jeon, O., Dang, P. N., Huynh, C. T., Varghai, D., Riazi, H., ... Alsberg, E. (2018). RNA interfering molecule delivery from in situ forming biodegradable hydrogels for enhancement of bone formation in rat calvarial bone defects. *Acta Biomaterialia*, 75, 105–114.

Oberoi, G., Nitsch, S., Edelmayer, M., Janjić, K., Müller, A. S., & Agis, H. (2018). 3D Printing: Encompassing the facets of dentistry. *Frontiers in Bioengineering and Biotechnology*, 6, 172.

Odelius, K., Plikk, P., & Albertsson, A.-C. (2008). The influence of composition of porous copolyester scaffolds on reactions induced by irradiation sterilization. *Biomaterials*, 29(2), 129–140.

Otsuki, B., Takemoto, M., Fujibayashi, S., Neo, M., Kokubo, T., & Nakamura, T. (2006). Pore throat size and connectivity determine bone and tissue ingrowth into porous implants: Three-dimensional micro-CT based structural analyses of porous bioactive titanium implants. *Biomaterials*, 27(35), 5892–5900.

Ozbolat, I. T., Peng, W., & Ozbolat, V. (2016). Application areas of 3D bioprinting. *Drug Discovery Today*, 21(8), 1257–1271.

Park, S. A., Lee, H.-J., Kim, K.-S., Lee, S. J., Lee, J.-T., Kim, S.-Y., ... Park, S.-Y. (2018). In vivo evaluation of 3D-printed polycaprolactone scaffold implantation combined with β-TCP powder for alveolar bone augmentation in a beagle defect model. *Materials*, 11(2), 238.

Patel, Z. S., Young, S., Tabata, Y., Jansen, J. A., Wong, M. E., & Mikos, A. G. (2008). Dual delivery of an angiogenic and an osteogenic growth factor for bone regeneration in a critical size defect model. *Bone*, 43(5), 931–940.

Pati, F., Song, T.-H., Rijal, G., Jang, J., Kim, S. W., & Cho, D.-W. (2015). Ornamenting 3D printed scaffolds with cell-laid extracellular matrix for bone tissue regeneration. *Biomaterials*, 37, 230–241.

Perez, J. R., Kouroupis, D., Li, D. J., Best, T. M., Kaplan, L., & Correa, D. (2018). Tissue engineering and cell-based therapies for fractures and bone defects. *Frontiers in Bioengineering and Biotechnology*, 6, 105.

Pham, Q. P., Kasper, F. K., Baggett, L. S., Raphael, R. M., Jansen, J. A., & Mikos, A. G. (2008). The influence of an in vitro generated bone-like extracellular matrix on osteoblastic gene expression of marrow stromal cells. *Biomaterials*, 29(18), 2729–2739.

Pilipchuk, S. P., Monje, A., Jiao, Y., Hao, J., Kruger, L., Flanagan, C. L., ... Giannobile, W. V. (2016). Integration of 3D printed and micropatterned polycaprolactone scaffolds for guidance of oriented collagenous tissue formation in vivo. *Advanced Healthcare Materials*, 5(6), 676–687.

Pisciotta, A., Carnevale, G., Meloni, S., Riccio, M., De Biasi, S., Gibellini, L., ... De Pol, A. (2015). Human dental pulp stem cells (hDPSCs): Isolation, enrichment and comparative differentiation of two sub-populations. *BMC Developmental Biology*, 15(1), 14.

Piskin, E. (1992). Biologically modified polymeric biomaterial surfaces: Introduction. In *Biologically Modified Polymeric Biomaterial Surfaces* (pp. 3–7): Springer.

Ponsford, M., & Glass, N. (2014). The night I invented 3D printing. *Cable News Network, 14.*

Porter, J. R., Ruckh, T. T., & Popat, K. C. (2009). Bone tissue engineering: A review in bone biomimetics and drug delivery strategies. *Biotechnology Progress, 25*(6), 1539–1560.

Prolo, D. (1990). Biology of bone fusion. *Clin Neurosurg, 36,* 135–146.

Qiao, F., Li, D., Jin, Z., Gao, Y., Zhou, T., He, J., & Cheng, L. (2015). Application of 3D printed customized external fixator in fracture reduction. *Injury, 46*(6), 1150–1155.

Rambhia, K. J., & Ma, P. X. (2015). Controlled drug release for tissue engineering. *Journal of Controlled Release, 219,* 119–128.

Rasperini, G., Pilipchuk, S., Flanagan, C., Park, C., Pagni, G., Hollister, S., & Giannobile, W. (2015). 3D-printed bioresorbable scaffold for periodontal repair. *Journal of Dental Research, 94*(9_suppl), 153S–157S.

Reed, S., & Wu, B. (2014). Sustained growth factor delivery in tissue engineering applications. *Annals of Biomedical Engineering, 42*(7), 1528–1536.

Riedl, G. E., & Valentin-Opran, A. (1999). Clinical evaluation of rhBMP-2/ACS in orthopedic trauma: A progress report. *Orthopedics, 22*(7), 663–665.

Ringeisen, B. R., Othon, C. M., Barron, J. A., Young, D., & Spargo, B. J. (2006). Jet-based methods to print living cells. *Biotechnology Journal: Healthcare Nutrition Technology, 1*(9), 930–948.

Ronca, A., Ambrosio, L., & Grijpma, D. W. (2013). Preparation of designed poly (D, L-lactide)/nanosized hydroxyapatite composite structures by stereolithography. *Acta Biomaterialia, 9*(4), 5989–5996.

Roseti, L., Parisi, V., Petretta, M., Cavallo, C., Desando, G., Bartolotti, I., & Grigolo, B. (2017). Scaffolds for bone tissue engineering: State of the art and new perspectives. *Materials Science and Engineering: C, 78,* 1246–1262.

Saijo, H., Igawa, K., Kanno, Y., Mori, Y., Kondo, K., Shimizu, K., … Anzai, M. (2009). Maxillofacial reconstruction using custom-made artificial bones fabricated by inkjet printing technology. *Journal of Artificial Organs, 12*(3), 200–205.

Salah, M., Tayebi, L., Moharamzadeh, K., & Naini, F. B. (2020). Three-dimensional bio-printing and bone tissue engineering: Technical innovations and potential applications in maxillofacial reconstructive surgery. *Maxillofacial Plastic and Reconstructive Surgery, 42*(1), 1–9.

Salgado, A. J., Coutinho, O. P., & Reis, R. L. (2004). Bone tissue engineering: State of the art and future trends. *Macromolecular Bioscience, 4*(8), 743–765.

Samorezov, J. E., & Alsberg, E. (2015). Spatial regulation of controlled bioactive factor delivery for bone tissue engineering. *Advanced Drug Delivery Reviews, 84,* 45–67.

Sándor, G. K., Numminen, J., Wolff, J., Thesleff, T., Miettinen, A., Tuovinen, V. J., … Miettinen, S. (2014). Adipose stem cells used to reconstruct 13 cases with cranio-maxillofacial hard-tissue defects. *Stem Cells Translational Medicine, 3*(4), 530–540.

Schultz, G. S., & Wysocki, A. (2009). Interactions between extracellular matrix and growth factors in wound healing. *Wound Repair and Regeneration, 17*(2), 153–162.

Seitz, H., Rieder, W., Irsen, S., Leukers, B., & Tille, C. (2005). Three-dimensional printing of porous ceramic scaffolds for bone tissue engineering. *Journal of Biomedical Materials Research Part B: Applied Biomaterials: An Official Journal of The Society for Biomaterials, The Japanese Society for Biomaterials, and The Australian Society for Biomaterials and the Korean Society for Biomaterials, 74*(2), 782–788.

Serra, T., Planell, J. A., & Navarro, M. (2013). High-resolution PLA-based composite scaffolds via 3-D printing technology. *Acta Biomaterialia, 9*(3), 5521–5530.

Sfeir, C., Ho, L., Doll, B. A., Azari, K., & Hollinger, J. O. (2005). Fracture repair. In *Bone Regeneration and Repair* (pp. 21–44): Springer.

Shah, N. J., Macdonald, M. L., Beben, Y. M., Padera, R. F., Samuel, R. E., & Hammond, P. T. (2011). Tunable dual growth factor delivery from polyelectrolyte multilayer films. *Biomaterials, 32*(26), 6183–6193.

Shen, C., Yang, C., Xu, S., & Zhao, H. (2019). Comparison of osteogenic differentiation capacity in mesenchymal stem cells derived from human amniotic membrane (AM), umbilical cord (UC), chorionic membrane (CM), and decidua (DC). *Cell & Bioscience*, *9*(1), 17.

Shen, C., Zhang, Y., Li, Q., Zhu, M., Hou, Y., Qu, M., ... Chai, G. (2014). Application of three-dimensional printing technique in artificial bone fabrication for bone defect after mandibular angle ostectomy. *Zhongguo xiu fu chong jian wai ke za zhi= Zhongguo xiufu chongjian waike zazhi= Chinese journal of reparative and reconstructive surgery*, *28*(3), 300–303.

Silindir, M., & Özer, A. Y. (2009). Sterilization methods and the comparison of e-beam sterilization with gamma radiation sterilization. *Fabad Journal of Pharmaceutical Sciences*, *34*(1), 43.

Skardal, A., Zhang, J., & Prestwich, G. D. (2010). Bioprinting vessel-like constructs using hyaluronan hydrogels crosslinked with tetrahedral polyethylene glycol tetracrylates. *Biomaterials*, *31*(24), 6173–6181.

Sobral, J. M., Caridade, S. G., Sousa, R. A., Mano, J. F., & Reis, R. L. (2011). Three-dimensional plotted scaffolds with controlled pore size gradients: Effect of scaffold geometry on mechanical performance and cell seeding efficiency. *Acta Biomaterialia*, *7*(3), 1009–1018.

Stoppato, M., Carletti, E., Sidarovich, V., Quattrone, A., Unger, R. E., Kirkpatrick, C. J., ... Motta, A. (2013). Influence of scaffold pore size on collagen I development: A new in vitro evaluation perspective. *Journal of Bioactive and Compatible Polymers*, *28*(1), 16–32.

Sukanya, V., Panigrahy, N., & Rath, S. N. (2021). Recent approaches in clinical applications of 3D printing in neonates and pediatrics. *European Journal of Pediatrics*, *180*(2): 323–332.

Sultana, N., & Wang, M. (2008). Fabrication of HA/PHBV composite scaffolds through the emulsion freezing/freeze-drying process and characterisation of the scaffolds. *Journal of Materials Science: Materials in Medicine*, *19*(7), 2555.

Sumida, T., Otawa, N., Kamata, Y., Kamakura, S., Mtsushita, T., Kitagaki, H., ... Takemoto, M. (2015). Custom-made titanium devices as membranes for bone augmentation in implant treatment: Clinical application and the comparison with conventional titanium mesh. *Journal of Cranio-Maxillofacial Surgery*, *43*(10), 2183–2188.

Suwanprateeb, J., Sanngam, R., Suvannapruk, W., & Panyathanmaporn, T. (2009). Mechanical and in vitro performance of apatite–wollastonite glass ceramic reinforced hydroxyapatite composite fabricated by 3D-printing. *Journal of Materials Science: Materials in Medicine*, *20*(6), 1281.

Suwanprateeb, J., Thammarakcharoen, F., Wongsuvan, V., & Chokevivat, W. (2012). Development of porous powder printed high density polyethylene for personalized bone implants. *Journal of Porous Materials*, *19*(5), 623–632.

Takahashi, K., & Yamanaka, S. (2006). Induction of pluripotent stem cells from mouse embryonic and adult fibroblast cultures by defined factors. *cell*, *126*(4), 663–676.

Takayama, K., Suzuki, A., Manaka, T., Taguchi, S., Hashimoto, Y., Imai, Y., ... Takaoka, K. (2009). RNA interference for noggin enhances the biological activity of bone morphogenetic proteins in vivo and in vitro. *Journal of Bone and Mineral Metabolism*, *27*(4), 402.

Tamimi, F., Torres, J., Gbureck, U., López-Cabarcos, E., Bassett, D. C., Alkhraisat, M. H., & Barralet, J. E. (2009). Craniofacial vertical bone augmentation: A comparison between 3D printed monolithic monetite blocks and autologous onlay grafts in the rabbit. *Biomaterials*, *30*(31), 6318–6326.

Tanaka, Y., Nakayamada, S., & Okada, Y. (2005). Osteoblasts and osteoclasts in bone remodeling and inflammation. *Current Drug Targets-Inflammation & Allergy*, *4*(3), 325–328.

Tang, M., Chen, W., Weir, M. D., Thein-Han, W., & Xu, H. H. (2012). Human embryonic stem cell encapsulation in alginate microbeads in macroporous calcium phosphate cement for bone tissue engineering. *Acta Biomaterialia, 8*(9), 3436–3445.

Tarafder, S., Balla, V. K., Davies, N. M., Bandyopadhyay, A., & Bose, S. (2013). Microwave-sintered 3D printed tricalcium phosphate scaffolds for bone tissue engineering. *Journal of Tissue Engineering and Regenerative Medicine, 7*(8), 631–641.

Tarafder, S., Banerjee, S., Bandyopadhyay, A., & Bose, S. (2010). Electrically polarized biphasic calcium phosphates: Adsorption and release of bovine serum albumin. *Langmuir, 26*(22), 16625–16629.

Tasnim, N., De la Vega, L., Kumar, S. A., Abelseth, L., Alonzo, M., Amereh, M., … Willerth, S. M. (2018). 3D bioprinting stem cell derived tissues. *Cellular and Molecular Bioengineering, 11*(4), 219–240.

Tayalia, P., & Mooney, D. J. (2009). Controlled growth factor delivery for tissue engineering. *Advanced Materials, 21*(32–33), 3269–3285.

Torres, J., Tamimi, F., Alkhraisat, M. H., Prados-Frutos, J. C., Rastikerdar, E., Gbureck, U., … López-Cabarcos, E. (2011). Vertical bone augmentation with 3D-synthetic monetite blocks in the rabbit calvaria. *Journal of clinical Periodontology, 38*(12), 1147–1153.

Trohatou, O., & Roubelakis, M. G. (2017). Mesenchymal stem/stromal cells in regenerative medicine: Past, present, and future. *Cellular Reprogramming, 19*(4), 217–224.

Tsai, K.-Y., Lin, H.-Y., Chen, Y.-W., Lin, C.-Y., Hsu, T.-T., & Kao, C.-T. (2017). Laser sintered magnesium-calcium silicate/poly-ε-caprolactone scaffold for bone tissue engineering. *Materials, 10*(1), 65.

Tsang, V. L., & Bhatia, S. N. (2004). Three-dimensional tissue fabrication. *Advanced Drug Delivery Reviews, 56*(11), 1635–1647.

Ullah, I. S., Subbarao, R. B., & Rho, G. J. (2015). RhoGJ. *Human Mesenchymal Stem Cells – Current Trends and Future Prospective, 35*(2), e00191.

Unger, R. E., Dohle, E., & Kirkpatrick, C. J. (2015). Improving vascularization of engineered bone through the generation of pro-angiogenic effects in co-culture systems. *Advanced Drug Delivery Reviews, 94*, 116–125.

Upton, Z., Cuttle, L., Noble, A., Kempf, M., Topping, G., Malda, J., … Kravchuk, O. (2008). Vitronectin: Growth factor complexes hold potential as a wound therapy approach. *Journal of Investigative Dermatology, 128*(6), 1535–1544.

van de Watering, F. C., Molkenboer-Kuenen, J. D., Boerman, O. C., van den Beucken, J. J., & Jansen, J. A. (2012). Differential loading methods for BMP-2 within injectable calcium phosphate cement. *Journal of Controlled Release, 164*(3), 283–290.

Vonau, R. L., Bostrom, M. P., Aspenberg, P., & Sams, A. E. (2001). Combination of growth factors inhibits bone ingrowth in the bone harvest chamber. *Clinical Orthopaedics and Related Research®, 386*, 243–251.

Vorndran, E., Klarner, M., Klammert, U., Grover, L. M., Patel, S., Barralet, J. E., & Gbureck, U. (2008). 3D powder printing of β-tricalcium phosphate ceramics using different strategies. *Advanced Engineering Materials, 10*(12), B67–B71.

Wada, T., Nakashima, T., Hiroshi, N., & Penninger, J. M. (2006). RANKL–RANK signaling in osteoclastogenesis and bone disease. *Trends in Molecular Medicine, 12*(1), 17–25.

Wang, Y., Tran, K. K., Shen, H., & Grainger, D. W. (2012). Selective local delivery of RANK siRNA to bone phagocytes using bone augmentation biomaterials. *Biomaterials, 33*(33), 8540–8547.

Whitaker, M. (2014). The history of 3D printing in healthcare. *The Bulletin of the Royal College of Surgeons of England, 96*(7), 228–229.

Williams, J. M., Adewunmi, A., Schek, R. M., Flanagan, C. L., Krebsbach, P. H., Feinberg, S. E., … Das, S. (2005). Bone tissue engineering using polycaprolactone scaffolds fabricated via selective laser sintering. *Biomaterials, 26*(23), 4817–4827.

Winkler, T., Sass, F., Duda, G., & Schmidt-Bleek, K. (2018). A review of biomaterials in bone defect healing, remaining shortcomings and future opportunities for bone tissue engineering: The unsolved challenge. *Bone & Joint Research*, 7(3), 232–243.

Wolff, J. (1986). The law of bone remodelling. Translated by P. Maquet and R. Furlong. *New York, S pringer*, 1(9), 8.

Wu, J. Q., Ma, S. H., Liu, S., Qin, C. H., Jin, D., & Yu, B. (2017). Safe zone of posterior screw insertion for talar neck fractures on 3-dimensional reconstruction model. *Orthopaedic Surgery*, 9(1), 28–33.

Wurm, M. C., Möst, T., Bergauer, B., Rietzel, D., Neukam, F. W., Cifuentes, S. C., & von Wilmowsky, C. (2017). In-vitro evaluation of Polylactic acid (PLA) manufactured by fused deposition modeling. *Journal of Biological Engineering*, 11(1), 1–9.

Xie, J., Peng, C., Zhao, Q., Wang, X., Yuan, H., Yang, L., … Zhang, Y. (2016). Osteogenic differentiation and bone regeneration of iPSC-MSCs supported by a biomimetic nanofibrous scaffold. *Acta Biomaterialia*, 29, 365–379.

Xing, L., Schwarz, E. M., & Boyce, B. F. (2005). Osteoclast precursors, RANKL/RANK, and immunology. *Immunological Reviews*, 208(1), 19–29.

Yamada, Y., Ueda, M., Naiki, T., Takahashi, M., Hata, K.-I., & Nagasaka, T. (2004). Autogenous injectable bone for regeneration with mesenchymal stem cells and platelet-rich plasma: Tissue-engineered bone regeneration. *Tissue Engineering*, 10(5–6), 955–964.

Yeon, Y. K., Park, H. S., Lee, J. M., Lee, J. S., Lee, Y. J., Sultan, M. T., … Park, C. H. (2018). New concept of 3D printed bone clip (polylactic acid/hydroxyapatite/silk composite) for internal fixation of bone fractures. *Journal of Biomaterials Science, Polymer Edition*, 29(7–9), 894–906.

Young, S., Patel, Z. S., Kretlow, J. D., Murphy, M. B., Mountziaris, P. M., Baggett, L. S., … Wong, M. (2009). Dose effect of dual delivery of vascular endothelial growth factor and bone morphogenetic protein-2 on bone regeneration in a rat critical-size defect model. *Tissue Engineering Part A*, 15(9), 2347–2362.

Yu, X., Khalil, A., Dang, P. N., Alsberg, E., & Murphy, W. L. (2014). Multilayered inorganic microparticles for tunable dual growth factor delivery. *Advanced Functional Materials*, 24(20), 3082–3093.

Zou, Y., Han, Q., Weng, X., Zou, Y., Yang, Y., Zhang, K., … Qin, Y. (2018). The precision and reliability evaluation of 3-dimensional printed damaged bone and prosthesis models by stereo lithography appearance. *Medicine*, 97(6).

12 Application of Additive Manufacturing (AM) Technology in the Medical Field
A Boon for the 21st Century

Sangita Agarwal
RCC Institute of Information Technology, Kolkata, India

Soumendra Darbar
Jadavpur University, Kolkata, India
Dey' Medical Stores (Mfg.) Ltd., Kolkata, India

Srimoyee Saha
Jadavpur University, Kolkata, India

CONTENTS

DOI: 10.1201/9781003301066-12

12.1 INTRODUCTION

The year 1980 marked the emergence of a new technique, the additive manufacturing (AM) technique, and it soon gained popularity because it could be designed and tailored according to the needs of the medical practitioner and his patients [1]. In 1987, the maiden variant of the 3D printer was commercially initiated, which led to the lowering of the cost of printers and helped to increase its applications [2]. After its launch, this technique found applications in many medicative and health disciplines, such as tissue engineering [3–9]; systems to deliver drugs [10,11]; probes in laboratory [12] and portable test tools [13].

AM is also used to design assistive tools for helping chronic patients in their day to day life [14]; in prefabrication and customising outhouses, which are used for many musculoskeletal problems and prostheses [15–17] and implants [18–20]. This technique is conveniently utilised in rare diseases where planning and training of surgical procedures are done through anatomical models [21,22], medical instruments for diagnosis and surgeries and also for surgical procedures for insertion of screws [24].

The introductory edition of guidelines for AM of medical instruments was released by the Food and Drug Administration (FDA) in 2017 [25].

With this background, we will be discussing the myriad applications of AM technique in medical science (Figures 12.1 and 12.2) for the benefit of the clinicians and their patients and can be a boon for humanity at large.

12.2 ADDITIVE MANUFACTURING FOR MEDICAL APPLICATIONS

Since the emergence of AM technique, it has been widely used in the biomedical sector, which is one of the fastest-growing industries reaping the benefits of AM. It is being used in the development of advanced medical tools, working models or functional prototypes, bioprinting and customisation of the implants depending on the needs and specifications of the patients (Figure 12.2).

The technique is relatively new, but more than 97 per cent of AM professionals (SME's 2017 Medical AM/3DP Survey) in the medical field are confident that it has enormous market potential and would be a dominating player in meeting the demands of medical sectors all over the world [25–28] (Figure 12.3).

12.3 DEVELOPMENTS IN MEDICAL ADDITIVE MANUFACTURING

AM has made significant developments and gained wide acceptance [29–31] in a number of medical areas like:

a. Functional prototype or working model and preoperative templating, which help surgeons in precise planning and performing procedures, especially in complicated cases
b. Fabricating functional patient-specific bone substitutes
c. Improved implant strength

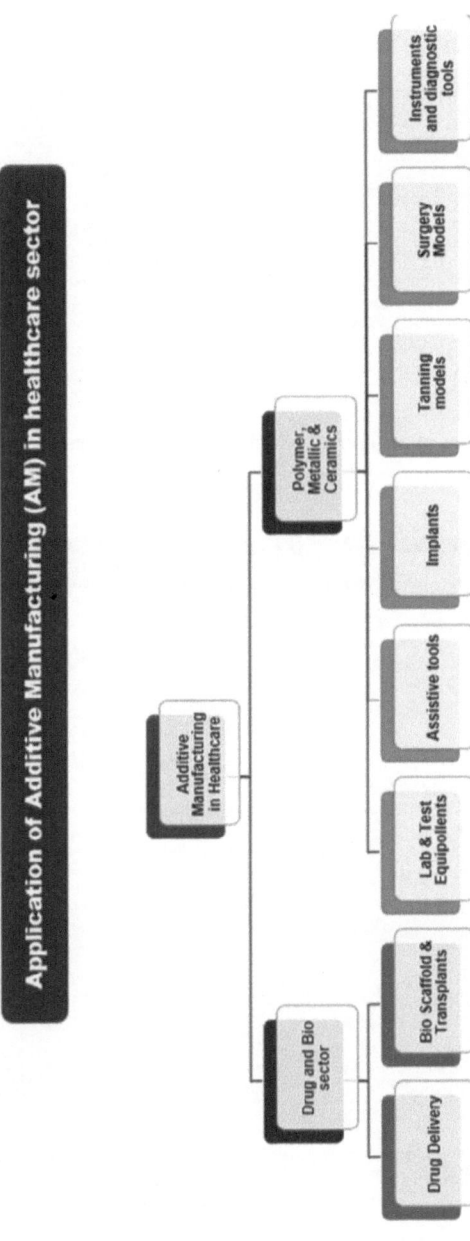

FIGURE 12.1   Applications of AM technique in various medical fields.

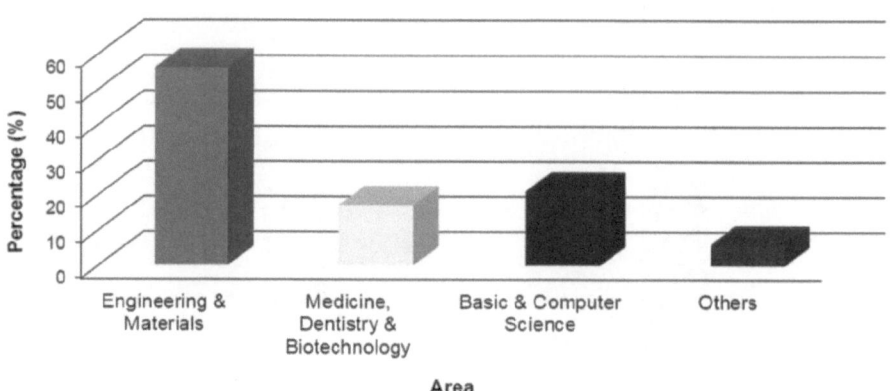

FIGURE 12.2 Differences of different 3D images extensively used for medical applications.

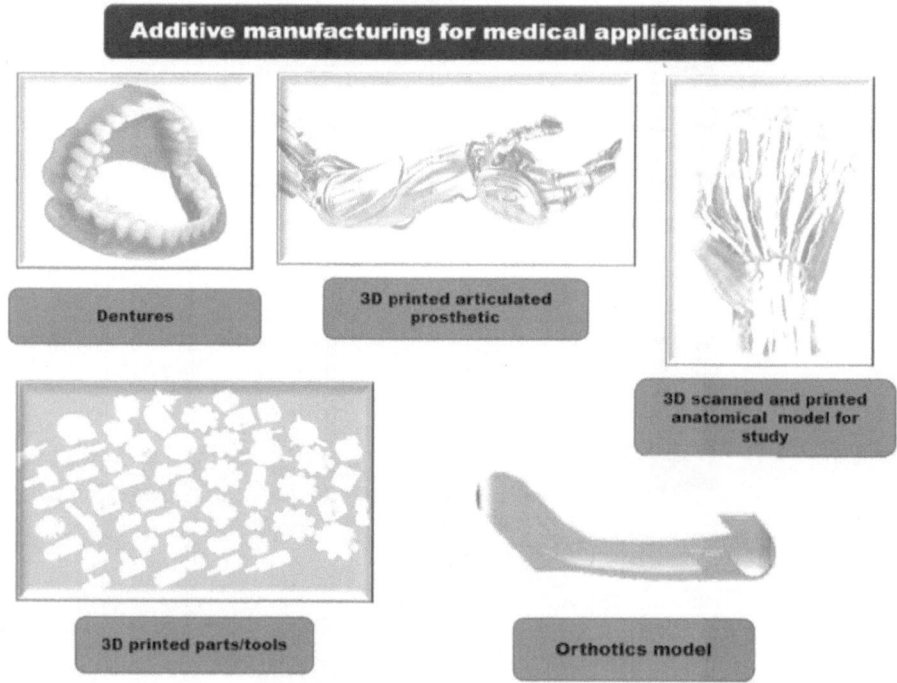

FIGURE 12.3 Photographs of different 3D images extensively used for medical applications.

d. Development and designing lightweight medical implants with improved quality
e. Better accuracy and precision
f. Reduction in operating time
g. Teaching tool and study aid to medical students
h. Aesthetic surgery and reconstructive surgery, even repairing of nose and skull
i. Cost reduction and waste minimisation
j. Fitting of different body parts precisely and accurately assisted by a realistic functional model using AM technology, and
k. Excellent surface quality.

12.4   3D TOOLS FOR MEDICAL TREATMENT

Medical 3D printing is now an indispensable part of medicine. With the advent of new tools and therapeutic models using 3D printing, the treatment of patients can be personalised, bringing new degrees of comfort. The newly developed and easily accessible technology is not only benefiting patients but also the doctors who use these tools for a greater understanding of complex cases, which leads to improvement in standard of care.

The following tools aid in medical treatment and hold great potential in AM for the healthcare sector:

12.4.1   3D-PRINTED DENTAL APPLICATIONS (DENTISTRY)

Presently, the market worth of the digital dentistry industry is $2.5 billion, which will double in a few years. People are now very much aesthetically inclined, and the field of dentistry and orthodontics would undoubtedly benefit from the evolution of AM. Traditionally orthodontics and dentistry require bridges, crowns, braces and dentures. The strength of 3D digital dentistry lies in the production of high resolution, customised, precise, patient-specific, one-of-a-kind objects. The 3D-printed dental appliances offer variability in the types of substrates that can be used, ranging from flexible polymers to rigid titanium. The 3D printers are specialised printers that use biocompatible resins, and these printers are also configured to use dental scanning software. One of the most significant advantages is that they can easily be accommodated in small spaces and, if required, can give an immediate result, thereby reducing the waiting time and anxiety associated with dental experience and the number of visits, saving time and money [27].

12.4.2   ANATOMICAL MODELS

The human body is arguably the most complex single structure, made up of billions of smaller structures, and each structure is unique. As individuals, we are unique, so for the patient-specific ailments related to a bone, an organ or a limb, or tumorous growth, an accurate anatomical model could help doctors and clinicians in the treatment process. This is a reality now that 3D printers can be used to design realistic and accurate models for investigations, using advances made in medical imaging technology and 3D scanning, assisted with sophisticated software [27]. These models are used to plan before surgery, train medical staff and students, and design implants and simulation for efficient treatment and healthcare practice. Patients can be educated on their exact condition with customised models.

12.4.3 GENERAL TOOLS

Auxiliary pieces of equipment like clamps or grips are called tools, which are used both by patients and clinicians. Clinicians use tools to help in investigations, therapy or operative procedures. Conventionally, manufacturing this auxiliary equipment is a time-consuming and costly affair. With the advances in AM, tools can be produced efficiently in short lead times and at low costs. AM is also being used to produce clamps which are non-specific, catheters and other low-cost fittings, especially in developing countries. The advantage is that manufacturing is rapid, fast, economical and high quality, and on-the-spot production can be done, as needed [28].

12.4.4 PROSTHETICS AND ORTHOTICS

Orthotic or prosthetic devices are assistive technologies, and these have been in existence for ages. Prosthetic devices are used internally or externally as a substitute for a body part. Conventionally, orthopaedic prosthetics were generic or expensive and were hand-crafted, time-consuming, required a lot of measurement and not accessible to all. Prosthetics are very much needed in regions facing military conflict [28]. Orthotic devices are used to support, correct, protect, and immobilise and treat injuries or dysfunctions of musculature and skeleton. With the advent of AM technology, there has been a paradigm shift in orthopaedic prosthetics and orthotics in terms of customisation, bringing sizing, fit, functionality and fashion. Moreover, orthotics prepared using 3D printing are not only lightweight but also strong, durable, attractive and comfortable.

12.5 HEALTH MONITORING AND DRUG DELIVERY

Medical microdevices are placed inside the body and function either to monitor patient's health or to deliver medicine, and this is possible because of AM. MIT and their collaborators have developed an ingestible and self-powered device, which can last for a month in the stomach. It can be used in the treatment of cancer or HIV, and it delivers calculated doses of drugs for patients requiring continuing care. These microdevices can revolutionize the procedure of health monitoring and can thus transmit internal data externally to a wearable medical device. Blood glucose levels, blood oxygenation and other parameters can be actively monitored by printed biosensors, which can be injected into the bloodstream, reducing the response time and thus improving the medical condition of patients [1,2] (Figure 12.4).

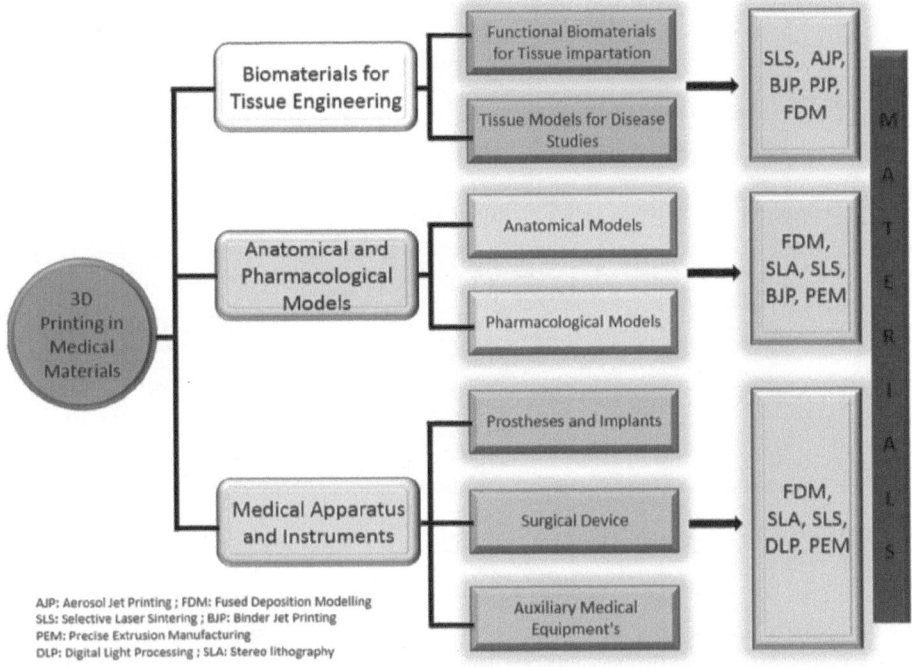

FIGURE 12.4   3D printing in medical materials.

12.6   APPLICATION IN MEDICAL MATERIALS

12.6.1   FUNCTIONAL BIOMATERIALS FOR TISSUE ENGINEERING

Three-dimensional (3D) printing offers great potential in tissue engineering, which uses tissue scaffold to fabricate functional and viable organs. In medical science, 3D printing with tissue engineering has focused on two aspects, one is biomaterials required for tissue implantation, and the other is tissue models for diseased states. Here, we will discuss biomaterials used to fabricate scaffolds that are assisted by AM technologies. Scaffolds are the external supports, and they are important for cell migration, attachment, proliferation and formation of new tissue.

An ideal tissue engineering scaffold should be bioactive, biocompatible, and have adequate mechanical properties. For filling tissue or fixation, basic medical scaffolds are usually used, and thus such scaffolds do not require bioactivity, but the implantable scaffolds used in tissue engineering should be biodegradable as palingenetic tissues would replace them eventually [2,4–6]. Moulding, freeze drying, and electrospinning techniques of the traditional method are still followed to activate tissue or growth of bone inside the scaffolds in the 3D-printing-enabled tissue engineering.

12.6.2   ANATOMICAL AND PHARMACOLOGICAL MODELS

All the studies undertaken to understand the mechanism of diseases, clinical trials of new drugs, preclinical therapy and their effectiveness, and anatomical structures

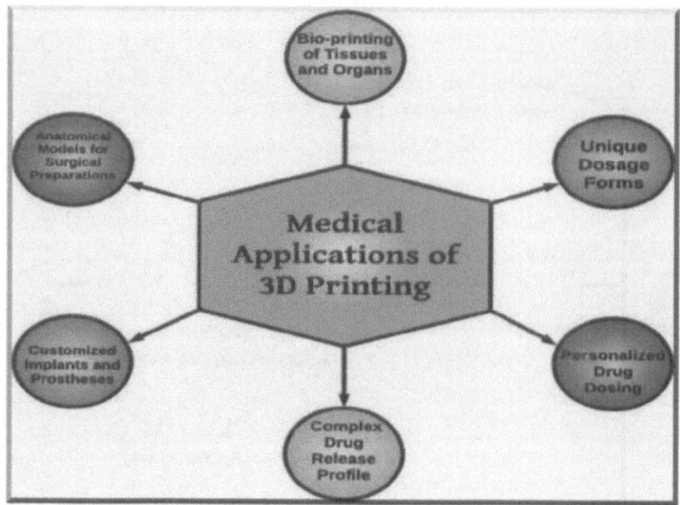

FIGURE 12.5 Different medical areas benefiting from 3D-printing technology.

of body parts and organs, have been transformed by three-dimensional (3D) printing models. In conventional methods, such studies are carried out on a number of mice and other experiment animals, which form the basis of animal modelling. For example, to study and understand patient-derived xenograft (PDX) models, we need to make many mice immune deficient to engraft diseased cells, which requires lots of time and money. These shortcomings were overcome by using tissue models using traditional fabrication, but the products exhibited inexact models with impracticable tissue status [7]. The biomimetic tissue models fabricated using 3D printing are much more cost efficient and have higher resolution than models developed using older techniques [8] (Figure 12.5).

12.6.3 MEDICAL APPARATUS AND INSTRUMENTS

AM is a novel technique when used in the production of healthcare devices and offers a number of advantages in comparison with traditional manufacturing techniques. The medical apparatus is fabricated and custom-designed through the clinical images of patients, making it more accurate and efficient [9]. One of the most significant advantages of this technique is that it gives anatomical fitness to patients and surgical safety to surgeons. With conventional techniques, complex microstructures cannot be manufactured, but this is possible through AM. With these advantages, AM allows rapid production with high resolution, along with a reduction in cost and wastage.

12.7 CONCLUSION

AM plays an exceptional role in developing products. It not only helps in the rapid development of products but is also useful in cutting costs and turnaround time. Using computer design and modelling, rapid fabrication of a physical part, model or assembly can be done. The potentiality of AM in applications such as reverse engineering, e-manufacturing processes, rapid tooling, product design and development in the field of medicine is immense. It also plays a significant role in imparting medical education and training, customising, designing and developing medical devices and implants, scaffolding, prostheses and orthotics, mechanical bone replicas, and forensics. AM can help resolve various medical problems with customised solutions and is thus a boon to humankind.

REFERENCES

1. Liaw CY, Guvendiren M. Current and emerging applications of 3D printing in medicine. *Biofabrication* 2017;9(2):024102.
2. Hoang D, Perrault D, Stevanovic M, Ghiassi A. Surgical applications of three-dimensional printing: A review of the current literature & how to get started. *Annals of Translational Medicine* 2016;4(23):456:1–19.
3. Hutmacher DW. Scaffolds in tissue engineering bone and cartilage. *Biomaterials* 2000;21 (24):2529–2543.
4. Singh S, Ramakrishna S, Singh R. Material issues in additive manufacturing: A review. *Journal of Manufacturing Processes* 2017;25:185–200.
5. Derakhshanfar S, Mbeleck R, Xu K, Zhang X, Zhong W, Xing M. 3D bioprinting for biomedical devices and tissue engineering: A review of recent trends and advances. *Bioactive Materials* 2018;3(2):144–156.
6. Nagarajan N, Dupret-Bories A, Karabulut E, Zorlutuna P, Vrana NE. Enabling personalized implant and controllable biosystem development through 3D printing. *Biotechnology Advances* 2018;36(2):521–533.
7. Placone JK, Engler AJ. Recent advances in extrusion-based 3D printing for biomedical applications. *Advanced Healthcare Materials* 2018;7(8):1701161.
8. Poomathi N, Singh S, Prakash C, Patil RV, Perumal PT, Barathi VA, Balasubramian KK, Ramakrishna S, Maheshwari NU. Bioprinting in ophthalmology: Current advances and future pathways. *Rapid Prototyping Journal* 2018;25(3):496–514.
9. Youssef A, Hollister SJ, Dalton PD. Additive manufacturing of polymer melts for implantable medical devices and scaffolds. *Biofabrication* 2017;9(1):012002.
10. Akmal JS, Salmi M, Mäkitie A, Björkstrand R, Partanen J. Implementation of industrial additive manufacturing: intelligent implants and drug delivery systems. *Journal of Functional Biomaterials* 2018;9(3):41.
11. Banga HK, Kalra P, Belokar RM, Kumar R. Customized design and additive manufacturing of kids' ankle foot orthosis. *Rapid Prototyping Journal*, Vol. ahead-of-print No. ahead-of-print. https://doi.org/10.1108/RPJ-07-2019-0194
12. Banga HK, Kalra P, Belokar RM, Kumar R. Design and fabrication of prosthetic and orthotic product by 3D printing online first. *IntechOpen* 2020. doi: 10.5772/intechopen.94846. Available from: https://www.intechopen.com/online-first/design-and-fabrication-of-prosthetic-and-orthotic-product-by-3d-printing.
13. Banga HK, Kalra P, Belokar RM, Kumar R (2020). 'Effect of 3D-Printed Ankle Foot Orthosis During Walking of Foot Deformities Patients'. In: Kumar H., Jain P. (eds) *Recent Advances in Mechanical Engineering*. Lecture Notes in Mechanical Engineering. Springer, Singapore, pp. 275–288.
14. Banga HK, Kalra P, Belokar RM, Kumar R. (2020). Role of finite element analysis in customized design of kid's orthotic product'. In: Singh S., Prakash C., Singh R. (eds) *Characterization, Testing, Measurement, and Metrology*, pp. 139–159 CRC Press Taylor & Francis Group, USA.

15. Banga HK, Kalra P, Belokar RM, Kumar R (2020). Improvement of human gait in foot deformities patients by 3D printed ankle–foot orthosis. In: Singh S., Prakash C., Singh R. (eds) *3D Printing in Biomedical Engineering*. Materials Horizons: From Nature to Nanomaterials. Springer, Singapore.

16. Banga HK, Kalra P, Belokar RM, Kumar R. Fabrication and stress analysis of ankle foot orthosis with additive manufacturing. *Rapid Prototyping Journal* 2018;24(2):300–312.

17. Banga HK, Kalra P, Belokar RM, Kumar R. Rapid prototyping applications in medical sciences. *International Journal of Emerging Technologies in Computational and Applied Sciences (IJETCAS)* 2014;5(8):416–420.

18. Banga HK, Belokar RM, Kumar R. A Novel Approach For Ankle Foot Orthosis Developed By Three Dimensional Technologies, *3rd International Conference on Mechanical Engineering and Automation Science (ICMEAS 2017)*, University of Birmingham, UK 2017, Vol. 8 No. 10, pp. 141–145.

19. Poukens J, Laeven P, Beerens M, Nijenhuis G, Sloten JV, Stoelinga P, Kessler P. A classification of cranial implants based on the degree of difficulty in computer design and manufacture. *The International Journal of Medical Robotics and Computer Assisted Surgery* 2008;4(1):46–50.

20. Xu N, Wei F, Liu X, Jiang L, Cai H, Li Z, Yu M, Wu F, Liu Z. Reconstruction of the upper cervical spine using a personalized 3D-printed vertebral body in an adolescent with Ewing sarcoma. *Spine* 2016;41(1):E50–E54.

21. Salmi M Possibilities of preoperative medical models made by 3D printing or additive manufacturing. *Journal of Medical Engineering* 2016;1–6.

22. Gibson I, Cheung LK, Chow SP, Cheung WL, Beh SL, Savalani M, Lee SH. The use of rapid prototyping to assist medical applications. *Rapid Prototyping Journal* 2006;12:53–58.

23. Jones DB, Sung R, Weinberg C, Korelitz T, Andrews R. Three-dimensional modeling may improve surgical education and clinical practice. *Surgical Innovation* 2016;23(2):189–195.

24. Randazzo M, Pisapia JM, Singh N, Thawani JP. 3D printing in neurosurgery: a systematic review. *Surgical Neurology International* 2016;7(Suppl 33):S801.

25. Guidance FD. *Technical Considerations for Additive Manufactured Medical Devices*. New Hampshire, NH, USA, Food and Drug Administration 2017.

26. Javaid M, Haleem A. Additive manufacturing applications in medical cases: A literature based review. *Alexandria Journal of Medicine* 2018;54(4):411–422.

27. Ahn DG, Lee JY, Yang DY. Rapid prototyping and reverse engineering application for orthopedic surgery planning. *Journal of Mechanical Science and Technology* 2006; 20(1):19.

28. Ahn SH, Lee CS, Jeong W. Development of translucent FDM parts by post-processing. *Rapid Prototyping Journal* 2004 Sep 1.

29. Azari A, Nikzad S. The evolution of rapid prototyping in dentistry: A review. *Rapid Prototyping Journal* 2009 May 29.

30. Balazic M, Kopac J. Improvements of medical implants based on modern materials and new technologies. *Journal of Achievements in Materials and Manufacturing Engineering* 2007;25(2):31–34.

31. Pham CB, Leong KF, Lim TC, Chian KS. Rapid freeze prototyping technique in bioplotters for tissue scaffold fabrication. *Rapid Prototyping Journal* 2008 Aug 1.

13 Additive Manufacturing Market Prognosis of Medical Devices in the International Arena

Soumendra Darbar
Jadavpur University, Kolkata, India
Deys Medical Stores (Mfg.) Ltd., Kolkata, India

Srimoyee Saha
Jadavpur University, Kolkata, India

Sangita Agarwal
RCC Institute of Information Technology, Kolkata, India

CONTENTS

13.1   INTRODUCTION

Three-dimensional (3D) printing is also known as additive manufacturing and as the name suggests it is used to create 3D pattern. The international market for additive manufacturing (AM) is expected to increase many times over. The market is expanding due to the adoption of process automation solutions and focus on emerging industries' on-demand manufacturing and customisation. The rapid growth and expansion in the automotive, healthcare, aerospace, defence, and consumer electronics industries

DOI: 10.1201/9781003301066-13

TABLE 13.1

Forecast: Countries Dominating the AM Market in Healthcare Between 2020 and 2027 (Wallis et al., 2020)

North America	Europe	Asia Pacific	Latin America	Middle East & Africa
a. The U.S.	a. UK	a. India	a. Brazil	a. South Africa
b. Cana	b. Germany	b. Japan	b. Mexic	b. Saudi Arabia
	c. France	c. China	c. Argentina	c. UAE
	d. Spain	d. Australia	d. Colombia	
	e. Italy	e. South Korea		

are propellers in the business growth of the AM market globally. There is a significant increase in demand for medical and dental care which is responsible for the boosting market of AM (Douroumis, 2019). It is projected that the AM market in the Asia Pacific region would grow at the rate of 15.7 per cent between 2019 and 2027, the reason being that these regions have a large consumer base with rising disposable income and untapped market (Report Linker, 2020). The market expansion potential of the AM in the developing Asia Pacific market may be attributed to automotive, direct healthcare and allied healthcare manufacturing industries (De Mori et al., 2018; Jamróz, et al., 2018). The forecast of countries which would be dominating the AM market in the healthcare sector between 2020 and 2027 is given in Table 13.1.

The segments of the AM market are based on end-user industry, material types, technology, and geographical regions. The AM market is classified into automotive, healthcare, dental and other industries based on end-user. Depending on the type of materials used in the production of components the global market is designated as plastic, metal alloy, ceramic, rubber, glass and others. Out of these material types, the use of plastic is unparalleled because of its cost-effectiveness in comparison with other material types (Gopinathan & Noh, 2018). The regions are differentiated as the United States, Canada, European territory, Asia Pacific, and the Rest of the World. The material-wise revenue share of the 3D-printing market in healthcare is given in Figure 13.1.

13.2 FUTURE MARKET FOR ADDITIVE MANUFACTURING (AM)

In the year 2018, the global AM market generated revenues amounting to $9.3 billion. As iterated by professionals working in the field of the healthcare market would grow unprecedentedly with an expected average expansion of 20-25 per cent by the year 2025 (Gnanasekaran et al., 2017). Healthcare sectors demand simple as well as complex designs which can be accomplished by this manufacturing technique. Conventional technology like milling, machining and others are being replaced by emerging simple and complex techniques of AM. It is a powerful and beneficial technology that can reduce wastage and hazards developed out of the older technique (Albanna et al., 2019; Ding & Chang, 2018). The substantial previous costs associated with the usual health and allied manufacturing processes are reduced by making prototypes using 3D CAD. The expansion of the wholesale AM international market over the years since 2015 is given in Figure 13.2.

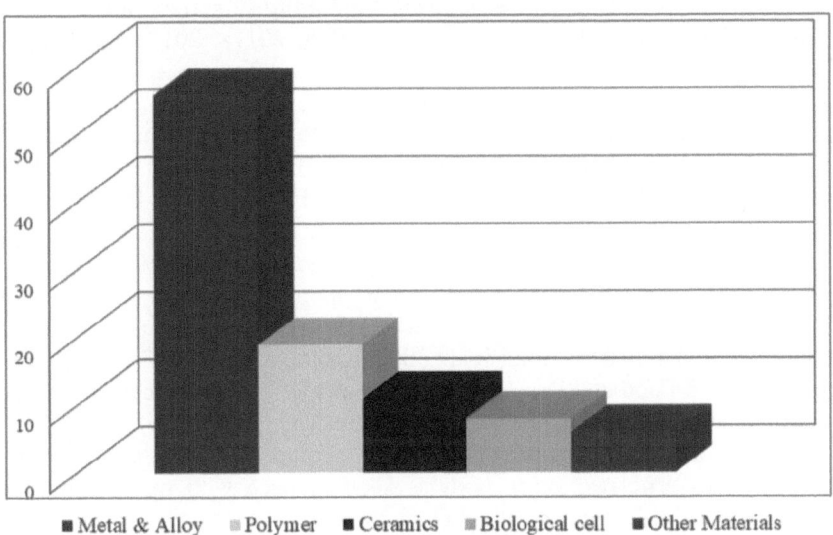

FIGURE 13.1 The material-wise revenue share of 3D-printing market in healthcare sector (Ricles et al., 2018).

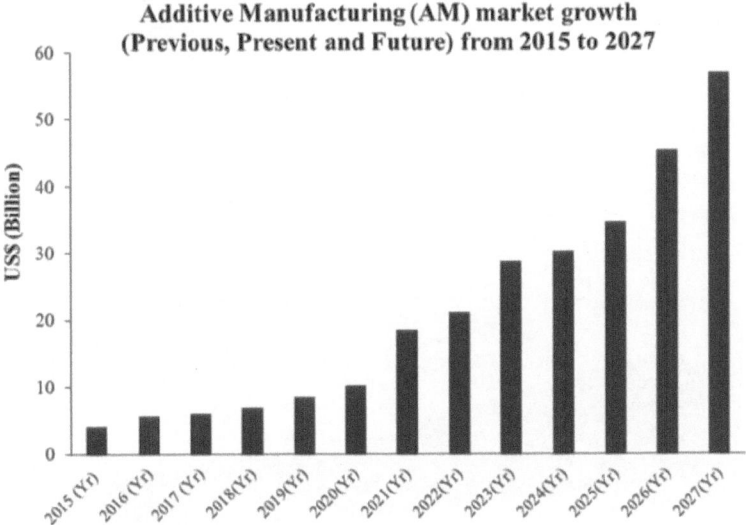

FIGURE 13.2 AM market growth (past, present and future) (Herderick 2016).

The field of medical tools manufacturing has been revolutionised by the usage of AM, which has created high demand, increased efficiency, and at a lower cost. The fabrication of outhouses, prostheses, dental implants, tissues, organs and other medical components now has switched over from conventional manufacturing to

3D-printing technology. The healthcare sector, which is ever demanding and has unfulfilled requirements because of the rise in new diseases, the pervasiveness of chronic disorders, and an increase in patients requiring surgeries, would be propelling the market growth (Banga et al., 2014, 2018, 2017a, 2017b, 2020a, 2020b, 2020c, 2020d, 2020e, 2021).

After patents expire, control of the original inventor is lost and the cost of the product is reduced, becoming affordable for all-both buyers and manufacturers. For example, in 2009 the fused deposition modelling (FDM) printing technique became off-patent, which led to a reduction in the price of FDM printers. User-friendly 3D printers were launched by Ultimaker and MakerBot at a low cost.

Technologies like liquid-based stereolithography, elective & selective lower sintering-2014 etc. are being used for multifarious applications of the same technology at a low cost. Hence the growth of the market is enhanced by the usage of 3D CAD (Derakhshanfar et al., 2018; Hölzl et al., 2016; Kirillova et al., 2017). The guidelines issued by the US Food and Drug Administration (FDA) on technical considerations specific to devices using AM, encompassing three-dimensional (3D) printing, outline considerations and recommendations for testing equipment and characterisation of medical devices. The regulatory body is keeping pace with rapid technological growth allows for efficient and safe manufacturing.

Classification of the global AM market is centred on applications, for use in the healthcare sector as medical devices, use in the automotive industry, and aerospace science. This manufacturing market is also categorised as concerned with the technology used such as 3D printing, laser sintering, stereolithography, fused modelling, electron beam melting (Figure 13.3) and tissue engineering (Invernizzi et al., 2018).

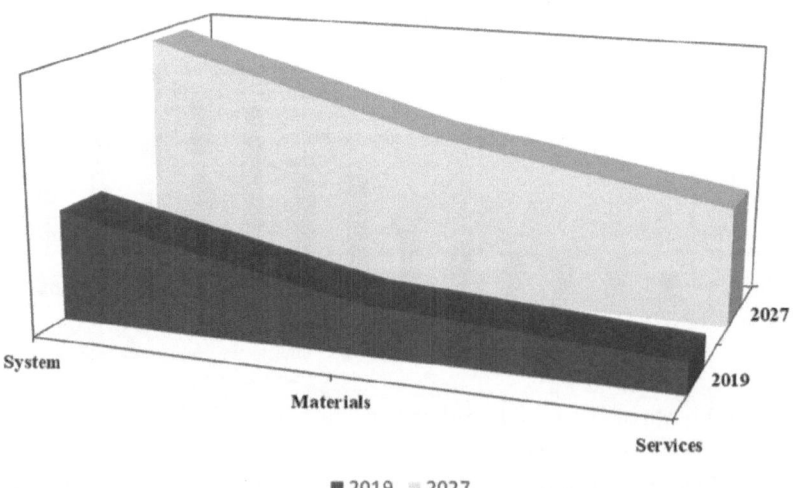

Global 3D Printing Healthcare Market (By Component)

FIGURE 13.3 Global 3D-printing healthcare market by component (2019 and 2027) (Hamdaoui et al., 2019).

Based on the type of material used in manufacturing, the global AM market is classified as homogeneous and heterogeneous. The global 3D-printing healthcare market by component is given in Figure 13.3 for the year 2019 and the year 2027 (predicted).

The global controlling authority US FDA takes an initiative to review the marketed products manufactured using 3D printers. The US FDA has been actively involved in understanding the technology to provide a broader regulatory pathway that keeps pace with the technological advancements and aids efficient access to safe and effective innovations enabled by AM (Belhouideg, 2020; Tarfaoui et al., 2020; Haq et al., 2020; Wesemann et al., 2020).

13.3   GLOBAL HEALTHCARE TRENDS AND OPPORTUNITIES OF 3D-PRINTING MARKET

The global AM market is classified based on applications such as medical devices, automotive and aerospace. This manufacturing market is further bifurcated based on technology such as 3D printing, stereolithography, fused deposition modelling, laser sintering, exposition modelling, electron beam melting and tissue engineering (Invernizzi et al., 2018). On the other hand, based on material type, the global AM market is segmented as homogeneous and heterogeneous with the support of systems and services (Figure 13.4).

3D-printing technology has played a pivotal role in the up-gradation of the existing healthcare sector, benefiting both medical professionals and patients. Globally, 3D-printing technology has gained popularity which has augmented its use in the medical field. Joint replacement remains the largest segment in the market of medical implants throughout the globe. The number of hip and knee replacements has increased rapidly worldwide which is the key factor in fuelling the demand for this

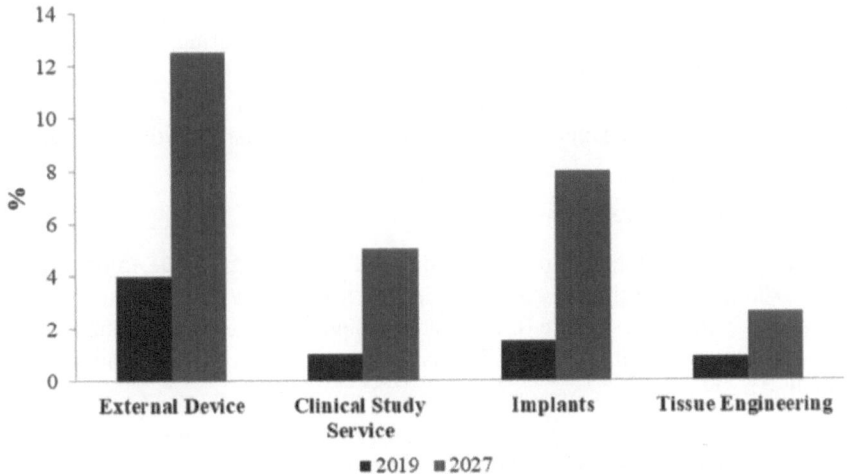

FIGURE 13.4   Global 3D-printing healthcare market by application (2019 and 2027) (Singh et al., 2020).

printing technology. Manufactures using this technology are customised based on individual needs with high-quality products at low cost and would be generating good revenues in the future (Gao et al., 2016).

13.4   GLOBAL HEALTHCARE MARKET POTENTIAL OF 3D-PRINTING MARKET

3D printing in the global healthcare market has created lots of opportunities and scope for improved research and development and testing within the medical field, which has caused a significant impact on the growth of the global healthcare 3D market. Moreover, the need to develop the blueprint using personalised digital data has also generated demand within the global healthcare 3D market (Wu, Huang, Zhao & Xie, 2018).

13.5   GLOBAL HEALTHCARE 3D-MARKET: COMPETITIVE LANDSCAPE

A scientific market survey report on various established companies like Bio-Rad Laboratories, SOLS, Organovo, Simbionix, Regen HU Ltd and Metamason threw light upon current and future growth prospects, untapped avenues, factors shaping their revenue potential, and demand and consumption patterns in the context of the world economy. Countries, mainly the United States of America, European territory, North America, Latin America, Asia Pacific, the Middle East and Africa, have the resources to flourish as the next generation marketing launch pads which solidify the economical pillars of medical tool manufacturing. (Haleem & Javaid, 2019; Miao et al., 2017).

13.5.1   Technology-Based Insights

The medical device AM market is segmented into laser sintering, stereolithography, electron beam melting, and extrusion-based on technology. The laser-sintering segment occupied the largest share of the market in2019; high mechanical performances and mature processing chains are responsible for spectacular growth in this segment.

13.5.2   Product-Based Insights

All implants and prosthetics, surgical guides and instruments, tissue engineering and other products are classified as products in the medical device jargon using AM. In the year 2019, the largest share of the medical device market was grabbed by surgical instruments but the highest CAGR was registered by the implants and prosthetics segment.

13.5.3   Application-Based Insights

The AM market for mainly medical devices is categorised into orthopaedic, dental, bioengineering and craniomaxillofacial surgical solutions based on this application.

TABLE 13.2

Different Segments Flourishing in the Healthcare Sector of AM Market Between 2020 and 2027

Technology	Products	Application	Material
1. Stereolithography	1. Implants and Prosthetics	1. Prosthetics	1. Polymers
2. Leaser Sintering	2. Surgical Instruments	2. Medical Implant	2. Biological Cells
3. Deposition Modelling	3. Surgical Guide	3. Tissue Engineering	3. Metal & Alloys
4. Electron Beam Melting	4. Tissue Engineering	4. Wearable Devices	4. Others
5. Laminated Object Manufacturing	5. Other products	5. Others	
6. Jetting Technology			
7. Others			

In the year 2019, the largest share of the medical device market was held by the orthopaedic segment which at the same time registered the highest CAGR (16.7 per cent) in the market. The global 3D-printing healthcare market by application is given in Figure 13.4 for the year 2019 and the year 2027 (predicted) (Banga et al., 2014, 2018, 2017a, 2017b, 2020a, 2020b, 2020c, 2020d, 2020e, 2021).

13.5.4 STRATEGIC INSIGHTS

Companies are expanding their global footprints and product portfolios by time-tested adopted strategies like new product launches, mergers and acquisitions which allows them to meet the growing consumer demand. Out of all major strategies undertaken by AM medical device makers, with new product launches (they are successfully able to enlarge their customer bases and continue to retain their presence globally) (Table 13.2).

13.6 CONCLUSION

AM and its newly developed technology dominate the medical field like regenerative medicine, diagnosis, implants, artificial tissues and organs in the future. Three-dimensional (3D) and four-dimensional (4D) printing technology can generate very effective innovative products, through R&D development, that are performance-based, low risk, and cost-effective. In this century, AM machinery and technology have grown enormously in the manufacture of innovative and high potential new drug formulations, biosensor-based feedback devices, personalised prostheses, implants, advanced diagnostics, and bioprinting of human organs and tissues and has demonstrated that it can play a key role in the advanced development of new equipment's and materials. The world is fully confident about the success of AM technology and holds out hope that in the future medical treatment will become highly personalised with patient-specific treatments, but more research and development are required.

REFERENCES

Albanna, Mohammed, Binder, Kyle W, Murphy, Sean V, Kim, Jaehyun, Qasem, Shadi A, Zhao, Weixin, Marco, Julie. (2019). In situ bioprinting of autologous skin cells accelerates wound healing of extensive excisional full-thickness wounds. *Scientific Reports*, 9(1), 1–15.

Banga, H.K., Belokar, R.M., & Kumar R. (2017b). A Novel Approach For Ankle Foot Orthosis Developed By Three Dimensional Technologies. *3rd International Conference on Mechanical Engineering and Automation Science (ICMEAS 2017)*, University of Birmingham, UK. Vol. 8 No. 10, pp. 141–145.

Banga H. K., Belokar, R.M., Madan, R., & Dhole S. (2017a). Three dimensional Gait assessments during walking of healthy people and drop foot patients. *Defence Life Science Journal*, 2, 14–20.

Banga, H.K., Kalra, P., Belokar, R.M. and Kumar, R. (2020a). Customized design and additive manufacturing of kids' ankle foot orthosis. *Rapid Prototyping Journal*, 26(10). https://doi.org/10.1108/RPJ-07-2019-0194

Banga, H.K., Kalra, P., Belokar, R.M. and Kumar, R. (2020b). Design and Fabrication of Prosthetic and Orthotic Product by 3D Printing [Online First], *IntechOpen*. doi:10.5772/intechopen.94846. Available from: https://www.intechopen.com/online-first/design-and-fabrication-of-prosthetic-and-orthotic-product-by-3d-printing.

Banga H.K., Kalra P., Belokar R.M., Kumar R. (2020c). Effect of 3D-printed ankle foot orthosis during walking of foot deformities patients. In: Kumar H., Jain P. (eds) *Recent Advances in Mechanical Engineering*. Lecture Notes in Mechanical Engineering. Springer, Singapore, pp. 275–288.

Banga H.K., Kalra P., Belokar R.M., Kumar R. (2020d) Role of finite element analysis in customized design of kid's orthotic product. In: Singh S., Prakash C., Singh R. (eds) *Characterization, Testing, Measurement, and Metrology*, pp. 139–159. CRC Press Taylor & Francis Group, USA.

Banga H.K., Kalra P., Belokar R.M., Kumar R. (2020e). Improvement of human gait in foot deformities patients by 3D printed ankle–foot orthosis. In: Singh S., Prakash C., Singh R. (eds) *3D Printing in Biomedical Engineering*. Materials Horizons: From Nature to Nanomaterials. Springer, Singapore.

Banga, H.K., Kumar P, Kumar H. (2021). Utilization of additive manufacturing in orthotics and prosthetic devices development. *IOP Conference Series: Materials Science and Engineering*. https://doi.org/10.1088/1757-899X/1033/1/012083

Banga, H.K., Parveen, K., Belokar, R.M., & Kumar R. (2014). Rapid Prototyping Applications in Medical Sciences. *International Journal of Emerging Technologies in Computational and Applied Sciences (IJETCAS)*, 5(8), 416–420.

Banga, H.K., Parveen, K., & Belokar, R.M., Kumar, R. (2018). Fabrication and stress analysis of ankle foot orthosis with additive manufacturing. *Rapid Prototyping Journal Emerald Publishing*, 24(2), 300–312.

Belhouideg, S. (2020). Impact of 3D printed medical equipment on the management of the Covid19 pandemic. *The International Journal of Health Planning and Management* 35(5), 1014–1022.

De Mori, A., Peña Fernández, M., Blunn, G., Tozzi, G., Roldo, M. (2018). 3D printing and electrospinning of composite hydrogels for cartilage and bone tissue engineering. *Polymers* 10(3), 285.

Derakhshanfar, S., Mbeleck, R., Xu, K., Zhang, X., Zhong, W., Xing, M. (2018). 3D bioprinting for biomedical devices and tissue engineering: A review of recent trends and advances. *Bioactive Materials* 3(2), 144–156.

Du, X., Yu, B., Pei, P., Ding, H., Yu, B., Zhu, Y. (2018). 3D printing of pearl/CaSO$_4$ composite scaffolds for bone regeneration. *Journal of Materials Chemistry* 6(3), 499–509.

Elouali, A., Kousksou, T., El Rhafiki, T., Hamdaoui, S., Mahdaoui, M., Allouhi, A., Zeraouli, Y. (2019). Physical models for packed bed: Sensible heat storage systems. *Journal of Energy Storage* 23:69–78.

Gao, Y., Gao, Z., Sun, W., Hu, Y. (2016). Selective flotation of scheelite from calcite: A novel reagent scheme. *International Journal of Mineral Processing* 154:10–15.

Gnanasekaran, K., Heijmans, T., Van Bennekom, S., Woldhuis, H., Wijnia, S., De With, G., Friedrich, H. (2017). 3D printing of CNT-and graphene-based conductive polymer nanocomposites by fused deposition modeling. *Applied Materials Today* 9, 21–28.

Gopinathan, J., Noh, I. (2018). Recent trends in bioinks for 3D printing. *Biomaterials Research* 22(1), 1–5.

Haleem, A., Javaid, M. (2019). Additive manufacturing applications in industry 4.0: A review. *Journal of Industrial Integration and Management* 4(04), 1–23.

Haq, M.I., Khuroo, S., Raina, A., Khajuria, S., Javaid, M., Haq, M.F., & Haleem, A. (2020). 3D printing for development of medical equipment amidst coronavirus (COVID-19) pandemic: Review and advancements. *Research on Biomedical Engineering* 1, 1–1.

Herderick, E.D. Additive manufacturing in the minerals, metals, and materials community: Past, present, and exciting future. *JOM* 2016 Mar 1;68(3):721–723.

Hölzl, Katja, Lin, Shengmao, Tytgat, Liesbeth, Van Vlierberghe, Sandra, Gu, Linxia, & Ovsianikov, Aleksandr. (2016). Bioink properties before, during and after 3D bioprinting. *Biofabrication*, 8(3), 032002.

Invernizzi, Marta, Turri, Stefano, Levi, Marinella, & Suriano, Raffaella. (2018). 4D printed thermally activated self-healing and shape memory polycaprolactone-based polymers. *European Polymer Journal*, 101, 169–176.

Jamróz, Witold, Szafraniec, Joanna, Kurek, Mateusz, & Jachowicz, Renata. (2018). 3D printing in pharmaceutical and medical applications–recent achievements and challenges. *Pharmaceutical Research*, 35(9), 176.

Kirillova, Alina, Maxson, Ridge, Stoychev, Georgi, Gomillion, Cheryl T, & Ionov, Leonid. (2017). 4D biofabrication using shape-morphing hydrogels. *Advanced Materials*, 29(46), 1703443.

Miao, Shida, Castro, Nathan, Nowicki, Margaret, Xia, Lang, Cui, Haitao, Zhou, Xuan, … Vozzi, Giovanni. (2017). 4D printing of polymeric materials for tissue and organ regeneration. *Materials Today*, 20(10), 577–591.

Report Linker, New York, Aug. 17, 2020 (GLOBE NEWSWIRE) https://www.reportlinker.com/p05896877/?utm_source=GNW

Ricles, L.M., Coburn, J.C., Di Prima, M., & Oh, S.S. (2018). Regulating 3D-printed medical products. *Science Translational Medicine* Oct 3;10(461), 1–6.

Singh, S., Urooj, S., Batra, N., & Kalathil, S. (2020). Healthcare Applications of 3D Printing in Human Implants: A Review. In *2020 IEEE 17th India Council International Conference (INDICON)* Dec 10 (pp. 1–6). IEEE.

Tarfaoui, M., Nachtane, M., Goda, I., Qureshi, Y., & Benyahia, H. (2020) 3D printing to support the shortage in personal protective equipment caused by COVID-19 pandemic. *Materials* Jan;13(15), 3339.

Wallis, M., Al-Dulimi, Z., Tan, D.K., Maniruzzaman, M., & Nokhodchi, A. (2020). 3D printing for enhanced drug delivery: current state-of-the-art and challenges. *Drug Development and Industrial Pharmacy* Sep 1;46(9), 1385–1401.

Wesemann, C., Pieralli, S., Fretwurst, T., Nold, J., Nelson, K., Schmelzeisen, R., Hellwig, E., & Spies, B.C. (2020). 3-D printed protective equipment during COVID-19 pandemic. *Materials* Jan;13(8), 1997.

Wu, Jing-Jun, Huang, Li-Mei, Zhao, Qian, & Xie, Tao. (2018). 4D printing: History and recent progress. *Chinese Journal of Polymer Science*, 36(5), 563–575.

14 Overview of 3D-printing Technology[1]
History, Types, Applications and Materials

Parth K. Patel
Thomas Jefferson University, Philadelphia, USA

CONTENTS

14.1 INTRODUCTION

Formative (moulds) and subtractive (machining) techniques are used in conventional manufacturing. As it involves multiple steps and expensive infrastructure, the ability to make timely changes to the final product is limited. Besides, it is extremely difficult, or even impossible, to create intricate and complex designs using traditional manufacturing techniques (Ahangar, Cooke, Weber, & Rosenzweig, 2019). However, since the last few decades, the advent of novel additive manufacturing (AM) technology has proved to be a boon to several industries to develop beneficial products for humankind AM is an umbrella that encompasses a wide array of technologies and is often known by several names, such as freeform fabrication, layer-based manufacturing, three-dimensional (3D) printing, solid freedom fabrication, rapid prototyping, additive layered manufacturing, rapid manufacturing and additive fabrication (Azam, Abdul Rani, Altaf, Rao, & Zaharin, 2018). According to the American Society for Testing and Materials (ASTM) F2792, AM is officially defined as the 'process of joining materials to make objects from three-dimensional (3D) model data, usually layer upon layer, as opposed to subtractive manufacturing methodologies' (ASTM International, 2013). In simple words, it unites materials layer by layer to form a 3D object. Computer-aided design (CAD) software is used to create the final design of a 3D-printed object (Gu, Fu, Lin, & He, 2020; Joshi & Sheikh, 2015; Tan, Maniruzzaman, & Nokhodchi, 2018). As the 3D-printing industry has progressed rapidly, it has gained more attention in the last decade in many fields, including engineering, medicine, education and manufacturing. To justify this, by glancing at Figure 14.1, it is pretty apparent that AM has been at the forefront for the last decade. Researchers and scientists from various domains have shifted their attention towards 3D-printing technology because of its versatile applications. 3D manufacturing

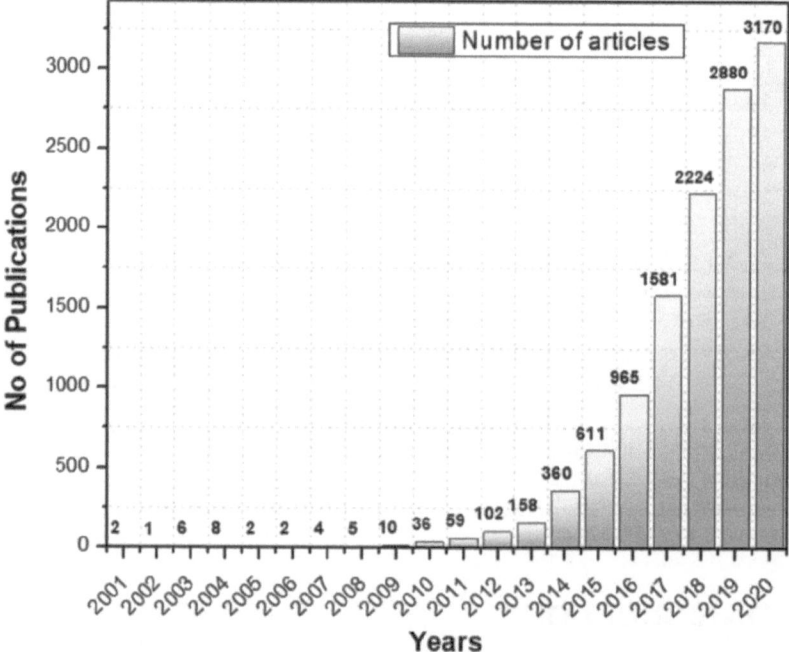

FIGURE 14.1   Number of publications in Web of Science database on additive manufacturing (Source: WoS).

techniques offer several advantages over conventional techniques, such as high precision, low cost, minimising the wastage of raw materials, fabrication of complex geometry, and personal customisation (Ngo, Kashani, Imbalzano, Nguyen, & Hui, 2018). Therefore, this chapter aims to provide an overview of several aspects of 3D printing, including the historical aspects of 3D printing, and highlighting the prominent inventions and advances that have taken place in 3D printing. The next section deals with the different techniques of 3D printing, followed by various types of material used, and finally, the applications of 3D printing in several industries.

14.2   HISTORY

In the late twentieth century, the development of advanced CAD software revolutionised design, computer-assisted fabrication, and prototyping (Savini & Savini, 2015). At the Nagoya Municipal Industrial Research Institute in Japan, Hideo Kodama developed the first rapid prototyping technique. In 1980 he filed a patent application for his work, but it expired before it could be pursued further in the patent process. He published several papers in 1980 and 1981 detailing the invention of methods for automatically fabricating three-dimensional models using UV rays and a photosensitive resin, later known as stereolithography (SLA) (Su & Al'Aref, 2018).

Finally, it came into the limelight in 1984, when the SLA apparatus was launched by Charles Hull. However, this concept was previously known and reported by experiments of Hideo Kodema and a French patent by Alain Le Méhauté and his colleagues (Jakus, 2019). He patented this SLA concept in 1986 that explained the process of polymerisation. When photopolymerisable resin was exposed to UV light, it resulted upon solidification in the formation of cross-sections of a 3D model. After two years, he co-founded 3D Systems Corporation, which is considered to be one of the most popular and largest organisations in both medical and nonmedical markets today (Madla, Trenfield, Goyanes, Gaisford, & Basit, 2018; Provaggi & Kalaskar, 2017; Su & Al'Aref, 2018). Further, Hull went on to develop the STL file format which would 'complete the electronic "handshake" from CAD software and transmit files for the printing of 3D objects'. 3D Systems and Hull produced the first commercial SLA printer in the world, SLA-250 (Gross, Erkal, Lockwood, Chen, & Spence, 2014). Carl Deckard, a graduate student at the University of Texas, invented and patented the selective laser sintering (SLS)"technique in 1988 after closely following Hull's patent. He established Desktop Manufacturing Corporation (DTM Corp) in 1992, which manufactured the first SLS printer (Olusegun et al., 2012).

The year 1988 also witnessed the invention of another technology called fused deposition modelling (FDM) by Scott Crump. FDM played an integral role in establishing the company known as Stratasys Ltd, which Crump co-founded with his wife Lisa in 1989. In 1992, he received a patent for his invention. In 2012, Stratasys collaborated with Objet Ltd, an Israeli 3D printer manufacturer (Matias & Rao, 2015; Savini & Savini, 2015). For the first time, MIT Professor Michael J. Cima used the term '3D printing' in 1993 and, along with his co-workers, developed and patented an inkjet-based 3D printer for printing ceramics, metals and polymers. Later this patent was commercialised by Z Corporation (Emanuel M. Sachs, Haggerty, & Cima, 1993; Savini & Savini, 2015). For nearly two decades during this period, 3D-printing

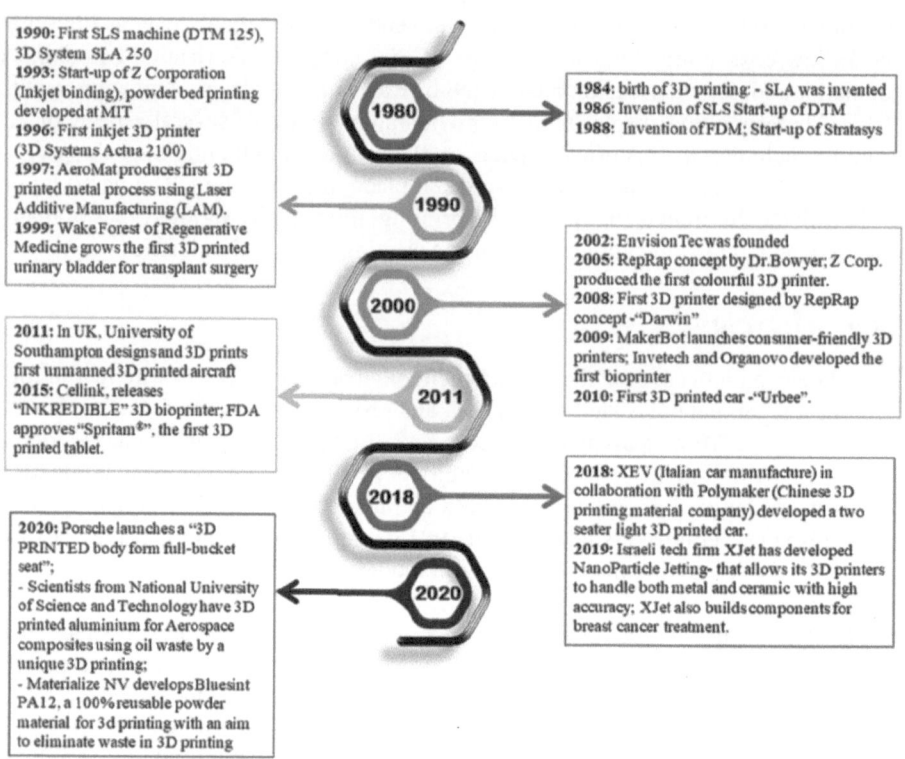

1990: First SLS machine (DTM 125), 3D System SLA 250
1993: Start-up of Z Corporation (Inkjet binding), powder bed printing developed at MIT
1996: First inkjet 3D printer (3D Systems Actua 2100)
1997: AeroMat produces first 3D printed metal process using Laser Additive Manufacturing (LAM).
1999: Wake Forest of Regenerative Medicine grows the first 3D printed urinary bladder for transplant surgery

2011: In UK, University of Southampton designs and 3D prints first unmanned 3D printed aircraft
2015: Cellink, releases "INKREDIBLE" 3D bioprinter; FDA approves "Spritam®", the first 3D printed tablet.

2020: Porsche launches a "3D PRINTED body form full-bucket seat";
- Scientists from National University of Science and Technology have 3D printed aluminium for Aerospace composites using oil waste by a unique 3D printing;
- Materialize NV develops Bluesint PA12, a 100% reusable powder material for 3d printing with an aim to eliminate waste in 3D printing

1984: birth of 3D printing: - SLA was invented
1986: Invention of SLS Start-up of DTM
1988: Invention of FDM; Start-up of Stratasys

2002: EnvisionTec was founded
2005: RepRap concept by Dr.Bowyer; Z Corp. produced the first colourful 3D printer.
2008: First 3D printer designed by RepRap concept -"Darwin"
2009: MakerBot launches consumer-friendly 3D printers; Invetech and Organovo developed the first bioprinter
2010: First 3D printed car -"Urbee".

2018: XEV (Italian car manufacture) in collaboration with Polymaker (Chinese 3D printing material company) developed a two seater light 3D printed car.
2019: Israeli tech firm XJet has developed NanoParticle Jetting- that allows its 3D printers to handle both metal and ceramic with high accuracy; XJet also builds components for breast cancer treatment.

FIGURE 14.2 Timeline chart of major events and advances in the history of 3D-printing technology from 1980 to 2020.

technology advanced rapidly, and the advances and inventions were mostly used by designers and engineers in the business world. However, in 2005, this trend shifted with the launch of Dr Adrian Bowyer's RepRap project, which aimed to make AM technology accessible to everyone. Another 3D-printing company, MakerBot®, was founded in 2009 by three ardent RepRap project participants, Bre Pettis, Adam Mayer, and Zach 'Hoeken' Smith, to familiarise and narrow the gap between consumers and emerging 3D-printing technology. It is the world's first 3D-printing company to produce and market consumer 3D printers that are affordable, accessible and simple to use. They introduced their first 3D printer, Cupcake CNC, in 2009, and after being acquired by Stratasys in 2013, they released their first Wi-Fi connected fifth generation desktop 3D printers in 2014, with a swappable smart extruder (MakerBot, 2016; Matias & Rao, 2015). Figure 14.2 illustrates the plethora of inventions and advances in 3D-printing technology over the years.

14.3 TECHNIQUES

After considering the broad historical background, it becomes essential to understand the common and emerging techniques in the field of AM. This section introduces

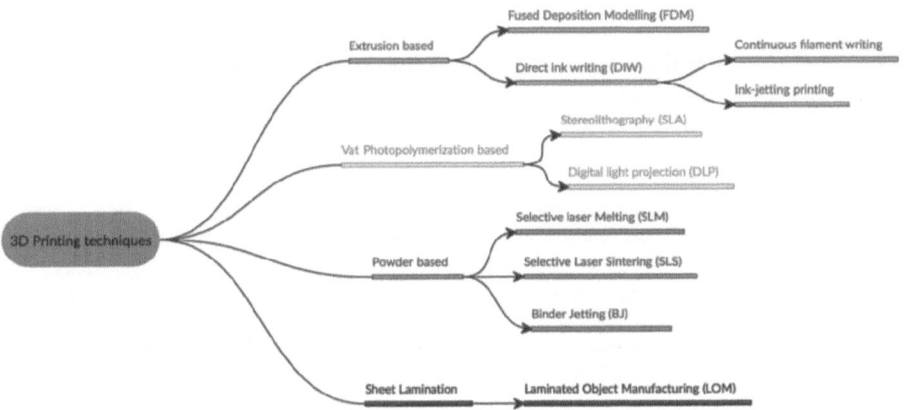

FIGURE 14.3 Schematic representation of various 3D-printing techniques.

the reader to different AM techniques and provides the fundamentals and functional understanding of the entire process to better understand the applications. However, there are many ways by which 3D-printing techniques can be classified, such as the physical state of the raw materials used, mechanism of layering,"and many more. One of the simplest classifications is illustrated in Figure 14.3 and discussed further. Table 14.1 summarises the advantages and disadvantages of AM techniques.

14.3.1 FUSED DEPOSITION MODELLING (FDM)

The FDM process involves melting the raw material or desired polymer and is passed through a heated movable nozzle and deposited layer by layer along the three axes (x-y-z). Once it gets solidified, desired shape object is formed, which was designed with the help of computer-aided models. Factors such as Raster thickness, space and angle play a crucial role in the porosity and shape of the object during the process (Ali, Ahmad, & Akhtar, 2020; Ameeduzzafar et al., 2018).

14.3.2 DIRECT INK WRITING (DIW)

DIW (also called robocasting) is the most flexible AM technique for the development of materials. It allows the production of complex 3D shapes using any raw material by preparing a paste with controlled rheology (Rocha, Saiz, Tirichenko, & García-Tuñón, 2020). It works on a similar principle and mechanism as that of FDM. Nevertheless, it differs from FDM in that it creates and maintains the shape and structure of objects using the rheological properties of inks, rather than drying or solidification when the ink leaves the nozzle. Good rheology for DIW is that of a pseudoplastic fluid, such as a Bingham fluid, which can be extruded at low pressure and maintains its shape after deposition. DIW is distinctive in that it can fabricate 3D-printed objects from almost any type of material, including hydrogels, metal alloys, polymers, biomaterials, ceramics and electronically functional materials. DIW is further classified into two categories: A) continuous filament writing and

TABLE 14.1

The Advantages and Disadvantages of Some Commonly Used 3D-Printing Techniques

Sr. No	3D-Printing Technique	Advantages	Disadvantages
1	SLA	High resolution, excellent print surface quality, nozzle free,	Extensive post-processing required, >1 day of printing time required
2	DLP	More accuracy for designing complex structures as compared to FDM or SLS, low cost as compared to SLA, less waste, rapid process, high resolution	Low drug loading, cytotoxicity due to polymer residues, resins are expensive, parts have worse mechanical properties also they are prone to degradation if left out in the sun
3	FDM	Low cost, open-source designs, a wide variety of thermoplastic materials for printing, minimal maintenance	Lower resolution, poor surface finish, involves manual removal of support structures after processing
4	DIW	Low cost, high volume production, fabrication of porous structures with precision	Poor resolution, low mechanical strength
5	SLS	Printability on metal and delicate structures, can produce complex parts, does not require support structures, excellent precession	Difficult to operate and calibrate, expensive, poor surface finish
6	Sheet lamination	Low cost, high speed	Limited material use, post-processing is required

B) inkjet printing. In continuous filament writing, the inks are continuously extruded from the nozzle, and the filament portion is patterned on a fixed platform for constructing objects, whereas, in inkjet printing, ink is injected drop-by-drop on demand. (Jiang, Ji, Zhang, Liu, & Wang, 2018; Ordoñez, Gallego, & Colorado, 2019)

14.3.3 SELECTIVE LASER SINTERING (SLS)

The substrate in this technique is a powdered material (powdered glass, nylon, polystyrene, ceramics, titanium). The fusion (sintering) of powder occurs when it is bombarded with a laser beam. As a result, each layer of powder is systematically constructed one at a time and the process continues until the final object is developed. The advantage of this technique is that the unsintered powder does not interfere with the process. However, it helps in the formation of the structure being printed by providing support and can later be used for other purposes (Lee Ventola, 2014; Prince, 2014).

14.3.4 VAT POLYMERISATION

Photopolymerisation involves the polymerisation of light-induced materials such as photopolymers, radiation curable resins and liquid. When these materials are exposed to a laser beam source, the liquid photopolymer in the vat or tank solidi-fies. As a result, a 2D patterned structure is formed by several layers one by one. This subfamily of 3D printing includes processes such as SLA and DLP (digital light projection) (Ali et al., 2020; Jakus, 2019; Madla et al., 2018)."A digital micro-mirror device (DMD) is used in DLP technology to reflect and focus UV light on the surfaces of photoreactive materials that polymerise in a layer-by-layer fashion. Using this principle, Kardy et al. successfully formulated modified-release theophyl-line (1 per cent) tablets by using PEGDA and PEGDMA as photoreactive polymers. Different types of tablets were printed with and without perforations. The release rate of the drug improved as the number of perforations increased (Kadry, Wadnap, Xu, & Ahsan, 2019).

14.3.5 SHEET LAMINATION

This technique involves printing a 3D model by stacking a layer of paper, metal or plastic sheet material onto a stage. The sheet is then traced and cut into the desired cross-section using a carbon dioxide laser beam or a razor, according to the (CAD) model. The excess material is discarded, the stage is lowered to deposit the second layer of sheet material, and the process is continued until the required 3D model is formed (Ashish, Ahmad, Gopinath, & Vinogradov, 2019; Gross et al., 2014).

14.4 MATERIALS

14.4.1 POLYMERS

Due to the versatility of polymers and ease of use in different 3D-printing processes, they are commonly used in AM. Photopolymers, resins, reactive monomers and ther-moplastic filaments are among the forms of polymers used for AM. The different types of polymers used for 3D printing are acrylonitrile-butadiene-styrene (ABS) (thermoplastic polymer), Eudragit® L-100, polybutylene terephthalate (PBT), poly-caprolactone (PCL), poly ethylene glycol (PEG), PEG-diacrylate (PEGDA) and polyurethane (PU) (Jang et al., 2018; Mukherjee, Rani, & Saravanan, 2019; Ngo et al., 2018; Tetsuka & Shin, 2020). As polyvinyl alcohol (PVA) has thermoplasticity, it is widely preferred to form polymer multilayers through inkjet printing during the AM process. Beck et al. had prepared a 3D-printed tablet by using poly (caprolac-tone) (PCL) and EudragitRL100 (Afsana, Jain, Haider, & Jain, 2019; Vogt, 2020). Hydrogels are solid polymers with liquid characteristics at the molecular level and are often used as hydrogel-based inks, functional hydrogel scaffolds or tissue-like structures for 3D printing (Azad et al., 2020; He et al., 2016; Heidarian, Kouzani, Kaynak, Paulino, & Nasri-Nasrabadi, 2019).

14.4.2 METALS AND ALLOYS

Stainless steel, austenitic stainless steels, precipitation hardenable stainless steels, and tools steels are among the metallic materials used in the AM process. Their alloys are also sometimes used to achieve high strength and improve the hardness for moulding applications. Aluminium possesses high thermal conductivity, which helps accelerate the 3D printing process; high reflectivity for the laser wavelengths and is widely used in 3D printing. AlSi10Mg and AlSi12 are commonly used alloys. Recently developed methods for printing metals include cold spraying, direct metal writing, and binder jetting (Gonzalez-Gutierrez et al., 2018; Ngo et al., 2018).

14.4.3 CERAMICS

Ceramic materials are made up of a combination of inorganic salts, including phosphate and calcium. They are mainly used for tissue engineering for preparing scaffolds for teeth and bones (Ahangar et al., 2019). Ceramic materials can be used to create complex-shaped lightweight objects. SLS is a common technique employed for 3D printing of ceramic models. The flowability, density, and resolution of the final 3D-printed object are greatly influenced by the particle size distribution, drying, liquid to solid ratio, temperature, air entrapment, and de-binding procedure of ceramics (Ngo et al., 2018).

14.4.4 CONCRETE

As concrete materials have unique properties such as viscosity, shear stress, buildability, extrudability and interlayer adhesion, they play a major role in the AM process. A new technique called contour crafting was developed to achieve smooth finishing instead of a layer-by-layer appearance of an object. The concrete paste is extruded using bigger nozzles and high pressure (Paul, van Zijl, & Gibson, 2018). The interlayer adhesion, on the other hand, is a problematic aspect of 3D-printed concrete structures.

14.5 APPLICATIONS

14.5.1 PHARMACEUTICAL INDUSTRY

- The pharmaceutical industry has benefited most from the advancement of 3D-printing technology, resulting in a significant shift in manufacturing processes. As a result, it is anticipated that it will be seen as a large-scale industry in the future (Warsi et al., 2018).
- Problem encountered in the traditional method of formulating tablets and dosage forms is that the drug can easily be degraded during the formulation process if proper guidelines and conditions are not practised. Consequently, the therapeutic value of the final formulation can be altered. By utilising 3D-printing technology, we can fabricate personalised pills that can be a combination of many active pharmaceutical ingredient (API) or are dispensed as multi-reservoir printed tablets (Ali et al., 2020).
- The first 3D-printed orodispersible tablet, Spritam®, was developed by Aprecia Pharmaceuticals. It contained levetiracetam, an epileptic agent and was approved in 2015 by FDA. Because of the soluble and porous matrix structure, the solubilisation time was significantly improved. In adults and children with epilepsy, it was used as an additional treatment for three

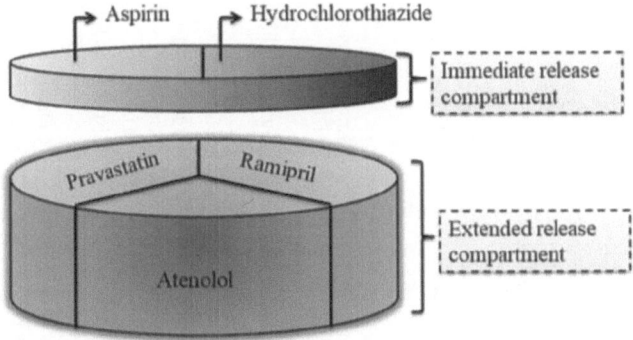

FIGURE 14.4   Schematic representation of a polypill having multiple drugs.

common forms of seizures: myoclonic, primary generalised tonic-clonic, and partial-onset (Kotta, Nair, & Alsabeelah, 2018; Warsi et al., 2018).

- The birth of the polypill concept, which refers to the combination of drugs in a single tablet, is because of 3D printing (see Figure 14.4) (Jose & Christoper, 2018). Recently Robles-Martinez et al. have developed a multilayered polypill that contains six drugs (prednisolone, paracetamol, naproxen, caffeine, chloramphenicol and aspirin) using a novel stereolithographic method. Table 14.2 provides the information on some recent 3D-printed tablets (Robles-Martinez et al., 2019).

14.5.2   Aerospace Industry

- According to Stratview Research, the aerospace industry presently holds 16.8 per cent of the 3D-printing market and is projected to expand at a magnetic CAGR of 16.9 per cent over the next seven years, reaching US\$ 6,717.4 million in 2027 (Stratview, 2020).
- The aerospace and defence (A&D) industry is increasingly utilising 3D-printing technology for both civil and military applications. With the assistance of 3D printing, it is easy to create stronger and lighter parts than those made using traditional manufacturing. Low volume production, material efficiency, part consolidation, maintenance and repair are some of the other advantages of AM in the aerospace industry (AMFG).
- Several spare parts of an aerospace engine are easily damaged and must be replaced regularly. Therefore, 3D-printing technology may be a viable option for procuring such spare parts. Also, as the use of materials used to produce aerospace components is reduced, this can lead to savings in fuel (Shahrubudin, Lee, & Ramlan, 2019).
- The NASA Aeronautics Research Institute has developed a non-metallic gas turbine engine by using 3D-printing technology (Grady et al., 2015). GKN Aerospace has designed the first advanced Ariane 6 nozzle (SWAN) (Figure 14.5) for the Vulcan 2.1 engine manufactured by Airbus Safran Launchers in France using the Direct Energy Deposition (DED) process

TABLE 14.2
Summary of Recent Studies for the Fabrication of Tablets Using 3D Printing

Sr. no	Dosage Form	Drug	Excipients	3D-printing Technique	Summary	References
1	Semi-solid tablet	Theophylline	HPMC K4M and E4M	Semi-solid extrusion	HPMC K4M 12% w/w hydrogel was ideal for the loading of theophylline, drug release was extended over 12 h, drug release profiles were well integrated into the first-order and Korsmeyer-Peppas release kinetic models	Yan et al. (2018)
2	IR Tablet	Itraconazole	Poly(vinyl alcohol), copovidone, crospovidone, magnesium stearate	FDM/HME	Itraconazole release from tablets that contained added copovidone was quicker than PVA alone, "good reproducibility during the object printing, superior drug dissolution"	Jamróz et al. (2020)
3	Tablets	Atomoxetine hydrochloride (ATH)	PEGDA 700, PEG 400	DLP (DLP printer Duplicator 7)	"Tablets with a higher quantity of suspended ATH had an improved drug release rate after 8 h, with increased tensile ability, mass and dimensions; a low amount of PEGDA increased the drug release rate"	Krkobabić et al. (2020)
4	Tablets	Levetiracetam (LEV)	HPC-M,croscarmellose sodium (CCMC-Na)	semi-solid extrusion	"High drug loading (96% w/w) of levetiracetam tablets in 3 geometrical shapes (cylinder, oval and torus); drug release (97.45% within 2 min) was observed in the torus tablets with 50% infill (cell size was 1.0 mm)"	Cui et al. (2020)
5	Tablets	Caffeine citrate	Eudragit EPO	FDM/HME	The concentrations of caffeine citrate released from the 3DP doughnut-shaped tablets were less than the tasting threshold of caffeine citrate after 1 min, and the tablets exhibited desired drug release rates in 0.1 N HCl, indicating a taste-masking ability; "immediate drug release profiles in gastric medium (10% infill, more than 80% release within 1 hour)"	Wang, Dumpa, Bandari, Durig, & Repka (2020)
6	IR Tablets	Pramipexole	Eudragit EPO and poly(ethylene) oxide	FDM/HME	"Good physico-pharmaceutical properties; more than 90% of the drug between 30 and 120 min;"by making physical changes such as decreasing thickness, creating space in tablets increases drug release rate and reduces drug release completion time to 5 min	Gültekin, Tort, & Acartürk (2019)
7	MR Tablets	Ibuprofen (IBF)	PEG 1500, PVP K12	HME	The ratio of IBF: PEG 1500: PVP K12- 5:75:20; the HME method demonstrated high reproducibility and precision in the preparation of dosage forms; Higher solubility and faster dissolution rate of IBF	Lee, Song, Noh, Song, & Rhee (2020)

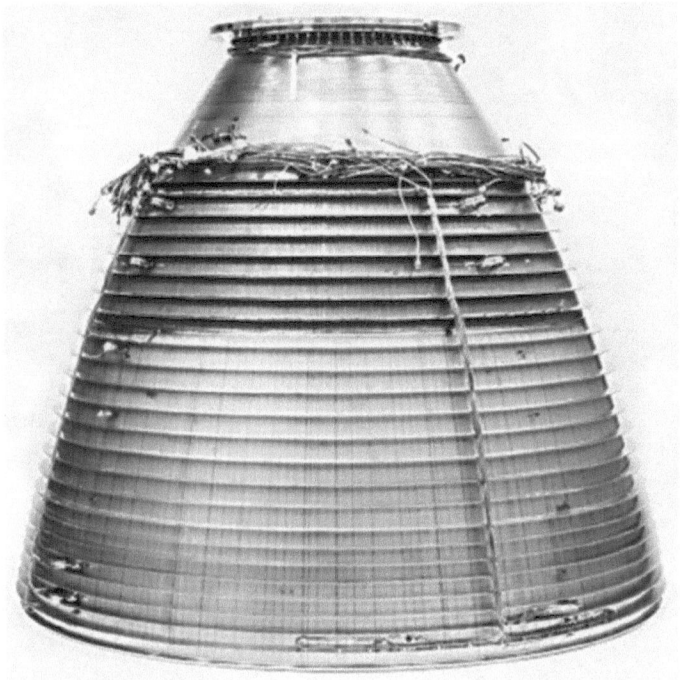

FIGURE 14.5   Ariane 6 nozzle for Vulcan 2.1 engine (AMFG) (Credits: GKN Aerospace).

of AM. The production of a 2.5 m diameter nozzle alleviated the cost (40%),"production time (30%) and usage of several parts [90% (1,000 parts to 100 parts)] (Aerospace GKN, 2017).

- "NASA's Rapid Analysis and Manufacturing Propulsion Technology project, or RAMPT, has recently used 'blown powder directed energy deposition' technique to 3D print a 40-inch diameter and 38-inch tall rocket engine nozzle with fully integrated cooling channels using lasers and metal powder. As a result, the most expensive and challenging rocket engine parts can now be produced at a lower cost than in the past (NASA, 2020) (see Figures 14.6 and 14.7). Overall, AM technology is a promising proposition for the aerospace industry in terms of hard benefits (Joshi & Sheikh, 2015).

14.5.3 CONSTRUCTION INDUSTRY

- For 3D printing of construction components, three major techniques have been developed. These techniques are D-shape, contour crafting and 3D concrete printing, each having its benefits and limitations (Avrutis, Nazari, & Sanjayan, 2019).
- The construction industry benefits from 3D concrete printing in terms of accuracy, optimising construction time, flexible design and customisation,

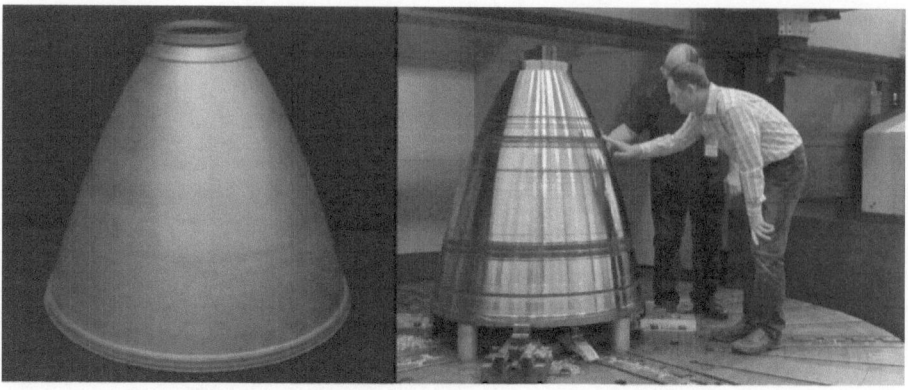

FIGURE 14.6 3D-printed engine nozzle by blown powder directed energy deposition technique within just 30 days (NASA, 2020) (Credit: NASA).

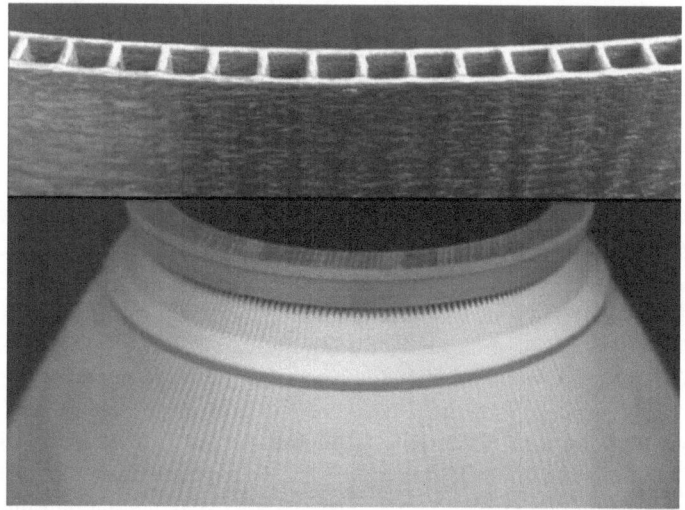

FIGURE 14.7 The sides of the 3D-printed nozzle and channel walls above are only the thickness of a few pieces of notebook paper (NASA, 2020) (Credit: NASA).

   cost, immediacy, error reduction, resource-saving, the applicability to extreme conditions as well as being environmentally friendly (Luo, Ma, & Yin, 2020; Malaeb, AlSakka, & Hamzeh, 2019).

- Across the construction industry, there are some records claiming innovative buildings which are 3D printed successfully (see Figure 14.8).
- For instance, in 2014, WinSun, a Chinese construction company, 3D printed 10 homes within 24 hours. According to Guinness World Records, the so-called 'Office of the Future', designed by architecture firm Gensler and 3D printed by Chinese company Winsun, is the first 3D printed commercially.

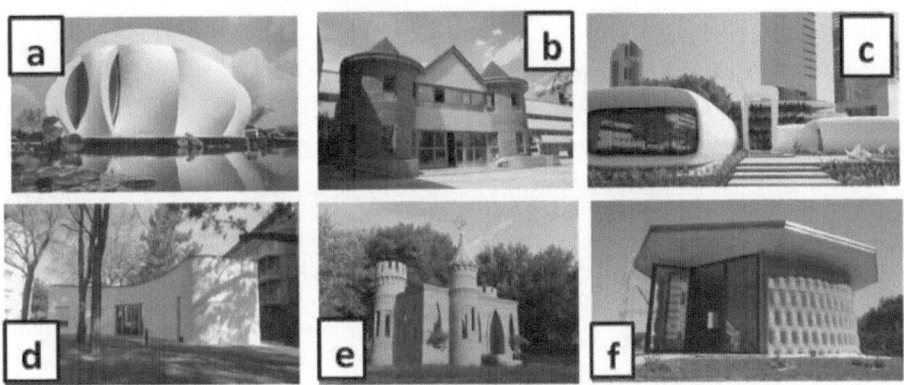

FIGURE 14.8 Remarkable 3DP structures in the world: a) 'Lotus House', b) 'Two-story Villa', c) 'Office of the future', d) 'Yhnova House', e) 'Mini castle', f) 'Gaia'.

It measures 240 m² and was designed by Gensler (see Figure 14.8.c). This project reduced construction waste (30–60%) and labour costs (50–80%) (Carolo, 2020; Labonnote, Rønnquist, Manum, & Rüther, 2016).

- Kamp C® recently constructed the first two-storey house with Europe's largest fixed 3D concrete printer in one piece, measuring 8 m² high and 90 m² in the area (KAMP C, 2020).
- Branch Technology, a company headquartered in Tennessee, is a leader in the field of 3DP, using its patented 'Cellular Fabrication' (C-Fab) technique for the prefabrication of interior walls and partitions (Kidwell, 2017). Some of the most recent 3D-printed construction projects are summarised in Table 14.3.

14.5.4 BIOMEDICAL INDUSTRY

- 3D printing in the biomedical sector is projected to be worth $3.5 billion by 2025, compared to $713.3 million in 2016 (Nawrat, 2020).
- Applications of AM in the biomedical industry can be categorised into the following areas: 1) customised manufacturing of permanent non- bioactive implants, 2) directly printing of organs and tissues with complete life functions, 3) manufacturing pathological organ models which can be helpful in planning treatments and analysis during preoperative surgeries, 4) fabrication of local scaffolds which are bioactive and biodegradable (Yan et al., 2018; Banga et al., 2017b, 2017a, 2020a, 2020b, 2020c, 2020d, 2020e, 2021).
- AM technology can be used to create bio-materials, cells, and cell-loaded biomaterials separately or in combination, layer by layer, directly forming 3D tissue-like structures (Lee Ventola, 2014). Bioprinting enables the construction of 3D structures with a specifically configured architecture, different cell types and a more physiologically appropriate microenvironment, compared with other biofabrication (Duan, 2017).

TABLE 14.3

Recent 3D-Printed Construction Projects

Sr. no	Name	Designed/3D Printed By	Description	Location	Year
1	Prvok (floating house)	Michal Trpak, Scoolpt	Walls are topped by green sustainable roofing, 43 m² house, printing process:48 hrs, 3 rooms, 3 times stronger than traditional concrete walls	Ceske Budejovice, Czech Republic	2020
2	Curve Appeal	WATG, Branch Technology	240 m² house, first prize in The Freeform Home Design Challenge, organic structures, exterior and interior walls 3D printed offsite	Chattanooga, Tennessee, USA	2020
3	Home for the Homeless	Logan Architecture, Icon	6 houses measuring 400-sq ft (38 m² house)	Austin, Texas, USA	2020
4	DFAB House	ETH Zurich	200 m² house, the ceiling is just 20 mm thick and weighs only half of what comparable structures usually do	Dübendorf, Switzerland	2019
5	Biggest house	SQ4D	1,900 sq ft house, 10 gallons of fuel used for every 500 square feet of construction, which is 70% reduction of construction costs in total	Long Island, USA	2019

- 3D-printing techniques such as inkjet 3D printing, vat photopolymerisation, fused filament fabrication (FFF), and SLS methods are very useful in the biomedical field (Estomba, González-Fernández, & Iglesias-Otero, 2017; Banga et al., 2014). Inkjet 3D-printing technique has been used to repair human articular cartilage (Ozbolat & Yu, 2013).
- Several industries, such as Helisys, Organovo and Ultimateker, utilise 3D-printing technology to produce living human tissue (Lee Ventola, 2014).
- As near-infrared (NIR) light possesses excellent tissue penetration power, a recent study designed a noninvasive AM technology-based process called digital NIR photopolymerisation (DNP) (see Figure 14.9). By *ex vivo* irradiation with the patterned NIR, the bio-ink was non-invasively injected via a subcutaneous route into customised tissue structures in situ. Without any surgery implantation, a customised ear-like tissue construct with chondrification and a repairable muscle tissue cell-loaded conformal scaffold was obtained *in vivo* (Chen et al., 2020). Figure 14.10 illustrates versatile applications of AM in the biomedical industry.
- Researchers have recently developed a new 3D-printing technique called 'cold spray' that creates a mechanically robust and porous structure using

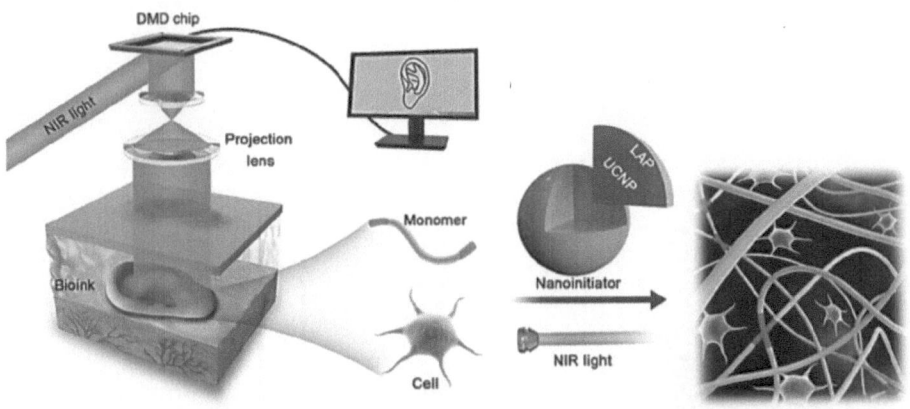

FIGURE 14.9   Schematic representation of DNP-based noninvasive 3D bioprinting (Chen et al., 2020).

a unique process that breaks down powder particles together at supersonic speeds. These porous structures can be used for artificial joints, facial and cranial implants, and they also allow the bone to grow inside the pores, resulting in a biological fixation (Moridi et al., 2020).

14.5.4.1   Market Demand for Additive Manufactured Biomedical Products

Since the last five years, AM has risen in popularity, and both applications and market size have exploded (Verhoef, Budde, Chockalingam, García Nodar, & van Wijk, 2018). The AM market for biomedical products is driven primarily by several factors such as increasing consumer demand, advances in technology, rapid innovation, easy production of customised biomedical products, and increasing applications in the healthcare sector. The global 3D-printing demand for biomedical devices is projected to rise by 17.5 %, from US\$ 0.84 billion in 2017 to US\$ 1.88 billion in 2022. Direct digital manufacturing, the expiry of vital patents in the upcoming years, rising demand for organ transplantation, and reconfiguration of supply chain models of biomedical device manufacturers are anticipated to pave the way for industry leaders by providing opportunities. Key players operating in the global additive manufactured biomedical products market include Stratasys Ltd, Evonik Industries AG, 3D Systems Inc., Formlabs Inc., Anatomics Ptv Ltd, Bioink Solution Inc., Biomedical Modelling Inc. and Sandvik AB. Among these, Stratasys is in the top position, while 3D Systems is in second position in the global AM market for biomedical materials. The demand for biocompatible additive manufactured products is anticipated to rise rapidly in the United States. "The presence of numerous manufacturers of 3D-printed biomedical materials as well as 3D printers in the United States has led to the widespread adoption of AM technology in the country. Consequently, their position in the global market has strengthened (Markets and Markets, 2017; Transparency Market Research, 2019).

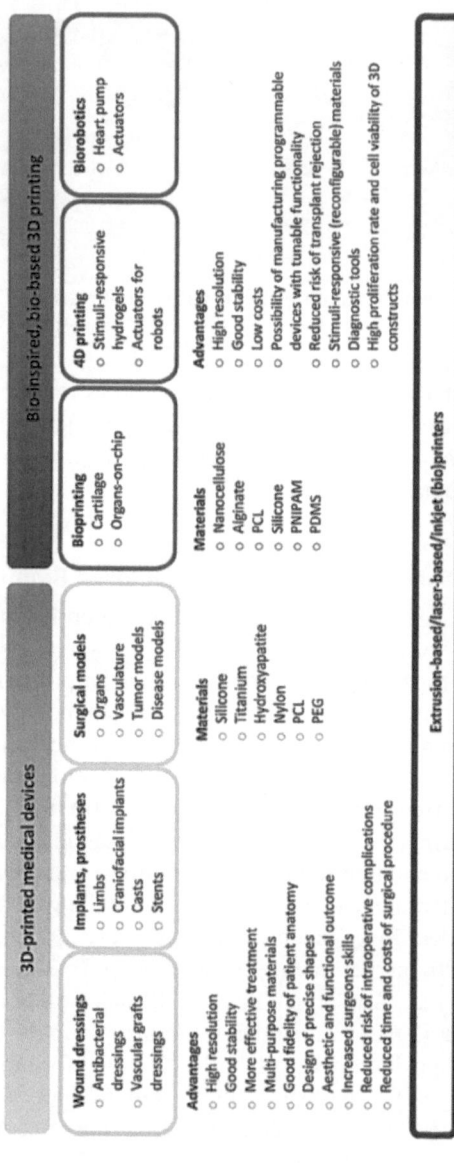

FIGURE 14.10   Various biomedical applications of 3D printing.

14.6 CONCLUSION AND FUTURE ASPECTS

AM has begun to permeate our daily routine due to its increasing versatile applications in many fields, including healthcare, engineering, construction and aerospace, as discussed in this chapter. However, 3D printing faces several challenges in biomedicine, drug delivery, education and electronics, where it is still in its infancy. But considering the rapid progress in 3D technology, hopefully, researchers will be able to develop novel advanced 3D-printing technologies to overcome these challenges. 3D printing also holds a lot of promises in developing smart sensors for monitoring, precision bio-scaffolds, mechanobiology, advanced miniature implantable devices and many more.

ANNEXURE FOR ABBREVIATIONS

3DP	3D printing
AM	additive manufacturing
ATH	atomoxetine hydrochloride
CAD	computer-aided design
DIW	direct ink writing
DLP	digital light projection
DMD	digital micromirror device
FDM	fused deposition modelling
HME	hot-melt extrusion
HPC	hydroxypropyl cellulose
HPMC	hydroxypropyl methylcellulose
IBF	ibuprofen"
LEV	levetiracetam
PEG	poly(ethylene glycol)
PEGDA	poly(ethylene glycol) diacrylate
PEGDA	poly(ethylene glycol) diacrylate
PEGDMA	poly(ethylene glycol) dimethacrylate
SLA	stereolithography
SLS	selective laser sintering

NOTE

1 Figures 14.9 and 14.10 are taken from open access articles distributed under the terms of the CC BY-NC 4.0 and CC BY licence, respectively.

REFERENCES

Aerospace GKN. (2017). GKN Aerospace delivers revolutionary ariane 6 nozzle to airbus safran launchers. Retrieved from https://www.gknaerospace.com/en/newsroom/news-releases/2017/gkn-delivers-revolutionary-ariane-6-nozzle-to-airbus-safran-launchers/ (accessed: 1 March 2021).

Ahangar, P., Cooke, M. E., Weber, M. H., & Rosenzweig, D. H. (2019). Current biomedical applications of 3d printing and additive manufacturing. *Applied Sciences (Switzerland)*, *9*(8). doi:10.3390/app9081713

Ali, A., Ahmad, U., & Akhtar, J. (2020). 3d printing in pharmaceutical sector: An overview. In U. Ahmad & J. Akhtar (Eds.), *Pharmaceutical Formulation Design – Recent Practices* (pp. 1–13): IntechOpen.

Ameeduzzafar, Alruwaili N. K., Rizwanullah, M., Abbas Bukhari, S. N., Amir, M., Ahmed, M. M., & Fazil, M. (2018). 3D printing technology in design of pharmaceutical products. *Current Pharmaceutical Design, 24*(42), 5009–5018.

Ashish Ahmad, N., Gopinath, P., & Vinogradov, A. (2019). 3D printing in medicine: current challenges and potential applications. In N. Ahmad, P. Gopinath, & R. Dutta (Eds.), *3D Printing Technology in Nanomedicine* (pp. 1–22): Elsevier.

ASTM International. (2013). *Standard terminology for additive manufacturing technologies.* (F2792 – 12a). Retrieved from https://web.mit.edu/2.810/www/files/readings/Additive ManufacturingTerminology.pdf.

Azad, M. A., Olawuni, D., Kimbell, G., Badruddoza, A., Hossain, M. S., & Sultana, T. (2020). Polymers for Extrusion-Based 3D Printing of Pharmaceuticals: A Holistic Materials-Process Perspective. *Pharmaceutics, 12*(2), 124. https://doi.org/10.3390/pharmaceutics12020124

Banga, H.K., Belokar, R.M., Kumar, R., (2017b). A Novel Approach For Ankle Foot Orthosis Developed By Three Dimensional Technologies, *3rd International Conference on Mechanical Engineering and Automation Science (ICMEAS 2017)*, University of Birmingham, UK, Vol. 8 No. 10, pp. 141–145.

Banga, H.K., Belokar, R.M., Madan, R., Dhole, S. (2017a). Three dimensional Gait assessments during walking of healthy people and drop foot patients. *Defence Life Science Journal, 2*, 14–20.

Banga, H.K., Kumar, P., & Kumar, H. (2021). Utilization of additive manufacturing in orthotics and prosthetic devices development. *IOP Conference Series: Materials Science and Engineering.* 10.1088/1757-899X/033/1/012083

Banga, H.K., Parveen, K., Belokar, R.M., Kumar, R. (2014). Rapid prototyping applications in medical sciences. *International Journal of Emerging Technologies in Computational and Applied Sciences (IJETCAS), 5*(8), 416–420. doi:10.1016/j.ijpharm.2020.119983

Banga, H.K., Parveen, K., Belokar, R.M., Kumar R, (2018)' Fabrication and stress analysis of ankle foot orthosis with additive manufacturing. *Rapid Prototyping Journal Emerald Publishing, 24*(2), 300–312.

Banga, H.K., Parveen, K., Belokar, R.M. and Kumar, R. (2020a). Customized design and additive manufacturing of kids' ankle foot orthosis. *Rapid Prototyping Journal, 26*, 10. doi:10.1108/RPJ-07-2019-0194

Banga, H.K., Parveen, K., Belokar, R.M. and Kumar, R. (2020b). Design and fabrication of prosthetic and orthotic product by 3D printing [Online First], *IntechOpen.* doi:10.5772/intechopen.94846. Available from: https://www.intechopen.com/online-first/design-and-fabrication-of-prosthetic-and-orthotic-product-by-3d-printing

Banga, H.K., Parveen, K., Belokar, R.M., Kumar, R. (2020c). Effect of 3D-printed ankle foot orthosis during walking of foot deformities patients. In: Kumar H., Jain P. (eds) *Recent Advances in Mechanical Engineering.* Lecture Notes in Mechanical Engineering. Springer, Singapore, pp 275–288.

Banga, H.K., Parveen, K., Belokar R.M., Kumar R. (2020d) Role of finite element analysis in customized design of kid's orthotic product'. In: Singh S., Prakash C., Singh R. (eds) *Characterization, Testing, Measurement, and Metrology*, pp. 139–159 CRC Press, Taylor & Francis Group, USA.

Banga H.K., Parveen, K., Belokar R.M., Kumar R. (2020e) Improvement of human gait in foot deformities patients by 3D printed ankle–foot orthosis. In: Singh S., Prakash C., Singh R. (eds) *3D Printing in Biomedical Engineering.* Materials Horizons: From Nature to Nanomaterials. Springer, Singapore.

Carolo, L. (2020). 3d printed house: 20 most important projects in 2020. Retrieved from https://all3dp.com/2/3d-printed-house-3d-printed-building/ (accessed: 2 March 2021).

Chen, Y., Zhang, J., Liu, X., Wang, S., Tao, J., Huang, Y., Wu, W., Li, Y., Zhou, K., Wei, X., Chen, S., Li, X., Xu, X., Cardon, L., Qian, Z., & Gou, M. (2020). Noninvasive in vivo 3D bioprinting. *Science Advances*, 6(23), eaba7406. doi:10.1126/sciadv.aba7406

Cui, M., Pan, H., Fang, D., Qiao, S., Wang, S., & Pan, W. (2020). Fabrication of high drug loading levetiracetam tablets using semi-solid extrusion 3d printing. *Journal of Drug Delivery Science and Technology*, 57(2020), 1–9. doi:10.1016/j.jddst.2020.101683

Duan, B. (2017). State-of-the-art review of 3d bioprinting for cardiovascular tissue engineering. *Annals of Biomedical Engineering*, 45(1), 195–209. doi:10.1007/s10439-016-1607-5

Estomba, C., González-Fernández, I., & Iglesias-Otero, M. (2017). 3d printing for biomedical applications: Where are we now? *European Medical Journal*, 2(March), 16–22.

Gonzalez-Gutierrez, J., Cano, S., Schuschnigg, S., Kukla, C., Sapkota, J., & Holzer, C. (2018). Additive manufacturing of metallic and ceramic components by the material extrusion of highly-filled polymers: A review and future perspectives. *Materials*, 11(5). doi:10.3390/ma11050840

Grady, J. E., Haller, W. J., Poinsatte, P. E., Halbig, M. C., Schnulo, S. L., Weir, D., … Mehl, J. (2015). A fully nonmetallic gas turbine engine enabled by additive manufacturing part i: System analysis, component identification, additive manufacturing, and testing of polymer composites. (May). NASA/TM—2015-218748. https://ntrs.nasa.gov/api/citations/20150010717/downloads/20150010717.pdf

Gross, B. C., Erkal, J. L., Lockwood, S. Y., Chen, C., & Spence, D. M. (2014). Evaluation of 3d printing and its potential impact on biotechnology and the chemical sciences. *Analytical Chemistry*, 86(7), 3240–3253. doi:10.1021/ac403397r

Gu, Z., Fu, J., Lin, H., & He, Y. (2020). Development of 3d bioprinting: From printing methods to biomedical applications. *Asian Journal of Pharmaceutical Sciences*, 15(5), 529–557. doi:10.1016/j.ajps.2019.11.003

Gültekin, H., Tort, S., & Acartürk, F. (2019). An effective technology for the development of immediate release solid dosage forms containing low-dose drug: Fused deposition modeling 3d printing. *Pharmaceutical Research*, 36(9), 1–13. doi:10.1007/s11095-019-2655-y

He, Y., Yang, F., Zhao, H., Gao, Q., Xia, B., & Fu, J. (2016). Research on the printability of hydrogels in 3d bioprinting. *Scientific Reports*, 6, 1–13. doi:10.1038/srep29977

Heidarian, P., Kouzani, A. Z., Kaynak, A., Paulino, M., & Nasri-Nasrabadi, B. (2019). Dynamic hydrogels and polymers as inks for three-dimensional printing. *ACS Biomaterials Science and Engineering* (May). doi:10.1021/acsbiomaterials.9b00047

Jain, V., Haider, N., & Jain, K. (2019). 3d printing in personalized drug delivery. *Current Pharmaceutical Design*, 24(42), 5062–5071. doi:10.2174/1381612825666190215122208

Jakus, A. E. (2019). *An Introduction to 3d Printing—Past, Present, and Future Promise.* Elsevier Inc.

Jamróz, W., Pyteraf, J., Kurek, M., Knapik-Kowalczuk, J., Szafraniec-Szczęsny, J., Jurkiewicz, K., … Jachowicz, R. (2020). Multivariate design of 3d printed immediate-release tablets with liquid crystal-forming drug—itraconazole. *Materials*, 13(21). doi:10.3390/ma13214961

Jamróz, W., Szafraniec, J., Kurek, M., & Jachowicz, R. (2018). 3d printing in pharmaceutical and medical applications. *Pharmaceutical Research*, 35(9), Article 176-Article 176.

Jang, T. S., Jung, H. D., Pan, H. M., Han, W. T., Chen, S., & Song, J. (2018). 3d printing of hydrogel composite systems: Recent advances in technology for tissue engineering. *International Journal of Bioprinting*, 4(1), 1–28. doi:10.18063/IJB.v4i1.126

Jiang, P., Ji, Z., Zhang, X., Liu, Z., & Wang, X. (2018). Recent advances in direct ink writing of electronic components and functional devices. *Progress in Additive Manufacturing*, 3(1), 65–86. doi:10.1007/s40964-017-0035-x

Jose, P., & Christoper, P. (2018). 3D printing of pharmaceuticals – A potential technology in developing personalized medicine. *Asian Journal of Pharmaceutical Research and Development*, 6(3), 46–54. doi:10.22270/ajprd.v6i3.375

Joshi, S. C., & Sheikh, A. A. (2015). 3d printing in aerospace and its long-term sustainability. *Virtual and Physical Prototyping*, *10*(4), 175–185. doi:10.1080/17452759.2015.1111519

Kadry, H., Wadnap, S., Xu, C., & Ahsan, F. (2019). Digital light processing (dlp) 3d-printing technology and photoreactive polymers in fabrication of modified-release tablets. *European Journal of Pharmaceutical Sciences*, *135*, 60–67. doi:10.1016/j.ejps.2019.05.008

KAMP C. (2020). World first: Kamp c is the first to print an entire house in one piece. Retrieved from https://www.kampc.be/c3po (accessed: 2 March 2021).

Kidwell, J. (2017). *Best Practices and Applications of 3d Printing In The Construction Industry*. Digital Commons @ Cal Poly, California Polytechnic State University, San Luis Obispo.

Kotta, S., Nair, A., & Alsabeelah, N. (2018). 3d printing technology in drug delivery: Recent progress and application. *Current Pharmaceutical Design*, *24*(42), 5039–5048. doi:10.2174/1381612825666181206123828

Krkobabić, M., Medarević, D., Pešić, N., Vasiljević, D., Ivković, B., & Ibrić, S. (2020). Digital light processing (dlp) 3d printing of atomoxetine hydrochloride tablets using photoreactive suspensions. *Pharmaceutics*, *12*(9), 1–17. doi:10.3390/pharmaceutics12090833

Labonnote, N., Rønnquist, A., Manum, B., & Rüther, P. (2016). Additive construction: State-of-the-art, challenges and opportunities. *Automation in Construction*, *72*, 347–366. doi:10.1016/j.autcon.2016.08.026

Lee, J., Song, C., Noh, I., Song, S., & Rhee, Y. S. (2020). Hot-melt 3d extrusion for the fabrication of customizable modified-release solid dosage forms. *Pharmaceutics*, *12*(8), 1–16. doi:10.3390/pharmaceutics12080738

Lee Ventola, C. (2014). Medical applications for 3d printing: Current and projected uses. *P and T*, *39*(10), 704–711.

Luo, W., Ma, X., & Yin, J. (2020). Application and research on building 3d printing. *Journal of Critical Reviews*, *7*(12), 564–578. doi:10.31838/jcr.07.12.103

Madla, C. M., Trenfield, S. J., Goyanes, A., Gaisford, S., & Basit, A. W. (2018). 3d printing technologies, implementation and regulation: An overview. *AAPS Advances in the Pharmaceutical Sciences Series*, *31*, 21–40. doi:10.1007/978-3-319-90755-0_2

MakerBot. (2016). Makerbot reaches milestone: 100,000 3d printers sold worldwide. Retrieved from https://www.makerbot.com/stories/news/makerbot-reaches-milestone-100000-3d-printers-sold-worldwide/

Malaeb, Z., AlSakka, F., & Hamzeh, F. (2019). 3D Concrete Printing: Machine design, mix proportioning, and mix comparison between different machine setups. In J. G. Sanjayan, A. Nazari, & B. Nematollahi (Eds.), *3D Concrete Printing Technology* (pp. 115–136): Butterworth-Heinemann.

Markets and Markets. (2017). *3d printing medical devices market by technology (3dp, ebm, lbm, photopolymerization and dd), component (3d printers, 3d bioprinters, material (plastic, metal, ceramic), software & services), product type (prosthetics, implant) - global forecast to 2022* (MD 3726). Retrieved from https://www.marketsandmarkets.com/Market-Reports/3d-printing-medical-devices-market-90799911.html

Matias, E., & Rao, B. (2015). 3d printing: On its historical evolution and the implications for business. In *Portland International Conference on Management of Engineering and Technology, 2015-September*, 551–558. doi:10.1109/PICMET.2015.7273052

Moridi, A., Stewart, E. J., Wakai, A., Assadi, H., Gartner, F., Guagliano, M., … Dao, M. (2020). Solid-state additive manufacturing of porous ti-6al-4v by supersonic impact. *Applied Materials Today*, *21*, 100865. doi:10.1016/j.apmt.2020.100865

Mukherjee, P., Rani, A., & Saravanan, P. (2019). *Polymeric Materials for 3d Bioprinting* Elsevier.

NASA. (2020). Future rocket engines may include large-scale 3d printing. Retrieved from https://www.nasa.gov/centers/marshall/news/releases/2020/future-rocket-engines-may-include-large-scale-3d-printing.html

Nawrat, A. (2020). 3d printing in the medical field: Four major applications revolutionising the industry. *Medical Device Network*. Retrieved from https://www.medicaldevice-network. com/features/3d-printing-in-the-medical-field-applications/

Nematollahi B., Xia, M. & Sanjayan, J. (2019) Post-processing methods to improve strength of particle-bed 3D printed geopolymer for digital construction applications. *Frontiers in Materials 6*:160. doi:10.3389/fmats.2019.00160

Ngo, T. D., Kashani, A., Imbalzano, G., Nguyen, K. T. Q., & Hui, D. (2018). Additive manufacturing (3d printing): A review of materials, methods, applications and challenges. *Composites Part B: Engineering, 143*(February), 172–196. doi:10.1016/j.compositesb.2018.02.012

Olusegun, A., Makun, H. A., Ogara, I. M., Edema, M., Idahor, K. O., Oluwabamiwo, B. F., & Eshiett, M. E. (2012). 3d-printed modified-release tablets: A review of the recent advances. *Intech*, 1–13.

Ordoñez, E., Gallego, J. M., & Colorado, H. A. (2019). 3d printing via the direct ink writing technique of ceramic pastes from typical formulations used in traditional ceramics industry. *Applied Clay Science, 182*, 1–11. doi:10.1016/j.clay.2019.105285

Ozbolat, I., & Yu, Y. (2013). Bioprinting towards organ fabrication: Challenges and future trends. *IEEE Transactions on Biomedical Engineering, 60*(3), 691–699.

Paul, S. C., van Zijl, G. P. A. G., & Gibson, I. (2018). A review of 3d concrete printing systems and materials properties: Current status and future research prospects. *Rapid Prototyping Journal, 24*(4), 784–798. doi:10.1108/RPJ-09-2016-0154

Prince, J. D. (2014). 3d printing: An industrial revolution. *Journal of Electronic Resources in Medical Libraries, 11*(1), 39–45. doi:10.1080/15424065.2014.877247

Provaggi, E., & Kalaskar, D. M. (2017). 3d printing families: Laser, powder, nozzle based techniques. In D. M. Kalaskar (Ed.), *3d Printing in Medicine* (pp. 21–42): Woodhead Publishing.

Robles-Martinez, P., Xu, X., Trenfield, S. J., Awad, A., Goyanes, A., Telford, R., … Gaisford, S. (2019). 3d printing of a multi-layered polypill containing six drugs using a novel stereolithographic method. *Pharmaceutics, 11*(6), 274. doi:10.3390/pharmaceutics11060274

Rocha, V. G., Saiz, E., Tirichenko, I. S., & García-Tuñón, E. (2020). Direct ink writing advances in multi-material structures for a sustainable future. *Journal of Materials Chemistry A, 8*(31), 15646–15657. doi:10.1039/D0TA04181E

Sachs, Emanuel M., Haggerty, J. S., Cima, M. J. & Williams, P. A. (1993). 5,204,055. U. S. Patent.

Savini, A., & Savini, G. G. (2015). A short history of 3d printing, a technological revolution just started. *Proceedings of the 2015 ICOHTEC/IEEE International History of High-Technologies and their Socio-Cultural Contexts Conference, HISTELCON 2015: The 4th IEEE Region 8 Conference on the History of Electrotechnologies*. doi:10.1109/HISTELCON.2015.7307314

Shahrubudin, N., Lee, T. C., & Ramlan, R. (2019). An overview on 3d printing technology: Technological, materials, and applications. *Procedia Manufacturing, 35*, 1286–1296. doi:10.1016/j.promfg.2019.06.089

Stratview, R. (2020). Aerospace 3d printing market size to reach us$ 6.7 billion in 2027. Retrieved from https://www.prnewswire.com/news-releases/aerospace-3d-printing-market-size-to-reach-us-6-7-billion-in-2027--says-stratview-research-300984367.html

Su, A., & Al'Aref, S. J. (2018). History of 3d printing. In *3d Printing Applications in Cardiovascular Medicine* (pp. 1–10): Elsevier Inc.

Tan, D. K., Maniruzzaman, M., & Nokhodchi, A. (2018). Advanced pharmaceutical applications of hot-melt extrusion coupled with fused deposition modelling (fdm) 3d printing for personalised drug delivery. *Pharmaceutics, 10*(4). doi:10.3390/pharmaceutics10040203

Tetsuka, H., & Shin, S. R. (2020). Materials and technical innovations in 3d printing in biomedical applications. *Journal of Materials Chemistry B, 8*(15), 2930–2950. doi:10.1039/d0tb00034e

Transparency Market Research (2019). *Biocompatible 3d printing materials market global industry analysis, size, share, growth, trends, and forecast 2019 – 2027* (TMRGL52266). Retrieved from https://www.transparencymarketresearch.com/biocompatible-3d-printing-materials-market.html

Verhoef, L. A., Budde, B. W., Chockalingam, C., García Nodar, B., & van Wijk, A. J. M. (2018). The effect of additive manufacturing on global energy demand: An assessment using a bottom-up approach. *Energy Policy, 112*, 349–360. doi:10.1016/j.enpol.2017.10.034

Vogt, B. D. (2020). A virtual issue of applied polymer materials: "3d printing of polymers". *ACS Applied Polymer Materials, 2*(6), 2102–2104. doi:10.1021/acsapm.0c00517

Wang, H., Dumpa, N., Bandari, S., Durig, T., & Repka, M. A. (2020). Fabrication of taste-masked donut-shaped tablets via fused filament fabrication 3d printing paired with hot-melt extrusion techniques. *AAPS PharmSciTech, 21*(7), 1–11. doi:10.1208/s12249-020-01783-0

Warsi, M. H., Yusuf, M., Al Robaian, M., Khan, M., Muheem, A., & Khan, S. (2018). 3d printing methods for pharmaceutical manufacturing: Opportunity and challenges. *Current Pharmaceutical Design, 24*(42), 4949–4956. doi:10.2174/1381612825666181206121701

Yan, Q., Dong, H., Su, J., Han, J., Song, B., Wei, Q., & Shi, Y. (2018). A review of 3d printing technology for medical applications. *Engineering, 4*(5), 729–742. doi:10.1016/j.eng.2018.07.021

15 Overview of 3D-printing Technology

Types, Applications, Materials and Post Processing Techniques

Rakesh Kumar
Auxein Medical Private Limited, Sonipat, Haryana, India

Santosh Kumar
Chandigarh Group of Colleges, Landran, Mohali, Punjab, India

CONTENTS

DOI: 10.1201/9781003301066-15

15.1   INTRODUCTION

3D printing is also referred to as solid freeform fabrication. In 2011, $642.6 million in revenue was reported for 3D printing goods worldwide. However, the United States accounts for $246.1 million or 38.3 per cent of global production [1]. About 62.8 per cent of all industrial or commercial units were manufactured using the top three producers of 3D manufacturing systems (Stratasys, 3D Systems and Z Corporation) in 2011. It is expected that 3D printing will manufacture 50 per cent of industrial/ commercial units from 2031 to 2038. However, in 2058–2065 this technology will produce 100 per cent industrial/commercial units [2].

Currently, this manufacturing technology is used to produce real-life components or models from digital computer-aided design (CAD) data in an additive fashion [3]. It offers several attractive properties such as customisation, low weight, less wastage, no need for skilled craftspeople, design flexibility, automation, part consolidation, and the ability to produce complicated shapes. However, this technology still has drawbacks such as poor part quality, high raw material costs, and more part processing time [4]. There are different 3D-printing techniques such as fusion filament fabrication (FFF), stereolithography (SLA), selective laser sintering (SLS), electron beam melting (EBM), inkjet printing (IJP) and selective laser melting (SLM). All these techniques use distinct materials such as powder, ceramics, plastic, liquid, metal alloy or even living cells [5]. Recently, 3D-printing methods have been extensively used to fabricate implants, bridges, food items, houses, rocket and automotive components. This technology encourages and drives innovation with unprecedented design freedom and a tool-less process that decreases product costs and waiting times. These technological varieties of components or machine parts can be designed specifically to avoid assembly needs with complicated shapes and features. Currently, AM has gone beyond being a fabricating process and industrial prototyping as the technology has become highly accessible to individuals and small-scale companies. Recent research and developments have diminished the cost of 3D-printing machines, thereby increasing their use in homes, labs and schools, etc. [6–11].

15.2   WHAT IS 3D PRINTING?

3D printing is an industrial standard term (ASTM F2792) given in 2009 [12]. It is an object-manufacturing technique by which three-dimensional components are fabricated by depositing materials in layers fashion from three-dimensional model data. It works by integrating photochemistry, laser, CAD modelling and control drives [13,14].

15.2.1   GENERIC PROCESS OF 3D PRINTING

The generic process of 3D printing is typically performed in the following basic steps, as depicted in Figure 15.1.

a. Creation of 3D CAD model

   The creation of a digital model is the first step in the 3D-printing process. Currently, numerous design software packages (SolidWorks, Autodesk, Catia, etc.) are used for the development of digital models. But, the extensively used technique for the development of a digital model is CAD. However, reverse engineering (back engineering) can also be utilised to produce a digital model via 3D scanning. It helps in considering the accurate size of the part and simulating to see that how the part will behave under distinct circumstances [15]

b. Conversion of STL file

   Once the CAD file is created, the next step is to transform this CAD model into a specific file format referred to as STL (stereolithography). This file format uses a series of triangles (polygons) to describe the surface geometry of a solid object.

c. File transfer to machine

   After the generation of STL files, these files are imported into the slicer program to convert them into G-code (numerical control programming language). These G-codes are further utilised in computer-aided manufacturing to control 3D printers.

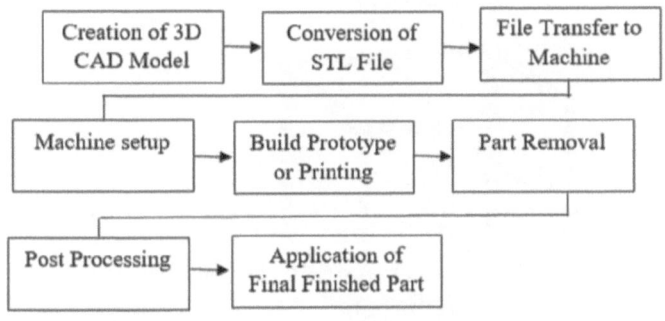

FIGURE 15.1   Basic steps of 3D printing [5].

d. Machine setup

The printing machine must be correctly set up before the part manufacturing. During this step, the print material (polymers and binder) is loaded into the printer, and the printer is set up with distinct printing parameters (printing orientation, filling ratio, filament feed rate and layer thickness, etc.).

e. Build prototype or printing

In this step, the 3D printer builds the model by adding material in layer fashion.

f. Part removal

In this step, the printed part is removed from the build base and its support structure.

g. Post-processing

Finally, distinct post-processing techniques (tumbling, polishing, painting, etc.) are utilised to prepare a print for an end-use. This will help make the part surface smooth and also add strength.

h. Application of the final finished part:

This is the last step in which parts for the particular application may now be ready to be used [16,17].

15.2.2 COMPARISON OF 3D PRINTING OVER CONVENTIONAL OR SUBTRACTIVE MANUFACTURING TECHNIQUES

The 3D-printing technique is different from conventional manufacturing in a distinct way such as no need for cutting tools, patterns, mould, coolant, automated, lightweight design, no need for skilled craftspeople, producing less noise, eco-friendly, etc., for the production of a part. A schematic diagram of subtractive vs additive manufacturing process is depicted in Figure 15.2.

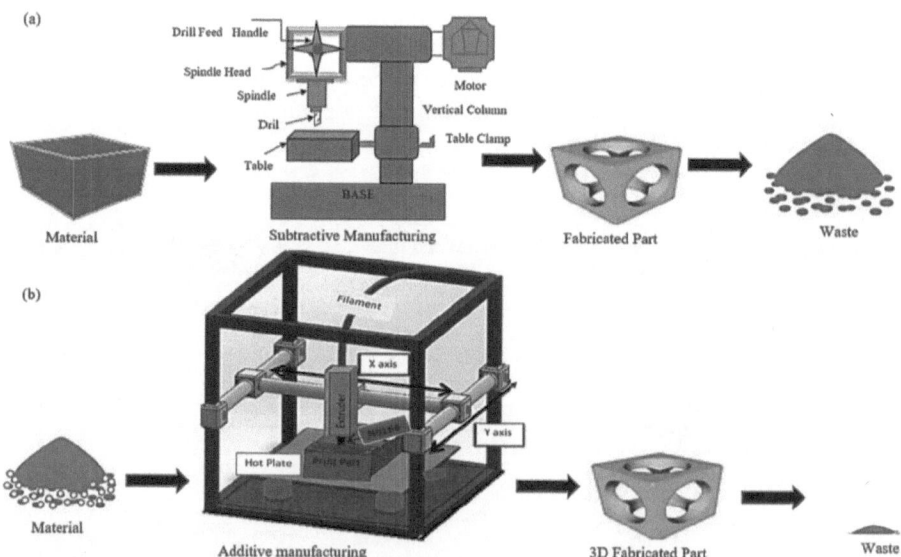

FIGURE 15.2   Subtractive manufacturing vs additive manufacturing [18].

TABLE 15.1
3D Printing vs Subtractive Manufacturing Techniques [19]

S.No.	3D Printing Technology	Subtractive Manufacturing
1	3D printing is a material addition process in layer fashion, to build a solid 3D component.	Subtractive manufacturing is a material removal method that can be used for solid metal irrespective of melting point.
2	It is used for generating prototypes since the weight of the part is easy to control.	It cannot control the material density or weight of the component.
3	The complicated parts can be easy to produce by using this technology.	Subtractive manufacturing processes have limited capacity in the manufacturing of complicated parts.
4	3D-printing methods are more costly and take more time because the material is deposited in successive thin layers.	Subtractive manufacturing methods are economical and time-consuming because the material is rapidly removed from the workpiece.
5	Much less wastage of material.	Subtractive manufacturing produces chips/scrap in large quantities. Hence, there is more wastage of material.
5	Common examples of these process technologies are FFF, FDM, SLA, SLS, etc.	Milling, grinding, lathe machine, etc. are the primary examples of this process technology.

The comparison between 3D printing and conventional manufacturing techniques is depicted in Table 15.1.

3D printing is also considered a genuinely innovative and versatile pillar of the third industrial revolution [20,21]. These techniques have gained the consideration of those in the pharmaceutical field because of their competence as a distinct medical implant from computed tomography (CT) replica [22]. In 2014, one architectural company called Win Sun printed a group of cost-effective houses in china within a day [23].

15.3   CURRENT COMPANIES AND THEIR PARAMETERS

Some researchers have provided information about 3D printer companies and their specifications which can be beneficial to future researchers for the proper selection of the process [24,25]. The comparison of consumer 3D printers and their specification is depicted in Table 15.2.

15.4   DECISION PARAMETERS FOR SELECTING 3D-PRINTING TECHNOLOGY

There are several types of decision parameters used to select the 3D-printing process. However, researchers cannot manufacture the right product without a deep knowledge of process parameters [26]. Hence, the knowledge of these parameters is essential. The primary decision parameters of 3D-printing technology are given in Figure 15.3.

TABLE 15.2
Comparison of Consumer 3D Printers

Company-Printer	Cost (US $)	Volume Build	Accuracy	Printing Speed
Ultimaker 2	2499	9 × 8.85 × 8	0.02 mm	30–300 mm/s
Felix	1749	10 × 8 × 9	0.05 mm	10–200 mm/s
Cube	1299	5.5 × 5.5 × 5.5	0.2 mm	15 mm/s
Orion Delta	1499	5 × 5 × 9	0.05 mm	40–300 mm/s
LulzBot TAZ4	2194	11.7 × 10.8 × 9.8	0.075 mm	200 mm/s
Printrbot Simple	349	3.9 × 3.9 × 3.9	0.1 mm	70 mm/s
MakerBot Replicator 5th gen.	2899	9.9 × 7.8 × 5.9	0.1 mm	150 mm/s

Available:-www.makershed.com/pages/3d-printer-comparison.

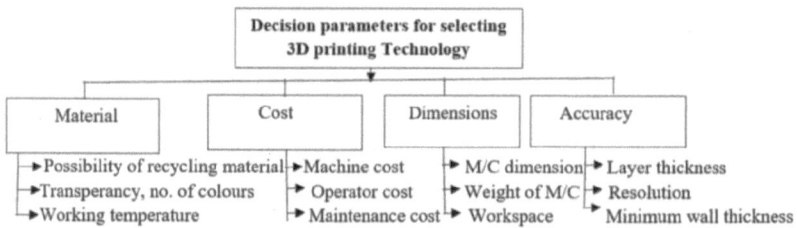

FIGURE 15.3   Parameters of 3D printing [26].

The selection of suitable 3D printing for each type of prototype depends upon the requirements such as functional, aesthetic, visual and investigational etc. Accordingly, different variables (software, manufacturing time, material, surface finish, resolution, cost, precision, size of model, etc.) are planned. The most important decision variables of 3D-printing technology are explained below:

a. Material: For the selection of particular material for a particular application, the following specifications should be considered. These include the possibility of recycling of material, transparency, colour, and working temperature.
b. Cost: This includes costs of the machine, operator, maintenance, etc.
c. Dimensions: These include the size and weight of the machine, and workspace.
d. Accuracy: It depends upon layer thickness, resolution and minimum wall thickness.

15.4.1   SELECTION OF AM PROCESS PARAMETERS

Generally, to enhance the mechanical characteristics and surface finish and reduce the defects of the 3D-printing components, it is highly important to know the interrelationship between the parameters and their effect on the material characteristics.

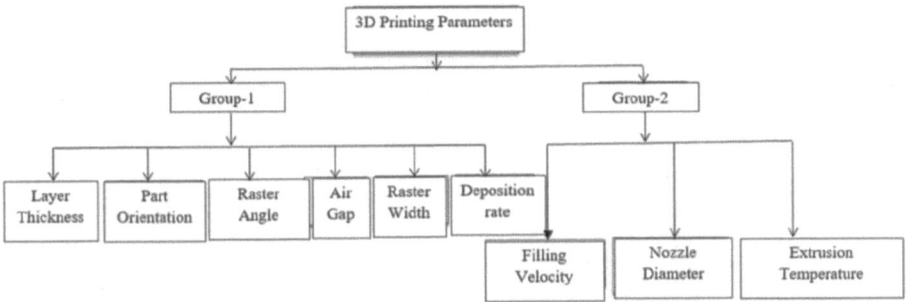

FIGURE 15.4 3D-printing parameters [27].

However, some parameters used during processing which greatly affect the mechanical features of 3D-printed objects/parts are depicted in Figure 15.4

The most important parameters (raster width, layer thickness, raster angle, orientation, gap between raster to raster, etc.) significantly affect the process output. The main process-parameter terms used in the 3D-printing process (FDM) are listed below.

a. Thickness of layers: This is the thickness of each layer sprayed by a nozzle and is always measured in the vertical (Z direction). In addition, the thickness of a layer depends on the size of the nozzle (diameter) used to construct/fabricate a 3D model.
b. Part orientation: This is the angle/inclination of a component in a build platform w.r.t. X, Y and Z-axis, where X and Y-axes are assumed to be parallel to the build base, and the Z-axis is along the direction of a component build.
c. Raster angle: The angle between two adjacent layers is called the raster angle.
d. Air gap: The gap between two adjacent rasters on the same layer.
e. Raster width: The distance across the raster pattern is called the raster width.
f. Deposition rate: This is also called filling velocity. It is the speed of the nozzle movement during component building action [28–30].

Most of the parameters given in the most recent research comprise the diameter of the nozzle, extrusion temperature, filling interval, extrusion velocity, filling pattern, filling velocity, etc. [31]. These parameters, called input control factors, help control the process to optimise the output response, such as build time and part quality [32]. A schematic representation of process parameters is given in Figure 15.5.

15.5 FABRICATION USING 3D PRINTING

According to the type of process and feedstock material used, 3D-printing technology is generally categorised in the following ways, as shown in Figure 15.6.

Techniques of 3D printing have been advanced to fulfil the requirement of printing complicated structures at good resolutions. The different 3D-printing process techniques are (a) fusion deposition modelling (FDM), (b) inkjet printing (IJP),

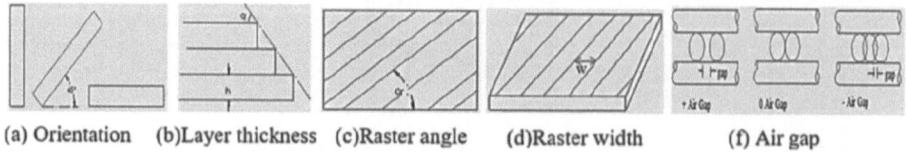

(a) Orientation   (b)Layer thickness   (c)Raster angle   (d)Raster width   (f) Air gap

FIGURE 15.5   Schematic representations of FDM process parameters [30].

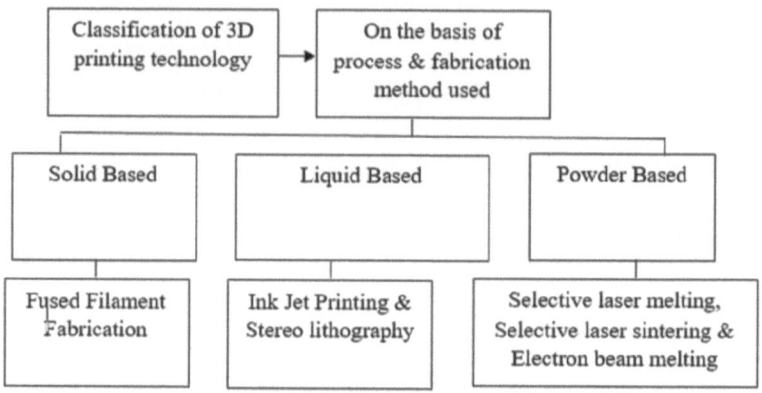

FIGURE 15.6   Classification of 3D-printing methods [33].

(c) selective laser sintering (SLS), (d) selective laser melting (SLM), (e) electron beam melting (EBM); (f) stereolithography (SLA) [33] used to manufacture 3D objects as described in the section below.

15.5.1   FUSION FILAMENT FABRICATION (FFF)

In 1988 Scott Crump developed a novel method known as FFF. This processing method utilised distinct materials such as thermoplastic polymer in a continuous filament type to print an object in a layer-by-layer fashion. Firstly the wire from a filament of diameter 1.75mm to 3mm is heated and then extruded on the base using a nozzle. The platform can move vertically (up and down) and the nozzle can move horizontally. In this way, the material is deposited onto a build base to produce a model as per the patient's requirement. The layer width, filament orientation, air gap and thickness are the major processing parameters that largely influence the mechanical characteristics of the printed components. Simplicity, high speed and low cost of the process are the major merits of the FFF process method, while the inferior quality of the surface and fewer mechanical properties are the main limitations of the FFF technique [34,35]. The schematics representation is represented in Figure 15.7.

15.5.2   SELECTIVE LASER SINTERING (SLS)

In the mid-1980s, Carl Deckard developed the SLS 3D-printing method for the development of 3D parts. This process technique mainly utilised CO_2 laser to heat

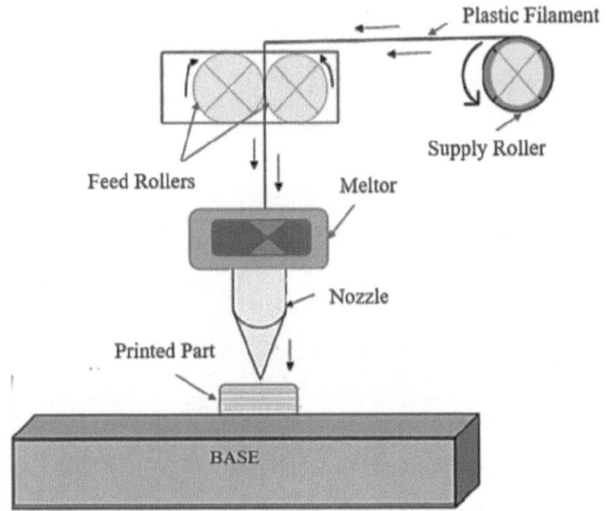

FIGURE 15.7 Schematic illustration of FDM technique [35].

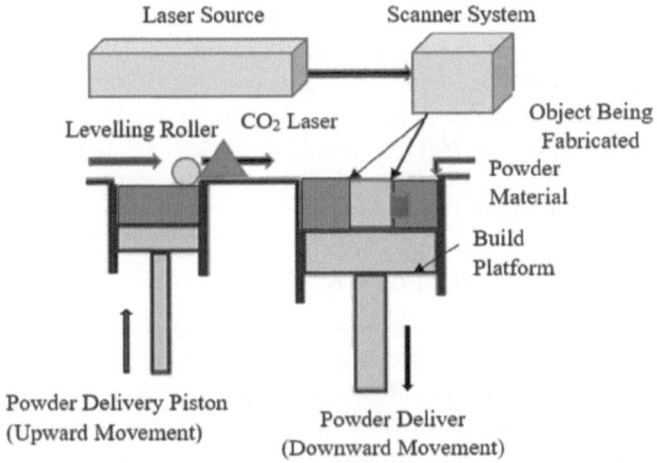

FIGURE 15.8 Schematic diagram of SLS method [43].

the powder materials that may be metals, polymers and ceramics, which are sprinkled on the base bed using a levelling roller in a layer fashion [36,37]. Finally, the piston is down, corresponding to a layer thickness and focuses the high power that heats the powder particles to develop a 3D component, as shown in Figure 15.8. In addition, superior mechanical properties, high quality, free form support material, high precision and better adhesion strength are the major merits of this technology. Internal porosity is the main drawback; therefore, post-processing is required [38–42].

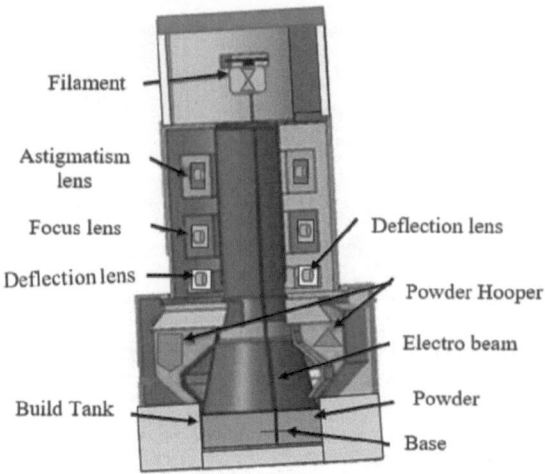

Filament

Astigmatism
lens

Focus lens

Deflection lens

Deflection lens

Powder Hooper

Electro beam

Build Tank

Powder

Base

FIGURE 15.9   Schematic diagram of EBM method [44].

15.5.3   Electron Beam Melting (EBM)

This was first commercialised by Arcam in Sweden, and is considered a low-cost technique compared to traditional manufacturing methods. This technology utilised an electron beam to melt the Ti powder. The electron gun extracts the electron from a filament of tungsten material under a vacuum. Finally, the laser melts the material and generates the layer of a part [44–49]. The process technique is repeated until the final part cannot be fully complicated. The schematic representation of the EBM process is depicted in Figure 15.9.

15.5.4   Selective Laser Melting (SLM)

This is a powder-based fusion process that started in 1995 and uses different materials (acrylonitrile butadiene styrene (ABS), polymers, etc.). The SLM process is extensively used in distinct industry domains (automotive, medical sector, aerospace and consumer products, etc.). This method utilises a high potential density laser to heat/melt the metallic material, and the laser beam moves away from the melt pool. Finally, the molten metal is cooled, and a dense structure is developed. After that, the powder material is injected onto the surface of the previously melted layer, and the object is completed. From the view of experiment, the SLM process control is not quite simple, but from the theoretical point of view, it is very simple. The limitation of this method is that it requires supporting material, which increases the cost. In addition, post-processing is also required [50–53]. The schematic diagram of SLM is represented in Figure 15.10.

15.5.5   Inkjet Printing (IJP)

IJP is an efficient, non-contact technique for the direct deposition of materials. The ink used in IJP is mainly composed of carbon materials, organic polymers and metal nanoparticles. Firstly the print head is positioned above the build platform and

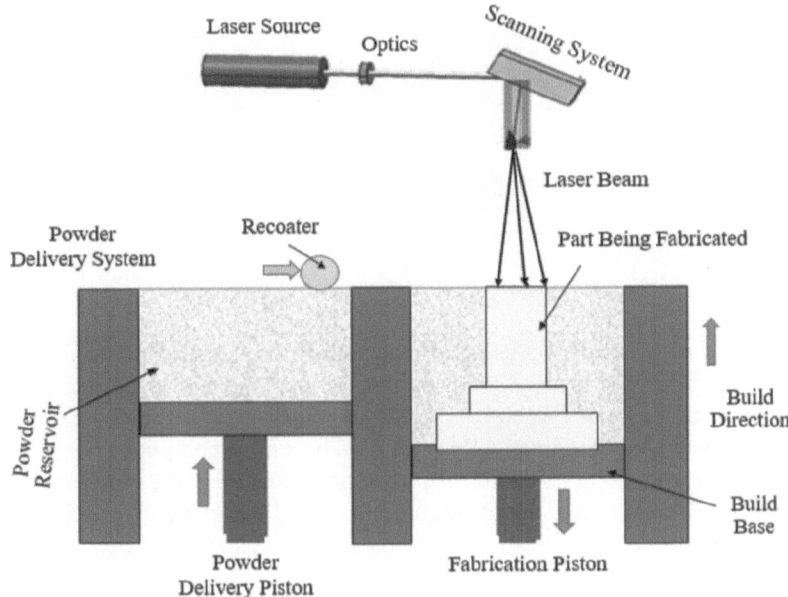

FIGURE 15.10 Schematic illustration of SLM method [50].

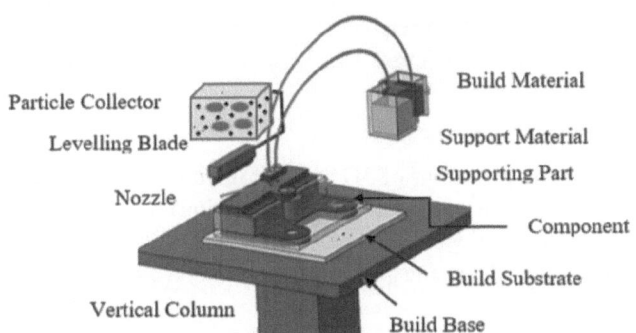

FIGURE 15.11 Schematic representation of IJP [56].

thermoplastic and wax held in a liquid state inside two heated tanks. These materials are supplied through shoot droplets, and IJP heads to the required region to form a layer of the component. Furthermore, these materials are cooled utilizing ultraviolet rays and generate a layer. If we compare this processing method to other types of AM method, no post-processing is needed [54–56]. The schematic illustration of IJP is depicted in Figure 15.11.

15.5.6 STEREOLITHOGRAPHY (SLA)

This is the first versatile, precise and high-speed printing technique developed by Hideo Kodama in 1981 and utilised for prototypes or model generation and

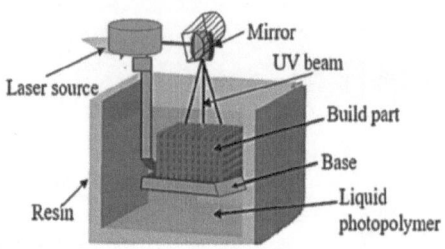

FIGURE 15.12   Schematic illustration of SLA method [57].

production of components by using photochemical processes. During this process, the laser draws the first layer of the print into the photo-sensitive resin. However, as heating by laser, the liquid solidifies. Further, this laser is directed to the coordinates as per need by a mirror automatically controlled by a mini-computer. The main merit of this technique is the non-requirement of supporting structure, superior resolution (10–150μm), no material wastage, high surface qualities (surface roughness 0.38–0.61μm) and less costly[57,58]. The schematic representation of SLA is presented in Figure 15.12.

15.6   APPLICATIONS OF 3D PRINTING

Recently, 3D-printing technology has been widely used in distinct industries (medical, aerospace, automotive, fashion, electronic, building, electric, architecture, medicine, construction, food etc.) (Figure 15.13).

15.6.1   MEDICAL

The primary medical applications of 3D printing include tissue and organ fabrication, surgical tool, anatomical models (surgical preparation), custom-made implants and prosthetics and pharmaceutical-related research linked with drug discovery. However, bioprinting is mainly used for transplantation generation and tissues [59,60].

15.6.2   AEROSPACE

3D printing is the next significant phenomenon in the aerospace sector. It has a lot of benefits and has been chiefly used in the aerospace industry for manufacturing

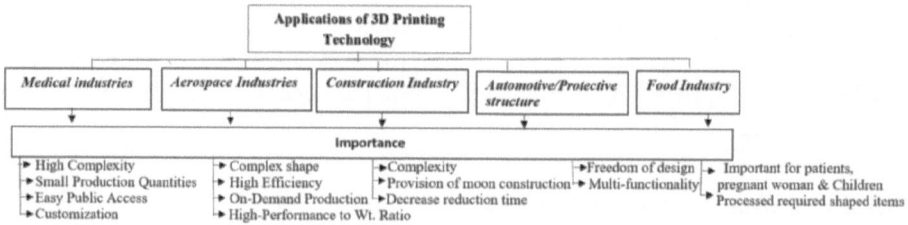

FIGURE 15.13   Applications of additive manufacturing.

and repairing aerospace parts, such as combustion chambers, fixtures, accessories, brackets and nozzles (Vulcan 2 demonstration nozzle) [61–63].

15.6.3 CONSTRUCTION/BUILDING

The application of 3D printing in distinct industries is to generate a physical model as well as end-use components. Architectural prototypes have been developed with this method for more than 10 years. [64]. AM has been used to develop the construction of whole buildings of cumbersome shape, shelters on the moon owing to the ability to process in situ materials, and printed houses by DusArchitects and Win Sun. The main challenges to the construction industry include worker safety during construction, reducing skilled workforce, manufacturing of waste material and working in harsh environments [65,66].

15.6.4 AUTOMOTIVE

This novel process technology in the automotive sector provides innovative, lighter, cleaner and safer products that lead to lower costs and shorter lead time [67].

The most common applications of 3D printing in the automobile industries are tooling, prototyping, jig and fixture, part manufacturing and assembly of automobile components. This technology produces a battery cover, air-conditioning ducting, alternator mounting bracket, bellows and headlight prototype, etc. In addition, aluminium-based alloys are of great interest mainly in the automotive and aeronautic industries because of their relatively superior strength, good wear and corrosion resistance [68,69].

15.6.5 FOOD

The good-quality food known as healthy food is generally needed for pregnant women, children, patients, athletes etc., for their proper growth [70]. By using this technology, a material of a particular type is mixed and processed into the required dimension and shape. The food items such as chocolate, pizza, sugar and pasta can be used to produce new food items with the required dimension [71–72]. To achieve precise printing, material characteristics (particle size, rheological properties), process parameters (printing speed, print distance and nozzle diameter) and post-processing methods (frying, baking, and cooking) should be kept in mind.

15.7 MATERIALS FOR 3D PRINTING

Recently, 3D printing has been a well-known process technology for fabricating 3D components with distinct materials (metals and alloy, composites, polymer, concrete and ceramics or combination). For high versatility and application, special consideration is needed to develop new advanced materials which can help in enhancing the mechanical properties, bioactivity and service life. The various materials used in 3D printing for manufacturing different parts and their applications are presented in Figure 15.14.

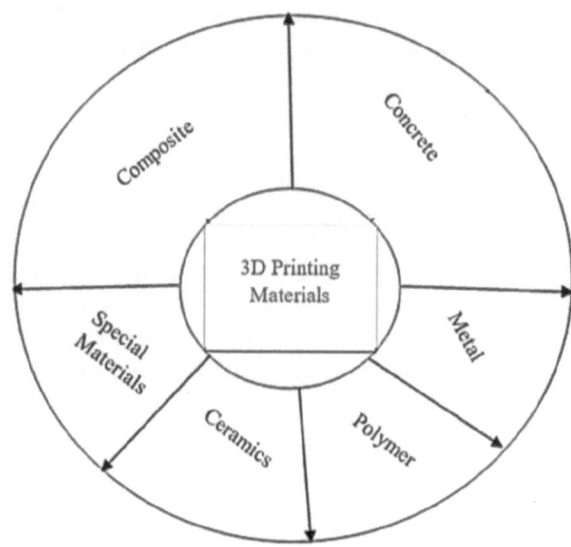

FIGURE 15.14   Classifications of additive manufacturing materials [73].

15.7.1 Composites

The capability of using three-dimensional printing of composites has been explored for many years in several industrial uses, such as medical fields, architecture, aerospace and toy manufacturing. The key characteristics of such material are versatility and being light in weight. Owing to its high strength and corrosion-resistant properties, composite material is used in the aerospace industry. Carbon fibre and glass fibre reinforced polymer composites are examples of composite materials [74]. Polylactic acid composite mixtures have recently been utilised to manufacture scaffolds for tissue engineering applications [75].

15.7.2 Concrete

The primary use of concrete is for construction and infrastructure. It is particularly helpful in space construction and harsh environment owing to less labour requirement. However, the threat involves the layer-by-layer appearance, its production having anisotropic mechanical characteristics, tailored concrete mixture design and a limited range of 3D-printing methods and tailored concrete mixture design.

15.7.3 Metals

Metals are primarily used in the automotive, biomedical and defence sectors [76,77]. They exhibit freedom for manufacturing complex configurations and possess superior physical properties, and are used for printing human organs or aerospace parts. The Al-based alloys, Co-based alloys, Ti-alloys and stainless steel are the main examples of materials. However, Co-based alloy is greatly recommended owing to high elongation, stiffness and resilience etc. In addition, some examples of 3D-printing techniques that use such material are binder jetting, powder bed fusion, direct energy deposition, and newly developed techniques such as friction stir welding (FSW) and cold spray (CS). Powder bed fusion produces parts with high accuracy of ± 0.02 mm and high mechanical properties [78,79].

15.7.4 POLYMER

Thermoplastics and thermosets are general types of polymers for three-dimensional printing. ABS and polycarbonate are examples of thermoplastic material. Photopolymer resins and polystyrene are examples of thermoset materials. These polymer materials are generally used in SLA, FDM, IJP and SLS 3D-printing techniques [80,81]. Owing to their ease of adoption and diversity, polymers are considered common materials in AM industries and are found in the form of powder, thermoplastic filaments and reactive monomers. However, nanocomposites have attracted the attention of distinct industries owing to many attractive characteristics (lightweight, better thermal conductivity, cost-effective, high strength, etc.) [82–86]. Polymers are used in orthopaedic implants, cartilage repair, biomaterials, medical devices and tissue engineering [87].

15.7.5 CERAMICS

3D printing has become an important technique for manufacturing biomaterials and tissue engineering. The primary benefits of ceramic materials for 3D printing include printing complicated structures, human organ scaffolds, and decreased part manufacturing time [88]. These materials are highly durable, fire resistant and robust and are beneficial for dental application, building construction and aerospace. There are different ceramics materials (bioactive glasses alumina, zirconia etc.), but alumina is generally used in distinct applications [89–92]. The distinct materials have been investigated, which enhances the mechanical characteristic of 3D-printed ceramic lattices more than conventional methods. In addition, SLS of powder is a technique for 3D printing of ceramic powders [93,94].

15.7.6 SPECIAL MATERIALS

Special materials include food materials such as pizza, meat and chocolate that can be processed and produced at the required size and shape by 3D-printing technology, and the material nutrients adjusted without diminishing the taste, so that high quality (healthy) food can be produced. Textiles and moon dust are other examples of special materials [95] (Table 15.3).

15.8 POST-PROCESSING TECHNIQUES

Additive manufacturing has several merits over traditional (subtractive) manufacturing technology, but it still has some drawbacks, such as surface quality, dimensional accuracy and staircase effect [111]. To overcome these drawbacks of AM, distinct post-processing is used. The distinct techniques that are commonly used for

TABLE 15.3

Summary of Distinct AM Materials and Their Process Methods [96–110]

Technology Used	Inventors	Initial State of Material	Power Source	Phase Change	Merits	Demerits	Types of Materials Used
FDM	S. Scott Crump	Filament	Thermal energy	Solidify by cooling	It is an economical method because of fewer machines, availability of components in many colours and durability over time.	Inferior mechanical characteristics, small temperature application, support is needed etc.	**Polymers:** ABS, PC, ULTEM, PC-ABS, PLA etc. **Composite:** Polymer-ceramic and short fibre reinforced composites etc. **Ceramics:** zirconia, Alumina.
SLM	Fockele and Schwarze	Powder	High powdered laser beam	Full melting	Economical, utilizes distinct material.	Used only for limited sizes part manufacturing application.	**Metals:** Stainless steel GP1, Titanium Ti6Al4V, PH1 & 17-4 & TiCP, steel MS1. **Composites:** polymer matrix.
SLA	Dr Hideo Kodama	Liquid	Ultraviolet laser	Photopoly-merisation	Fabricate superior quality parts, more resolution, and large-sized components can be easily manufactured.	More machine cost, less durability and strength, build process is very slow and more expensive.	**Ceramic:** Alumina, silica. **Polymers:** Photo-curable polymers.
SLS	Dr Carl Deckard	Powder	High powdered laser beam	Partial melting	Post-processing needed, No need for support, fabricated complex structure easily.	Poor structural property metal parts can be printed only; need for post-processing.	Polymers: Polyamide 12, polystyrene. Composites: Ceramic-ceramic.
EBM	Arcam	Powder	Electron beam	Full melting	Economical and small technology.	Limited sizes and slow processing.	Metals: Ti6Al4V, Co –Cr etc.

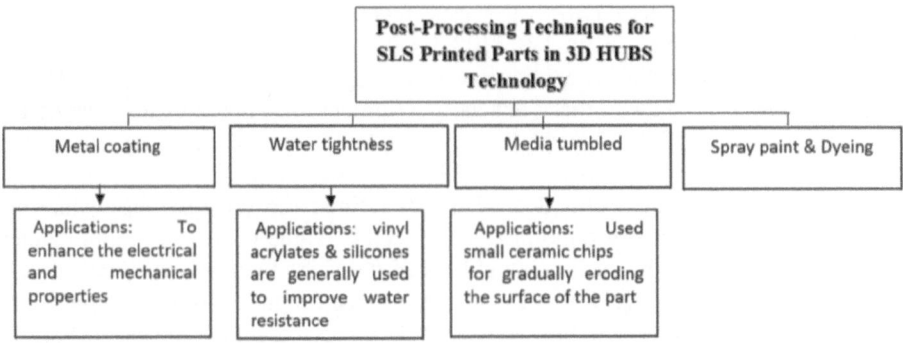

FIGURE 15.15   Post-processing techniques used in 3D-printing technology [112].

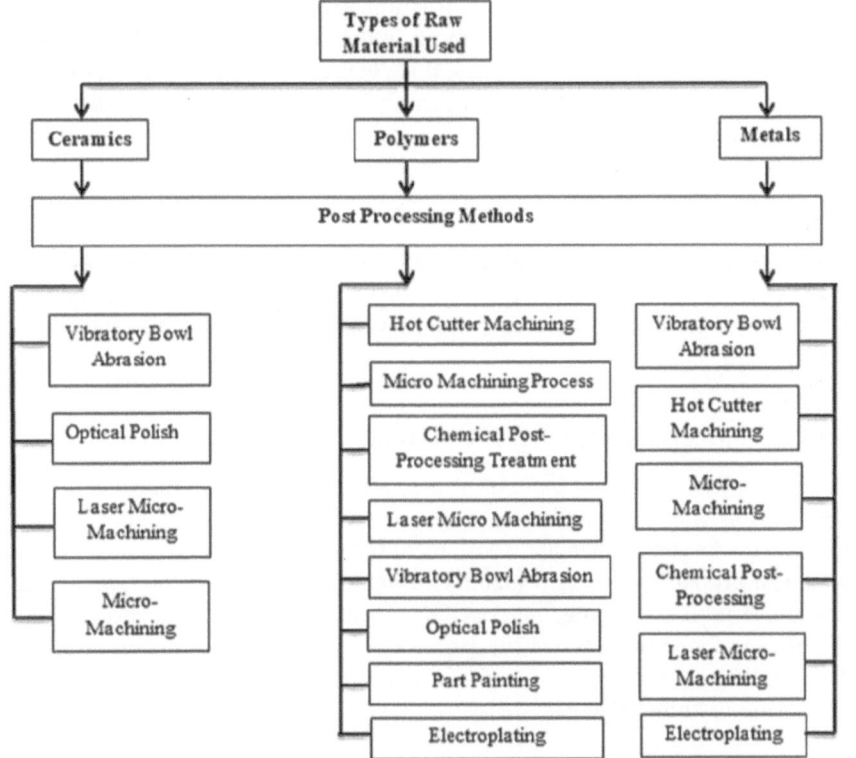

FIGURE 15.16   Distinct post-processing methods based on raw material [115].

the post-processing of distinct materials are vibro polish, lacquering/painting, dyeing, water tightness, metal coating, etc. [112–114]. The particular post-processing techniques used for SLS parts are shown in Figure 15.15.

However, based on the raw material used, post-processing methods can be categorised, as shown in Figure 15.16.

Spencer et al. [116] used two post-processing techniques (vibratory bowl abrasion finishing) on parts made from XB 5143 (general purpose resin) and Ciba-Geigy XB5081-1 (durable resin) to enhance surface roughness. The results of SEM and surface topography showed that both the post-processing method can enhance the surface finish of a model. However, the vibratory bowl abrasion finishing process has gained a superior surface finish which is about 74 per cent improvement over ultrasonic abrasion finishing. Schmid et al. [117] refined the selective laser sintering (SLS) parts using vibratory grinding and reduced R_a value from 11 to 2μm. Pandey et al. [118] improved the surface roughness of the parts built by the FDM process using hot cutter machining. It was found that surface roughness of 0.3 μm has 87 % confidence levels. However, this technique is restricted to flat surfaces. Various researchers [119–121] used different lasers to improve surface finish. However, carbon dioxide laser is most commonly used for industrial applications (marking, drilling, cutting, engraving, annealing and heat treatment of industrial materials) owing to its high efficiency and rugged construction. However, among distinct post-processing techniques, laser micromachining is the most widely used method [122]. From the results of various researchers, it is clear that the surface finish of the additive manufacturing parts can be significantly enhanced by utilising distinct post-processing methods.

15.8.1 APPLICATION OF POST-PROCESSING

The post-processing methods are generally utilised to improve parts quality and to overcome 3D-printing demerits. They improve surface texture, aesthetic look, mechanical properties and geometric accuracy and eliminate the need for supporting material [122].

15.9 CHALLENGES OF 3D PRINTING

AM has many merits, such as ease of use, ability to print complicated structures, design flexibility and customisation of products. However, AM technology still has some drawbacks and challenges. These include the limit on the part size, anisotropic mechanical properties, low part manufacturing efficiency, high costs, low accuracy, pillowing, stringing, warping, under and over extrusion, mass production and demerits in the use of materials [123–125]. However, the significant challenges in 3D printing are (a) this technology is not standardised; (b) high product and equipment costs; (c) 3D-printing knowledge gap.

15.10 CONCLUSION

AM plays an important role in particular manufacturing industries, such as the food, automobile, fashion and medical sectors. AM has several applications in today's world with the capability to revolutionise the embraced sector and generate innovative ideas. 3D printing is the most attractive area in engineering, metallurgy and science. It has many process techniques dealing with distinct materials to process, and each technique has particular materials to use. Conventional manufacturing methods are generally limited by complicated shape and design customisation of the components to be manufactured. In each field of application, we can achieve low weight, ergonomic and multi-material products and fewer assembly errors because of lower tooling investment costs and best use of materials. The technology selection is dependent on the specific application being planned: first the application, then the technology. Laser systems are being increasingly utilised, mainly in final finished part production. However, the future of AM lies in the advancement of 3D printing of a wide range of materials.

ACKNOWLEDGEMENTS

The authors are grateful to the RIC Department of Chandigarh University, CGC Landran and Auxein Medical Private Limited, Sonipat, India, for giving them the opportunity to carry out this book chapter.

REFERENCES

1. Monzón, M.D., Ortega, Z., Martínez, A., and Ortega, F. (2014). Standardization in additive manufacturing: Activities carried out by international organizations and projects. *The International Journal of Advanced Manufacturing Technology*, 76(5–8), 1111–1121. doi:10.1007/s00170-014-6334-1
2. Thomas, D. (2016). Costs, benefits, and adoption of additive manufacturing: A supply chain perspective. *The International Journal of Advanced Manufacturing Technology*, 85, 1857–1876. doi:10.1007/s00170-015-7973-6
3. Zhou, C., Chen, Y., Yang, Z., and Khoshnevis, B. (2011). Development of a Multi-material Mask-Image-Projection-based Stereolithography for the Fabrication of Digital Materials, *Solid Freeform Fabrication Symposium*. Austin, Texas, USA, 65–80.
4. Kumar, R. and Kumar, S. (2020). Trending applications of 3D printing: A study. *Asian Journal of Engineering and Applied Technology*, 9(1), 1–12.
5. Jiménez, M., Romero, L., Dominguez, I.A., Espinosa, M.M. and Dominguez, M. (2019). Additive manufacturing technologies: An overview about 3D printing methods and future prospects. *Complexity*, 1–30. doi:10.1155/2019/9656938.
6. Torabi, K., Farjood, E., and Hamedani, S. (2015). Rapid prototyping technologies and their applications in Prosthodontics, a review of literature. *Journal of Dentistry*, 16(1), 1–9.
7. Dawood, A., Marti, B.M., Sauret-Jackson, V., and Darwood, A. (2015). 3D printing in dentistry. *British Dental Journal*, 219(11), 521–529. doi:10.1038/sj.bdj.2015.914
8. Shahrubudin, N., Lee, T.C., and Ramlan, R. (2019). An overview on 3D printing technology: Technological, materials and applications. *Procedia Manufacturing*, 35, 1286–1296.
9. Keles, O., Blevins, C.W., and Bowman K. (2017). Effect of build orientation on the mechanical reliability of 3D printed ABS, *Rapid Prototyping Journal*, 23, 320–328.
10. Beaman, J.J., Barlow, J.W., Bourell, D.L., and McAlea, K.P. (1997). *Production & Process Engineering, Research and Applications in Thermal Laser Processing*, Springer Science+ Business Media, New York.
11. Wong, K.V. and Hernandez, A. (2012). A Review of additive manufacturing. *Mechanical Engineering*, Article ID 208760, 1–10. doi:10.5402/2012/208760
12. Standard Terminology for Additive Manufacturing Technologies (2013). Available: https://wohlersassociates.com/additive-manufacturing.html (accessed: 12 May 2022).

13. Chua, S.K., Teh, S.H., and Gay, K.L. (1999). Rapid prototyping versus virtual prototyping in product design and manufacturing. *Advanced Manufacturing Technology*, 15, 597–603.

14. Chua, C.K., Leong, K.F., and Lim, C.S. (2010). Rapid prototyping: Principles and applications. *Assembly Automation*, 30 (4), doi:10.1108/aa.2010.03330dae.001

15. Chua, C.K., Leong, K.F., and Lim, C.S. (2003). *Rapid Prototyping: Principles and Application*, 2nd ed., World Scientific, New Jersey, NJ.

16. Gibson, I., Rosen, D., and Stucker, B. (2015). Additive manufacturing technologies 3d printing, rapid prototyping, and direct digital manufacturing second edition ISBN 978-1-4939-2112-6 ISBN 978-1-4939-2113-3 (eBook) doi 10.1007/978-1-4939-2113-3 Springer New York Heidelberg Dordrecht London, 1–18.

17. Page, D., Koschan, A., Voisin, S., Ali, N., and Abidi, M. (2005). 3D CAD model generation of mechanical parts using coded-pattern projection and laser triangulation systems. *Assembly Automation*, 25 (3), 230–238. doi:10.1108/01445150510610953

18. Jamie, D. (2018). 3D Printing vs CNC Machining: Which is best for prototyping? Available: https://www.3dnatives.com/en/3d-printing-vs-cnc-160320184/

19. Pintu (2021). Difference Between Additive and Subtractive Manufacturing. Available: http://www.difference.minaprem.com/machining/difference-between-additive-and-subtractive-manufacturing/

20. Yang, Y., Fuh, J.Y.H., Loh, H.T., and Wong Y.S. (2003). A volumetric difference-based adaptive slicing and deposition method for layered manufacturing. *Journal of Manufacturing Science and Engineering* 125(3), 586 doi:10.1115/1.1581887.

21. Long, Y., Pan, J., Zhang, Q., and Hao, Y. (2017). 3D printing technology and its impact on Chinese manufacturing. *International Journal on Production Research*, 55 (5), 1488–1497.

22. Stansbury, J.W. and Idacavage, M.J. (2016). 3D Printing with polymers: Challenges among expanding options and opportunities. *Dental Materials*, 32(1), 54–64. doi:10.1016/j.dental.2015.09.018.

23. Wu, P., Wang, J., and Wang, X. (2016). A critical review of the use of 3D printing in the construction industries. *Automation in Construction*, 68, 21–31.

24. Barnatt, C. (2013). 3D printing, the next industrial revolution. Available: https://www.explainingthefuture.com/3dp_chapter1.pdf

25. Lipson, H. and Kurman, M. (2013). *Fabricated, the New World of 3D Printing*. John Wiley & Son, Hoboken, Indianapolis, ISBN: 978-1-118-35063-8.

26. Mariano J., Luis R., Iris A., and Manuel D. (2019). Additive manufacturing technologies: An overview about 3D printing methods and future prospects, *Hindawi Complexity*, 1–30. doi:10.1155/2019/9656938

27. Mohamed, O. A., Masood, S.H., and Bhowmik, J.L.(2015). Optimization of fused deposition modeling process parameters: A review of current research and future prospects. *Advances in Manufacturing*, 3, 42–53. doi:10.1007/s40436-014-0097-7

28. Mahmood, S., Qureshi, A.J., and Talamona, D. (2018). Taguchi based process optimization for dimension and tolerance control for fused deposition modelling. *Additive Manufacturing*, 21, 183–190.

29. Nancharaiah, T. D., Ranga, R., and Raju, R. (2010). An experimental investigation on surface quality and dimensional accuracy of FDM components. *International Journal on Emerging Technologies*, 1(2), 106–111.

30. Nancharaiah, T. (2011). Optimization of process parameters in FDM process using design of experiments. *Optimize*, 2, 100–102.

31. Wong, K. V. and Hernandez, A. (2012). A review of additive manufacturing. *ISRN Mechanical Engineering*, 2, 1–10.

32. Peng, A., Xiao, X., and Yue R. (2014). Process parameter optimization for fused deposition modeling using response surface methodology combined with fuzzy inference system. *The International Journal of Advanced Manufacturing Technology*, 73, 87–100.

33. Bhushan, B. and Caspers M. (2017). An overview of additive manufacturing (3D printing) for micro fabrication. *Microsystem Technology*, 23(4), 1117–1124.

34. Tagore, G.R.N., Anjikar, S.D., and Venu Gopal, A. (2007). Multi objective optimization of build orientation for rapid prototyping with fused deposition modeling (FDM). In: *Seventeenth Solid Freeform Fabrication (SFF) Symposium*, Austin, 246–255.

35. Masood, S. H. (2014). Advances in fused deposition modeling, *Comprehensive Materials Processing*, 69–91. doi:10.1016/b978-0-08-096532-1.01002-5

36. Deckard, C., (1989). Method and apparatus for producing parts by selective sintering, U.S. Patent 4,863,538, filed October 17, 1986, published September 5, 1989.

37. Lou, A. and Grosvenor, C. (2013). Selective laser sintering, birth of an industry, *The University of Texas*, 7, 3–22.

38. Ventola, C.L. (2014). Medical applications for 3D printing: Current and projected uses. *Medical Devices*, 39 (10), 704–711.

39. Eshraghi, S. and Das, S. (2010). Mechanical and microstructural properties of polycaprolactone scaffolds with one-dimensional, two-dimensional, and three-dimensional orthogonally oriented porous architectures produced by selective laser sintering. *Acta Biomater*, 6(7), 2467–2476. doi:10.1016/j.actbio.2010.02.002.

40. Vaezi, M., Seitz, H., and Yang, S. (2013). A review on 3D micro-additive manufacturing technologies. *International Journal of Advance Manufacturing Technology*, 67, 1721–1754 doi:10.1007/s00170-012-4605-2.

41. Salmoria, G.V., Klauss, P., Paggi, R.A., Kanis, L.A., and Lago, A. (2009). Structure and mechanical properties of cellulose based scaffolds fabricated by selective laser sintering, *Polymer Testing*, 28, 648–652.

42. Raja, M., Mussawib, A.A., Faridc, F., Alkhafagyd, M.T., and Shafiei, F. (2016). Prosthodontic using rapid prototyping. *American Scientific Research Journal of Engineering Technology*, 26(1), 271–285.

43. Negi, S., Nambolan, A.A., Kapil, S., Joshi, P.S., Manivannan, R., Karunakaran, K.P., and Bhargava, P. (2019). Review on electron beam based additive manufacturing, *Rapid Prototyping Journal*, 26 (3), 485–498. doi:10.1108/RPJ-07-2019-0182.

44. Murr, L., Gaytan, S., Ramirez, D. et al. (2012). Metal fabrication by additive manufacturing using laser and electron beam melting technologies. *Journal of Materials Science and* Technology, 28(1), 1–14. doi:10.1016/S1005-0302(12)60016-4

45. Lu, L., Fuh, J., and Wong, Y.S. 2001. *Laser Induced Materials and Processes for Rapid Prototyping*, Kluwer Academic Publishers, Dordrecht.

46. Heinl, P., Rottmair, A., Korner, C., and Singer, R.F. (2007). Cellular titanium by selective electron beam Melting. *Adcance Engineering Materials*, 9 (5), 360–364. doi:10.1002/adem.200700025

47. Rafi, H.K., Karthik, N.V., Gong, H., Starr, T.L., and Stucker, B. E. (2013). Microstructures and mechanical properties of Ti6Al4V parts fabricated by selective laser melting and electron beam melting *Journal of Materials Engineering and Performance*, 22, 3872–3883. doi:10.1007/s11665-013-0658-0.

48. Parthasarathy, J., Starly, B., Raman, S., and Christensen, A. (2010). Mechanical evaluation of porous titanium (Ti6Al4V) structures with electron beam melting (EBM*). Journal of the Mechanical Behavior of Biomedical Materials*, 3, 249–259. doi:10.1016/j.jmbbm.2009.10.006

49. Razvan, P., and Ancuta, P. (2016). Applications of the selective laser melting technology in the industrial and medical fields, new trends in 3D printing, Igor V Shishkovsky, *Intech Open*. doi:10.5772/63038.

50. Gokuldoss, P. K., Kolla, S., and Eckert, J. (2017). Additive manufacturing processes: Selective laser melting, electron beam melting and binder jetting-selection guidelines. *MDPI*, 10(6), 1–12. doi:10.3390/ma10060672

51. Kumar, S. (2014). 10.05-selective laser sintering/melting, *Comprehensive Materials Processing*, 10, 93–134. doi:10.1016/B978-0-08-096532-1.01003-7

52. Santos, E.C., Osakada, K., Shiomi, M., Kitamura, Y., and Abe, F. (2004). Microstructure and mechanical properties of pure titanium models fabricated by selective laser melting. *Journal of Mechanical Engineering Science*, 218, 711–720. doi:10.1243%2F09544 06041319545.

53. Nayak, L., Mohanty, S., Nayak, S.K., and Ramadoss, A. (2019). A review on inkjet printing of nanoparticle inks for flexible electronics. *Journal of Material Chemistry-C*, 7(29), 8771–8795.

54. Dou, R., Wang, T., Guo, Y., and Derby, B. (2011). Ink jet printing of zirconia: Coffee staining and line stability. *Ceramic Society*, 94(11), 3787.

55. Jang, T.S., Jung, H.D., Pan, H. M., and Tun, H.W. (2018). 3D printing of hydrogel composite systems: Recent advances in technology for tissue engineering. *International Journal of Bio Printing*, 4, 1–28. doi:10.18063/ijb.v4i1.126.

56. Attaran, M. (2017). The rise of 3-D printing: The advantages of additive manufacturing over traditional manufacturing. *Business Horizons*, 60, doi:10.1016/j.bushor.2017.05.011.

57. Ligon, S.C., Liska, R., Stampfl, J., Gurr, M., and Mülhaupt, R. (2017). Polymers for 3D printing and customized additive manufacturing. *Chemical Reviews*, 117(15), 10212–10290.

58. Kumar, R., Kumar, M., and Chohan, J.S. (2021). The role of additive manufacturing for biomedicalapplications: A critical review. *Journal of Manufacturing Processes*, 64, 828–850.

59. Sharma, S. and Goal, S.A. (2018). Three dimensional printing and its future in medical world. *Journal of Medical Research and Innovation*, 3(1), 1–8.

60. Mohd Yusuf, S., Cutler, S., and Gao, N. (2019). Review: The impact of metal additive manufacturing on the aerospace industry. *Metals*, *9*, 1286.

61. Kumar, L. J. and Krishnadas Nair, C. G. (2016). Current trends of additive manufacturing in the aerospace industry. *Advances in 3D Printing & Additive Manufacturing Technologies*, 39–54. doi:10.1007/978-981-10-0812-2_4

62. Joshi, S.C. and Sheikh, A.A. (2015). 3D printing in aerospace and its long term sustainability. *Virtual and Pphysical Prototyping*, 10, doi:10.1080/17452759.2015.1111519.

63. Kumar, L.J. and Nair, C.K. (2017). Current trends of additive manufacturing in the aerospace industry. In Wimpenny, D., Pandey, P. and Kumar, L. (eds), *Advances in 3D Printing and Additive Manufacturing Technologies*. Springer, Singapore, 39–54. doi:10.1007/978-981-10-0812-2_4

64. Freaeson, A. (2016). DUS Architects builds 3D-printed micro home in Amsterdam. Available: https://www.dezeen.com/2016/08/30/dus-architects-3d-printed-micro-home-amsterdam-cabin-bathtub/

65. Levy, K. (2014). A Chinese company 3D printed 10 house in a day. Available: https://www.businessinsider.com/a-chinese-company-3d-printed-10-houses-in-a-day-2014-4?IR=T

66. Giff, C.A., Gangula, B., and Illinda, P. (2014). *3D Opportunities in the Automotive Industry: Additive Manufacturing Hits the Road*. Deloitte University Press.

67. Bill Artley. Automotive 3D printing application. Avaiilable: https://www.3dhubs.com/knowledge-base/automotive-3d-printing-applications/

68. Singh, H., Kumar, S., and Kumar, R. (2021). Overview of corrosion and its control: A critical review. *Proceedings on Engineering Sciences*, 3 (1), doi:10.24874/PES03.01.002.

69. Liu, Z., Zhang, M., Bhandari, B., and Wang, Y. (2017). 3D printing: Printing precision and application in food sector. *Trends in Food Science & Technology*, 69, 83–94. doi:10.1016/j.tifs.2017.08.018

70. Dankar, I., Pujola, M., Omar, F. E., Sepulcre, F., and Haddarah, A. (2018). Impact of mechanical and microstructural properties of potato puree-food additive complexes on extrusion-based 3D printing. *Food and Bioprocess Technology*, 1, 1–11.

71. Kumar, R., Kumar, R., Kumar, S., and Goyal, N. (2020). Trending applications and mechanical properties of 3D printing: A review, *I Manager Journal on Mechanical Engineering*, 11(1), 17–34.

72. Benjamin, V., Frédéric, V., and François, F. (2012). Metallic additive manufacturing: State-of-the-art review and prospects. *Mechanics and Industry*, 13, 89–96. 10.1051/meca/2012003.

73. Sathishkumar, T.P., Satheeshkumar, S., and Naveen, J. (2014). Glass fiber-reinforced polymer composites- A review. *Journal of Reinforced Plastics and Composites*, 33, 1. doi:10.1177%2F0731684414530790

74. Senatov, F.S., Niaza, K.V., Zadorozhnyy, M.Y., Maksimkin, A.V., Kaloshkin, S.D., and Estrin Y.Z. (2016). Mechanical properties and shape memory effect of 3D-printed PLA-based porous scaffolds. *Journal of Mechanical Behaviour Biomed. Mater* 57, 139–148.

75. Brien, M.O. and Alues, A.L.V. (2018). Existing standards as the framework to qualify additive manufacturing of metals. In *Proceedings of the 2018 IEEE Aerospace Conference*, Big Sky, MT, USA, 3–10, 1–10.

76. Bedi, T.S., Kumar S., and Kumar, R. (2019). Corrosion performance of hydroxyapatite and hydroxyapatite/titania bond coating for biomedical applications, *Materials Research Express*, 7, 42–52.

77. Gibson, I., Rosenc, D., Stucker, B., and Khorasani, M. (2021). *Powder Bed Fusion in Additive Manufacturing Technologies*. Springer, Cham. doi:10.1007/978-3-030-56127-7_5

78. Kumar, S., Kumar, M., and Jindal, N., (2020). Overview of cold spray coatings applications and comparisons: A critical review. *World Journal of Engineering*, 17(1), 27–51. doi:10.1108/WJE-01-2019-0021.

79. Ngo, T.D., Kashani, A., Imbalzano, G., Nguyen, K.T.Q., and Hui, D, (2018). Additive manufacturing (3D printing): A review of materials, methods, applications and challenges, *Composites Part B: Engineering*, 143(15), 172–196.

80. Park, S., Lih, E., Park, K., Ki, Y., and Keun, D. (2017). Progress in polymer science biopolymer-based functional composites for medical applications. *Progress in Polymer Science*, 68, 77–105

81. Gundrati, N.B., Chakraborty, P., Zhou, C., and Chung, D.D.L. (2018). Effects of printing conditions on the molecular alignment of three-dimensionally printed polymer. *Composites Part B: Engineering*, 134, 164–168.

82. Postiglione, G., Natale, G., Griffini, G., Levi, M., and Turri, S. (2015). Conductive 3D microstructures by direct 3D printing of polymer/carbon nanotube nanocomposites via liquid deposition modeling. *Composites Part A: Applied Science and Manufacturing*, 76, 110–114.

83. Kumar, R., and Kumar, S. (2018). Comparative parabolic rate constant and coating properties of nickel, cobalt, iron and metal oxide based coating: A review. *I-Manager's Journal on Material Science*, 6(1), 45–56. doi:10.26634/jms.6.1.14379.

84. Caminero, M.A., Chacon, J.M., Garcia-Moreno, I., and Rodriguez, G.P. (2018). Impact damage resistance of 3D printed continuous fibre reinforced thermoplastic composites using fused deposition modelling. *Composite Part B: Engineering*, 148(1), 93–103.

85. Williams, J.M., Adewunmi, A., Schek, R.M., Flanagan, C.L., Krebsbach, P.H., Feinberg, S.E., Hollister, S.J., and Das, S. (2005). Bone tissue engineering using polycaprolactone scaffolds fabricated via selective laser sintering. *Biomaterials*, 26(23), 4817–4827. doi:10.1016/j.biomaterials.2004.11.057.

86. Hallab, N.J. and Jacobs, J.J. (2020). *2.5.4 – Orthopedic Applications, Biomaterials Science* (Fourth Edition), Academic Press, pp. 1079–1118, ISBN 9780128161371, doi:10.1016/B978-0-12-816137-1.00070-2.

87. Regassa, Y., Lemu, H.G., and Sirabizuh, B. (2019). Trends of using polymer composite materials in additive manufacturing. *IOP Conferences Series: Materials Science and Engineering*, 659, 1–8 doi:10.1088/1757-899X/659/1/012021

88. Hagedorn, Y.C., Balachandran, N., Meiners, W., Wissenbach, K., and Poprawet, R. (2011). SLM of net shaped high strength ceramics: New opportunities for producing dental restorations. In: *SFF Symposium Internet.*. Austin, TX, USA: University of Texas at Austin; Available from: https://sffsymposium.engr.utexas.edu/Manuscripts/2011/2011-42-Hagedorn.pdf

89. Wen, Y., Xun, S., Haoye, M., Baichuan, S., Peng, C., Xuejian, L., Kaihong, Z., Xuan, Y., and Jiang, P. (2017). 3D printed porous ceramic scaffolds for bone tissue engineering: A review. *Biomaterial Science*, 9, 1690.

90. Travitzky, N., Bonet, A., Dermeik, B., Fey, T., Filbert-Demut, I., Schlier, L., Schlordt, T., and Greil, P. (2014). Additive manufacturing of ceramic-based materials. *Advance Engineering Material*, 16, 729–754.

91. Withell, A., Diegel, O., and Grupp, I., Reay, S., and Potgieter, J. (2012). Porous ceramic filters through 3D printing. Innovative developments in virtual and physical prototyping. *Proceedings of the 5th International Conference on Advanced Research and Rapid Prototyping*, 313, 1–8.

92. Liu, F.H., Shen, Y.K., and Liao, Y.S. (2011). Selective laser generation of ceramic–matrix composites. *Composites Part B: Engineering*, 42(1), 57–61.

93. Wang, X., Jiang, M., Zhou, Z., Gou, J., and Hui, D. (2017). 3D printing of polymer matrix composites: A review and prospective. *Composites Part B: Engineering*, 110, 442–458. doi:10.1016/j.compositesb.2016.11.034.

94. Kazemian, A., Yuan, Xiao, Eva, C., and Khoshnevis, B. (2017). Cementitious materials for construction-scale 3D printing: Laboratory testing of fresh printing mixture. *Construction and Building Materials*. 145, 639–647. doi:10.1016/j.conbuildmat.2017.04.015.

95. Griffith, M.L. and Halloran, J.W. (1966). Freeform fabrication of ceramics via stereo lithography. *Journal of the American Ceramic Society*, 79(10), 2601–2608.

96. Dufaud, O. and Corbel, S. (2002). Stereo lithography of PZT ceramic suspensions. *Rapid Prototyping Journal*, 8(2), 83–90.

97. Rangarajan, S., Venkataraman, N, Safari, A., and Danforth, S.C. (2000). Powder processing, rheology, and mechanical properties of feedstock for fused deposition of Si3N4 ceramics. *Journal of the American Ceramic Society*, 83(7), 1663–1669.

98. Agarwala, M.K., Weeren, R., Bandyopadhyay, A., Whalen, P.J., Safari a Danforth, S.C. (1996). Fused deposition of ceramics and metals: An overview. In: *Proceeding of Solid Freeform Fabrication Symposium*. Austin, TX.

99. Leu, M.C., Pattnaik, S., and Hilmas, G.E. 2010. Optimization of selective laser sintering process for fabrication of zirconium diboride parts. In: *Proceeding of International Solid Freeform Fabrication Symposium*. Austin, TX.

100. Guo, N., and Leu, M.C. (2010). Effect of different graphite materials on electrical conductivity and flexural strength of bipolar plates fabricated by selective laser sintering. In: *Proceedings of the Solid Freeform Fabrication Symposium*. Austin, TX.

101. Goodridge, R.D., Dalgarno, K.W., and Wood, D.J. (2006). Indirect selective laser sintering of an appetite-mullite glass-ceramic for potential use in bone replacement applicationsProceedings of the Institution of Mechanical Engineers. Part H. *Journal of Engineering in Medicine*, 220(1), 57–68.

102. Nikzad, M., Masood, S.H., Sbarski, I., and Groth, A. (2010). Rheological properties of a particulate-filled polymeric composite through fused deposition process. *Materials Science Forum*, 654–656, 2471–2474.

103. Zhong, W., Li, F., Zhang, Z., Song, L., and Li, Z. (2001). Short fiber reinforced composites for fused deposition modeling. *Materials Science and Engineering*, 301, 125–130.

104. Shofner, M.L., Lozano, K., Rodriguez-Macias, F.J., and Barrera, E.V. (2003). Nanofiberreinforced polymers prepared by fused deposition modeling. *Journal of Applied Polymer Science*, 89, 3081–3090.

105. Kumar, S. and Kruth, J.P. (2010). Composites by rapid prototyping technology. *Materials and Design*, 31(2), 850–856.

106. Wiria, F.E., Leong, K.F., Chua, C.K., and Liu, Y. Poly-epsiloncaprolactone/hydroxyapatite for tissue engineering scaffold fabrication via selective laser sintering. *Acta Biomaterial*, 3(1), 1–12.

107. Eosoly, S., Lohfeld, S., and Brabazon, D. (2009). Effect of hydroxyapatite on biodegradable scaffolds fabricated by SLS. *Key Engineering Materials*, 396–398, 659–662.

108. Leong, C.C., Lu, L., Fuh, J.Y.H., and Wong, Y.S. (2002). In-situ formation of copper matrix composites by laser sintering. *Materials Science and Engineering*, 338(1–2), 81–88.

109. Stevinson, B.Y., Bourell, D.L., and Beaman, J.J. (2008). Over-infiltration mechanisms in selective laser sintered Si/SiC preforms. *Rapid Prototyping Journal*, 14(3), 149–154.

110. Kumbhar, N.N. and Mulay, A.V. (2018). Post processing methods used to improve surface finish of products which are manufactured by additive manufacturing technologies: A review. *Journal of The Institution of Engineers (India): Series C*, 99, 481–487. doi:10.1007/s40032-016-0340-z.

111. Redwood, B. (2021). Post processing for SLS parts. Available: https://www.3dhubs.com/knowledge-base/post-processing-sls-printed-parts/.

112. Kumar, S., Kumar, R.., Singh, S., Singh, H., and Handa, A. (2020). The role of thermal spray coating to combat hot corrosion of boiler tubes: A study, *Journal of Xidian University*, 14 (5), 229–239. doi:10.37896/jxu14.5/024.

113. Kumar, R., and Kumar, S. (2018). Thermal spray coating process: A study. *International Journal of Engineering Science and Research Technology*, 7 (3), 610–617.

114. Kumbhar, N. and Mulay, A. (2016). Post processing methods used to improve surface finish of products which are manufactured by additive manufacturing technologies: A review. *Institution of Engineers (India):* Series C. 99. 10.1007/s40032-016-0340-z.

115. Spencer, J.D., Cobb, R.C., and Dickens, P.M., (1993). Vibratory finishing of stereo lithography parts, Department of Manufacturing Engineering and Operations Management, University of Nottingham, UK. Available: http://sffsymposium.engr.utexas.edu/Manuscripts/1993/1993-03-Spencer.pdf

116. Schmid, M., Simon, C., and Levy, G.N. (2009). Finishing of SLS-parts for rapid manufacturing (RM): A comprehensive approach.. Available: http://utwired.engr.utexas.edu/lff/symposium/proceedingsArchive/pubs/Manuscripts/2009/2009-01-Schmid.pdf

117. Pandey, P.M., Reddy, N.V., and Dhande, S.G.(2003). Improvement of surface finish by staircase machining in fused deposition modeling. *Journal of Materials Processing Technology*, 132, 323–331.

118. Berrie, P.G. and Birkett, F.N. (1980). The drilling and cutting of polymathic methacrylate (Perspex) by CO_2 laser. *Optics and Lasers in Engineering*, 1(2), 107. ISSN:0143-8166.

119. Crane, K.C.A. and Brown, J.R., (1981). Laser-induced ablation of fibre/epoxy composites. *Journal of Physics D: Applied Physics*, 14(1), 2341–2349.

120. Crane, K.C.A. (1982). Steady-state ablation of aluminum alloys by a CO_2 laser. *Journal of Physics D: Applied Physics*, 15(10), 2093–2098.

121. Abdulhameed, O., Al-Ahmari, A., Ameen, W., and Mian, S.H. (2019). Additive manufacturing: Challenges, trends and applications. *Recent Trend in Design and Additive Manufacturing*, 11(2), 1–27.

16 Using Additive Manufacturing Techniques for Product Design and Development
Case Study on Biomaterials

Najla Bentrad
University of Sciences and Technology Houari Boumediene
(USTHB), Algiers, Algeria

Asma Hamida-Ferhat
University Hospital Center Mustapha, Pierre and Marie
Curie Center (CPMC), Algiers, Algeria

CONTENTS

DOI: 10.1201/9781003301066-16

16.1   INTRODUCTION

The concept of regenerative medicine and tissue engineering focuses mainly on the development of usable tissues and organs to regenerate diseased or weakened tissues and organs, or to create new tissues and organs (Figure 16.1). The integration of three-dimensional printing/bioprinting, big data and computer algorithms with regenerative medicine and tissue engineering is revolutionising medical treatment (Dzobo et al., 2019). Significant attention has been paid to the latest developments in 3DP technologies and the application of this technology to the construction of bionic structures of many tissues and organs, including blood vessels, heart, liver, and cartilage (Zhang et al., 2017). Using different configurations and combinations of extracellular matrix (ECM), cells and inductive biomolecules, the damaged and diseased tissues and organs can potentially be regenerated or formed (Dzobo et al., 2019). The various formats used in the tissue bioengineering area are summarised in this book chapter and demonstrate the difference between *in vitro* 3D-printing models and standard cell culture techniques.

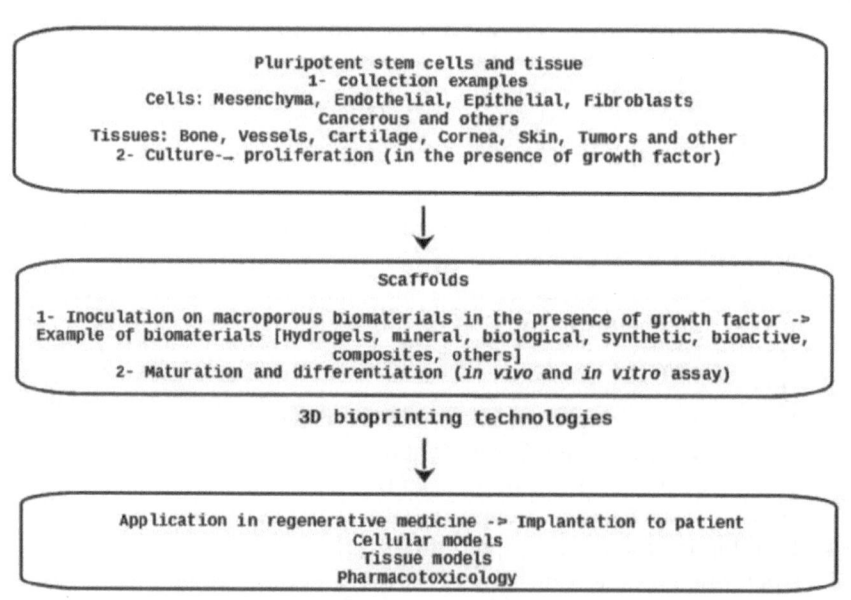

FIGURE 16.1   A diagram showing the principle of tissue engineering. Autologous cells are amplified, differentiated, and seeded on a macroporous material (scaffold) in the presence of growth factors. Before implanting into the patient of the neo-tissue, an in *vitro* or *in vivo* maturation phase is often used.

The progress in material science, cell biology, mechanobiology, and bioreactor technology will be crucial to continue progress in this complex field (Parveen et al., 2006; Kimlin et al., 2013). Several approaches using cells to replicate in tissues have been created to regulate *in vitro* the particular micro-environment of each tissue, growth and organic or inorganic substrate.

The osteochondral defects (i.e. defects affecting articular cartilage and subchondral bone) are frequently associated with the mechanical failure of the joints and are often at risk of induction of degenerative changes for osteoarthritis (Martin et al., 2007). For continued progress in this diverse area, advances in material science, cell biology, mechanobiology and bioreactor technology are important. For example, for osteochondral composites resulting from the cells grown in single-component or composite scaffolds with a broad variety of compositions and biomechanical properties, different engineering methods have been described (Parveen et al., 2006; Kimlin et al., 2013).

Moreover, by automating and standardising the development process within a structured setting, bioreactors can minimise production costs, optimising the therapeutic impact of the artificial osteochondral graft (Wendt et al., 2005). After an appropriate maturation time, the tissue can be reimplanted into the patient. (Hollister, 2005). *In vivo* studies recently proposed the use of scaffold design to refine tissue engineering therapies and to merge this design with cell printing, in order to create a hybrid designer (Sodian et al., 2000; Visconti et al., 2010).

The variable shape of the solid scaffold must allow for the dispersion and vascularisation of the cells. Due to its excellent mechanical properties and biocompatibility, polyether ketone (PEEK) is the perfect alternative material for orthopaedic implants.

In vitro results revealed that the PEEK porous scaffold is biocompatible for cell adhesion, proliferation and osteogenic differentiation; the PEE-450 scaffold is particularly useful. Also, *in vivo* studies indicate that the PEEK-450 form has a preferential prospect for bone growth and vascular perfusion (Feng et al., 2020).

Frequently differentiated stem cells that are pluripotent, isolated from patients, are considered for tissue engineering because their phenotypes can target multiple cell lines. For example, mesenchymal stem cells (MSC) derived from adipose tissue can be differentiated into osteoblasts or chondroblasts (Ohgushi, 2014). So, the combination cell/matrix/ceramic arrangement can automatically indicate bone formation in the body and can be used for bone reconstructive surgery (Krawiec et al., 2017). By developing MSC in an osteogenic medium, various osteoblasts may be distinguished, such as osteoblasts after differentiation on the ceramic surface. This chapter aims to conduct a non-exhaustive study of these various complementary aspects of additive manufacturing in regenerative medicine or tissue engineering.

16.2   BIOMATERIAL SCIENCE AND BIOFABRICATION CONCEPTS

The current 3D-printing techniques are called 'biofabrication', which aims to spatially superimpose and combine various cells, biological materials and molecules in the matrix to compromise the directional sophistication of artificial tissues. Many

3D-printing prototype models have been produced in production processes using many different rapid prototyping methods, such as stereolithography and laser sintering, as well as several chemical materials (Nakamura et al., 2010). These bioprinting methods have distinct positive and negative impacts on cells and proteins (Horch et al., 2018).

Biomaterial science has focused mainly on tissue regeneration to sustain the development period of the cell and to serve as a substitute for tissue regeneration (Gauvin et al., 2010; Tondreau et al., 2016). A wide variety of polymer materials and the most advanced approaches have been used to build structures called scaffolds (Perez-Puyana et al., 2020).

A synthetic polyester that is very useful in tissue engineering is polylactic acid (PLA). The PLA is synthesised by ring-opening polymerisation or polycondensation, making it suitable for medicinal applications. Besides, nanofibre PLA scaffolds have broad potential as drug delivery vectors, where processing parameters and drug-PLA compatibility directly impact drug delivery kinetics (Santoro et al., 2016).

There is another 3D-printing plastic scaffold with multifunctional therapeutic properties that has multiple advantages for the regeneration of complex contaminated bone defects over allogeneic or xenogeneic bone grafts. A polylactide-co-glycolide (PLGA)/hydroxyapatite (HA) grafted to a chitosan scaffold shows improved *in vitro* antimicrobial and osteoconductive properties and good *in vivo* biocompatibility using radiographic, micro-computed tomography, microbiological and histopathological tests.

Overall, grafting PLGA/HA scaffolds have enhanced anti-infectious and bone regeneration functionality in different models of infected bone defects. This point offers significant opportunities to create dual-function 3DP bone scaffolds for use in future plastic and orthopaedic surgery in polluted bone defects (Griffith and Naughton, 2002; Caneparo et al., 2020).

During cell culture, hypoxic dermal fibroblast medium (DF-Hx) results in increased proliferation of endothelial cells compared to normoxic dermal fibroblast DF-Nx medium (Caneparo et al., 2020). The DF-Hx endothelial cell proliferation period decreased by 10.4 per cent after one week of conditioning and by 20.3 per cent after two weeks compared to DF-Nx. As a result, dermal fibroblasts (2 per cent O_2) were grown under hypoxia to influence their medium cell culture (Caneparo et al., 2020).

Modern tissue engineering techniques based on cells in scaffolds have also been investigated in 3D-printing processes for vascular construction. For the delivery of nutrients and oxygen, as well as for waste disposal, the vascularisation of bone tissue is important. An analysis shows that extracellular cartilage matrix/gelatin methacrylate/exosome using a 3D-printing scaffold can be a promising method for early osteoarthritis treatment and cartilage regeneration (Chen et al., 2019). However, further research is required to better demonstrate the efficacy of this technology in the laboratory and its clinical application. It can improve the survival of implanted artificial tissues and their integration. Microfluidic technologies are progressively being used in 3D printing to design living structures to address the disadvantages of extrusion printing (Davoodi et al., 2020).

16.3 APPLICATION OF 3D PRINTING FOR TISSUE ENGINEERING

Most tissue engineering research focuses on the use of a solid, biodegradable scaffold combined with cells. Many approaches have been identified to facilitate the cellular penetration of the material, such as the use of a bioreactor or the alteration of the scaffold form (Chu et al., 2002). Some inherent drawbacks of conventional scaffolding methods, such as lack of control over pore morphology and design and reproducibility, can be recorded.

The extrusion technique extrudes the molten polymer through the platform layer by layer in the form of fine fibre, forming a 3D-printing scaffold. This technique allows the architecture and pore-scale to be fully regulated. However, the pore height is determined by the extrusion die's diameter and not by the technique itself (Hoque et al., 2012).

To create a variety of transplanted tissues, including skin, cartilage and bone, the use of 3D-printing technology has gained interest in orthopaedic spine surgery as well as regenerative medicine (Mandrycky et al., 2016). The blood vessels must also be implanted to allow the tissue to extend and mature into the host organism (Chu et al., 2002). Also, cells printed on tissue scaffolds model (such as the hydrogel layer) have shown that about 95 per cent of the cells survived and remained viable through the metastasis phase, suggesting that the neuronal and muscular pathways have efficiently distinguished (Ringeisen et al., 2004).

The 3D tissue models, together with the latest advances in human pluripotent stem cell technology, can serve as a blueprint for predictive, high-throughput drug screening and more successful regenerative therapy using living tissues or artificial organs, integration of biodegradation, and systemic approaches (Mandrycky et al., 2016). Therefore, research in this area is still mainly limited to case reports and small cohort studies, and it is clear that there are many opportunities for 3D-printing advances in this area. Further research is needed to clarify how it can influence spinal surgery (Tong et al., 2020).

16.3.1 RAPID PROTOTYPING (RP)

The rapid prototyping (RP) technique offers a remarkable opportunity to build dynamic 3D structures to solve these constraints that could potentially be applied to real patient applications. Organic printing uses the RP technique to print cells, biomaterials and cell-loaded biomaterials, independently or in combination, layer by layer, specifically producing 3D tissue structures (Ozbolat and Yu, 2013). This method may be used to reproduce the matrix of the micro-environment of tumour cells to study the development and growth of tumours, metastases, angiogenesis, and the regulation of related processes (Horch et al., 2018).

Using RP techniques, researchers were able to refine scaffolds to replicate the biomechanical properties of the repaired/replaced organ or tissue (in terms of structural integrity, strength, and micro-environment) (Hoque et al., 2012).

16.3.2 STEREOLITHOGRAPHY (SLA)

Stereolithography remains one of the most effective available technologies. Due to their low cost and good quality performance, biomedical applications of stereolithography and biodegradable resin materials are used for the preparation of porous materials in tissue engineering (Melchels et al., 2010) and the production of microfluidic devices.

This improvement in absorbance allows the printing of SLA microdevices with a resolution of sub-pixels, using commercial office printers, without reducing clarity or biocompatibility.

A low absorption of small hydrophobic molecules and Microflex labelling of mammalian cells grown in 3D-printed poly(ethylene glycol) diacrylate with a molecular weight of 258 (PEG-DA-258) microdevices have demonstrated the potential for the development of PEG-DA-based cell assays for drug discovery (Kuo et al., 2019). However, there is still a shortfall of 3D-printing resins with high clarity, high biocompatibility and high resolution at the same time. The photosensitiser isopropyl thioxanthone has been shown to improve resin penetration (containing PEG-DA-258 and photoinitiator Irgacure-819) by more than an order of magnitude in a concentration-dependent manner.

16.3.3 Selective Laser Sintering (SLS)

In the industrial processing of plastic, metal and ceramic articles, three-dimensional selective laser sintering (SLS) is currently used. Overall this study has shown that SLS is a functional and realistic technique that can be extended to the pharmaceutical industry (Fina et al., 2017). Permanent samples were printed effectively; the 3D-printed tablets were durable and there was no evidence of degradation of the substance (Fina et al., 2017).

Pharmaceutical thermoplastic polymers, Kollicoat IR (75% polyvinyl alcohol and 25% polyethylene glycol copolymer) and Eudragit L100-55 (50% methacrylic acid copolymer and 50% ethyl acrylate), and about 3% Candurin® with golden highlights were added to each powder formulation to promote the sintering process (Fina et al., 2017).

Some reports provide recommendations on the SLS process and post-treatment polymer technology, using epoxy resin diffusion to strengthen the mechanical properties of polystyrene (Zeng et al., 2019).

16.3.4 Extrusion Printing

Comprehensive printing technologies, such as 3D extrusion monitoring, help biological materials to be integrated to increase the ability to regenerate tissues. Microcomputer tomography revealed that, during the two-phase scaffold, the exact orientation of the strands and combined pore spaces were also measured as hydrogel strands in the swollen state of the alginate and alginate-gellan mixture (Ahlfeld et al., 2017).

The application of phosphate glass increased the in vitro scaffolds degradation and demonstrated strong biocompatibility of the tricalcium phosphate ceramic scaffolds. Spherical polymer scaffolds, prepared by bonding adjacent spheres or by quenching randomly filled spheres, have a homogeneous pore structure, full 3D linkage, and substantial mechanical power (He et al., 2017).

16.3.5   ENGINEERING APPLICATIONS OF ELECTROSPINNING

Applications for electrospinning are under development in regenerative medicine, tissue engineering, managed delivery of drugs, biosensors and cancer diagnostics. Electrospun nanofibres have been used in medical device coatings, *in vitro* 3D modelling of cancer, and membrane filtration (Liu et al., 2020). The electrospinning method allows micro to nanometric topography scaffolds to be generated with a high porosity compared to ECM. Electrospun scaffolds can improve cell adhesion, drug loading, and transformation properties. For example, drugs can be inserted into electrospinning scaffolds, ranging from antibiotics and anti-cancer agents to proteins, DNA, and RNA (Sill and Von Recum, 2008). This technique was tested by polymer processing, demonstrating that the electrospinning device proposed is suitable for producing repeatable and homogeneous electrospinning fibres for tissue engineering applications (Liu et al., 2020).

16.3.6   BIOPRINTING AND ORGAN PRINTING

Bioprinted structures can survive with adequate *in vivo* vascularisation and expand into tissues. Each printed cell type maintained its regular viability and growth rates, phenotypic expression, and physiological roles within the heterogeneous framework (Xu et al., 2013). Organ printing occurs in the form of cells in a modular scaffold using a single interface in a computer-aided design cells model, which facilitates the exact alignment of cells and proteins in 3D hydrogel structures. This advance not only increases the possibility of spatial regulation of the scaffold structure, but also the type and thickness of the tissue (e.g. capillaries and vessels) must further be built into a scaffold (Boland et al., 2006).

Recent advances and future 3D printing implemented using organ-on-chip microfluidics provide insights into the convergence of both technologies in developing efficient, modularly designed, and scalable organ-on-chip systems (Mi et al., 2018). Also, organ-on-chip engineering would facilitate the creation of different microorganisms, the ideal configuration of 3D cells, tissue-specific functions, or inside a microfluidic device (Yi et al., 2017).

The application of 3D printing and microfluidic technologies in organ-on-chip offers a more efficient solution for the production of complex functional organ or tissue structures (Mi et al., 2018). The organ chip is primarily focused on poly(dimethylsiloxane) microfluidic devices, whereas conventional soft lithography requires a cumbersome manufacturing technique, and the chip or organ chip relies on the complicated loading process of cells and biomaterials, and other micro-environmental factors to understand physiological or pathological processes (Mi et al., 2018). The alginate and fibrin hydrogel materials play a crucial role in biomanufacturing and in biometrics in manufacturing technology (Nakamura et al., 2010). For 3D dental printing, the most widely used materials are polydimethylsiloxane coatings filled with chlorhexidine on the surface microstructure for its antibacterial action using mesoporous silica nanoparticles to encapsulate chlorhexidine (Mai et al., 2020).

16.3.7 Inkjet Printing and Collagen Bio-Ink

For instance, stem cells derived from human amniotic fluid, canine smooth muscle cells, and bovine aortic endothelial cells were combined separately with ion-crosslinked calcium chloride ($CaCl_2$), put in various ink cartridges, and printed using an adapted thermal inkjet printer (Xu et al., 2013). The 3D porous cell block is composed mainly of a biocompatible collagen bio-ink and genipin, a cross-linking agent. Various biocompatible synthetic and natural biopolymer hydrogels have been used in the cell printing process. The analysis revealed that the collagen bio-ink manufacture will be an innovative platform for the designing of highly biocompatible and effect-based cell blocks using osteoblast and human adipose stem cells. Under these treatment conditions, a macroscopic 3D-printing collagen-based cell block and cell viability of more than 95 per cent were achieved (Kim et al., 2016).

16.3.8 Laser-Assisted Bioprinting (LAB)

In regenerative medicine and tissue engineering, the construction of complex, three-dimensional living cells and biomaterials involves computer-assisted biomanufacturing of fully functioning living tissues (Koch et al., 2013). Laser-assisted bioprinting (LAB) has been an alternative method for developing two-dimensional materials (Schiele et al., 2010). Laser printing parameters for two and three-dimensional modelling and assembly of nano-hydroxyapatite and human osteoprotector showed that cell printers would be deposited at a microscopic resolution at a speed of 5 kHz and with computer-assisted geometric control (Guillotin et al., 2010). These experiments can now demonstrate almost 100 per cent cell viability that creates heterogeneous structures for tissue engineering applications (Barron et al., 2004a; Devillard et al., 2014). The laser printing assembly shows that nano-hydroxyapatite (nHA) and human osteoprotector can be printed and organised by LAB in two and three dimensions. The physicochemical properties of nHA or the viability, proliferation, and phenotype of human osteoprotector over time (up to 15 days) have not been altered by LAB (Catros et al., 2011).

16.4 CELL PRINTING FOR MEDICAL APPLICATION

Different requirements for these issues have been highlighted for the development of engineered tissues/organs of native significance, including complex, high-volume composition, tissue-specific micro-environments and functional vasculatures. Current experiments have shown that a cardiac patch with human umbilical vein cells and human MSC has been added with the laser-induced-forward-transfer (LIFT) that may treat myocardial infarctions, and increase wound healing and functional preservation. Besides, improved capillary density and human cell integration could be seen in functionally related vessels of the murine vascular system (Gaebel et al., 2011; Sorkio et al., 2018). The development of tissue-engineered bone structures with an efficient vascular system has considerable potential for *in vitro* biostimulation of natural bone tissue and for enhancing *in vivo* bone regeneration (Xing et al., 2020). MSC have been associated with some weaknesses, despite their promising properties (Kim et al., 2020).

By combining cellular solutions with materials capable of forming stable gels, the LAB approach may be used to build scaffold-free 3D cell systems using a layer-by-layer method. It has been shown that the printed cells are not disrupted by the laser printing process and that the differentiation of the printed stem cells is not induced (Koch et al., 2013). Thebioinque and 3D cell printing technologies of the decellularised skeletal muscle extracellular matrix allow the imitation of the structural and functional properties of the native muscle and are very promising for the development of clinically important artificial muscles for the treatment of muscle injuries (Choi et al., 2016). Current evidence suggests ways to reduce patient risks following the widespread expansion of 3D imaging in the medical field (Belk et al., 2020).

Effective tissue/organ structures have been developed that fulfil these criteria and can facilitate the *in vivo* regeneration of damaged tissues (Kim et al., 2020).

16.5   APPLICATION OF MICROREACTOR ARRAY (μRA) AND BIOPRINTING OF CANCER CELLS

16.5.1   MICROREACTOR ARRAY (μRA)

Various proteomics experiments are based on bioprinting techniques or feather matrices that have been developed for the development of cDNA chips. However, these strategies often do not fit the requirements for effective protein measurement in high-throughput matrix-based proteomic profiling (Barron et al., 2004b). The manufacture of a chip based on the microreactor array (μRA) allows *in situ* synthesis into high-density molecules. For example, a single-amplified microarray DNA pattern can be self-assembled, transformed into an RNA messenger or immobilised into a μRA (Biyani and Ichiki, 2015). These reports show that the laser emission tested with normal fluorescence does not affect the active locations of the delivered proteins to produce effective protein chips (Ringeisen et al., 2002). For example, the printing of the alkaline phosphatase enzyme accompanied by a positive reaction with a colourimetric substrate indicates that this laser printer can be used to detect the functional protein (Barron et al., 2004b).

A system for the treatment of bacterial colony arrays and specific patterns using commercially available inkjet printers has been developed. Adapting the concentration of bacterial suspensions culminated in the formation of particular colonies of viable bacteria. Bacterial colony arrays with a density of 100 colonies/cm were obtained by directly ejecting *Escherichia coli* into an agar-coated substrate at a rapid arraying rate of 880 spots per second. Also, dynamic models of viable bacteria and bacterial density gradients have been developed using basic digital printers (Xu et al., 2004).

16.5.2   3D-BIOPRINTING APPLICATIONS FOR CANCER CELLS

3D-bioprinting applications can explore the transition from 2D modelling to 3D scaffolding for the implementation of biophysical and modelling the micro-environment of cancer cells which were classified into two groups (Belgodere et al., 2018; Dzobo et al., 2019) as follows: biochemical factors that modulate breast cancer cell-ECM interactions and 3D-printing methods and implementation for micro-environment simulation for breast cancer.

16.6 APPLICATION OF PRINTING FOR DRUG MANUFACTURING

Pharmaceutical technology and scientific developments are continually evolving and give different possibilities to fulfil the needs of customised drug therapy (Alhnan et al., 2016; Souto et al., 2019; Zhang et al., 2018). Since the first acceptance of the use of 3D-printed drugs by the Food and Drug Administration (FDA) in 2015, people have been highly involved in this technology for drugs manufacturing (Norman et al., 2017; Warsi et al., 2018), which allows the prototype production of personalised drugs (Palo et al., 2017; Kim et al., 2020). The recent approval of Spritam® and the announcement of the Food and Drug Administration's 'Technical Guidelines for the Additive Manufacture of Medical Devices' have contributed to comprehensive studies in various fields of drug delivery systems and bioengineering (Jacob et al., 2020).

Their uses are suitable for manufacturing capsules, implants, and nanoparticles (Warsi et al., 2018). 3D printing has a competitive edge as a platform technology in complex and customisable products, and multi-pill drug tablets (Norman et al., 2017; Ameeduzzafar et al., 2018; Warsi et al., 2018). It has the inherent potential to overcome multiple drug formulation and distribution challenges, usually related to medicines that are poorly soluble in water, because of its invention and special features (Jacob et al., 2020). As a result, personalised treatment tends to improve the efficacy of medications and reduce adverse effects, such as individual human toxicity associated with the excessive dosage of drugs (Alam et al., 2018).

16.7 CONCLUSION

Additive processing related to regenerative medicines, including 3D printing and biofabrication, involves a number of fashionable innovations that draw researchers' interest in biomaterials and tissue engineering. Current techniques do not regulate cell density and biomaterial organisation or facilitate the survival and incorporation of implanted artificial tissues. Analysis has included numerous methods and resources used to regenerate specific organs in order to understand physiological and pathological mechanisms and to change and build damaged cells and tissues. Promising advances in the field of tissue engineering are innovative 3D-printing technologies and various functional bio-inks that have made it possible to construct complex 3D living tissues/organs. It allows heterogeneous biocompatible structures made up of different cell types, biomaterials and biomolecules to be bioproduced. Further experiments are required to further demonstrate the efficacy and therapeutic application of this technology.

CONFLICTS OF INTEREST

The authors declare no conflicts of interest.

ANNEXURE FOR ABBREVIATIONS

3D   three-dimensional
DF-Hx   hypoxic dermal fibroblast medium

ECM	extracellular matrix
FDA	Food and Drug Administration.
HA	hydroxyapatite
LAB	laser-assisted bioprinting
LIFT	laser-induced-forward-transfer
MSC	mesenchymal stem cells
nHA	nano-hydroxyapatite
PEEK	polyether ketone
PEG-DA-258	poly (ethylene glycol) diacrylate with a molecular weight of 258
PLA	polyactic acid
PLGA	polylactide-co-glycolide
RP	rapid prototyping
SLA	stereolithography
SLS	selective laser sintering
μRA	microreactor array

REFERENCES

Ahlfeld, T., Akkineni, A.R., Förster, Y., Köhler, T., Knaack, S., Gelinsky, M., & Lode, A. (2017). Design and Fabrication of Complex Scaffolds for Bone Defect Healing: Combined 3D Plotting of a Calcium Phosphate Cement and a Growth Factor-Loaded Hydrogel. *Ann Biomed Eng*, 45(1), 224–236. https://doi.org/10.1007/s10439-016-1685-4

Alam, M.S., Akhtar, A., Ahsan, I., & Shafiq-Un-Nabi, S. (2018). Pharmaceutical product development exploiting 3D printing technology: Conventional to novel drug delivery system. *Curr Pharm Des*, 24(42), 5029–5038. https://doi.org/10.2174/138161282566 6190206195808

Alhnan, M.A., Okwuosa, T.C., Sadia, M., Wan, K.W., Ahmed, W., & Arafat, B. (2016). Emergence of 3D printed dosage forms: Opportunities and challenges. *Pharm Res*, 33(8), 1817–32. https://doi.org/10.1007/s11095-016-1933-1

Ameeduzzafar, A. N.K., Rizwanullah, M., Abbas Bukhari, S.N., Amir, M., Ahmed, M.M., & Fazil, M. (2018). 3D printing technology in design of pharmaceutical products. *Curr Pharm Des*, 24(42), 5009–5018. https://doi.org/10.2174/1381612825661901161046320

Barron, J.A., Rosen, R., Jones-Meehan, J., Spargo, B.J., Belkin, S., & Ringeisen, B.R. (2004a) Biological laser printing of genetically modified Escherichia coli for biosensor applications. *Biosens Bioelectron*, 20(2), 246–52. https://doi.org/10.1016/j.bios.2004.01.011

Barron, J.A., Wu, P., Ladouceur, H.D., & Ringeisen, B.R. (2004b). Biological laser printing: A novel technique for creating heterogeneous 3-dimensional cell patterns. *Biomed Microdevices*, 6(2), 139–47. https://doi.org/10.1023/b:bmmd.0000031751.67267.9f

Belgodere, J.A., King, C.T., Bursavich, J.B., Burow, M.E., Martin, E.C., & Jung, J.P. (2018). Engineering breast cancer microenvironments and 3D bioprinting. *Front Bioeng Biotechnol*, 6, 66. https://doi.org/10.3389/fbioe.2018.00066

Belk, L., Tellisi, N., Macdonald, H., Erdem, A., Ashammakhi, N., & Pountos, I. (2020). Safety considerations in 3D bioprinting using mesenchymal stromal cells. *Front Bioeng Biotechnol*, 8, 924. https://doi.org/10.3389/fbioe.2020.00924

Biyani, M., & Ichiki, T. (2015). Microintaglio printing for soft lithography-based in situ microarrays. *Microarrays*, 4, 311–13. https://doi.org/10.3390/microarrays4030311

Boland, T., Xu, T., Damon, B., & Cui, X. (2006). Application of inkjet printing to tissue engineering. *Biotechnol J*, 1(9), 910–17. https://doi.org/10.1002/biot.200600081

Caneparo, C., Baratange, C., Chabaud, S., & Bolduc, S. (2020). Conditioned medium produced by fibroblasts cultured in low oxygen pressure allows the formation of highly structured capillary-like networks in fibrin gels. *Sci Rep*, 10(1), 9291. https://doi.org/10.1038/s41598-020-66145-z

Catros, S., Fricain, J.C., Guillotin, B., Pippenger, B., Bareille, R., Rémy, M., Lebraud, E., Desbat, B., Amédée, J., & Guillemot, F. (2011). Laser-assisted bioprinting for creating on-demand patterns of human osteoprogenitor cells and nano-hydroxyapatite. *Biofabrication*, 3(2), 025001. https://doi.org/10.1088/1758-5082/3/2/025001

Chen, P., Zheng, L., Wang, Y., Tao, M., Xie, Z., Xia, C., Gu, C., Chen, J., Qiu, P., Mei, S., Ning, L., Shi, Y., Fang, C., Fan, S., & Lin, X. (2019). Desktop-stereolithography 3D printing of a radially oriented extracellular matrix/mesenchymal stem cell exosome bioink for osteochondral defect regeneration. *Theranostics*, 9(9), 2439–2459. https://doi.org/10.7150/thno.31017

Choi, Y.J., Kim, T.G., Jeong, J., Yi, H.G., Park, J.W., Hwang, W., & Cho, D.W. (2016). 3D cell printing of functional skeletal muscle constructs using skeletal muscle-derived bioink. *Adv Healthc Mater*, 5(20), 2636–2645. https://doi.org/10.1002/adhm.201600483

Chu, T.G., Orton, D.G., Hollister, S.J., Feinberg, S.E., & Halloran, J.W. (2002). Mechanical and in vivo performance of hydroxyapatite implants with controlled architectures. *Biomaterials*, 23(5), 1283–1293.

Davoodi, E., Sarikhani, E., Montazerian, H., Ahadian, S., Costantini, M., Swieszkowski, W., Willerth, S., Walus, K., Mofidfar, M., Toyserkani, E., Khademhosseini, A., & Ashammakhi, N. (2020). Extrusion and microfluidic-based bioprinting to fabricate biomimetic tissues and organs. *Adv Mater Technol*, 5(8), 1901044. https://doi.org/10.1002/admt.201901044

Devillard, R., Pagès, E., Correa, M.M., Kériquel, V., Rémy, M., Kalisky, J., Ali, M., Guillotin, B., & Guillemot, F. (2014). Cell patterning by laser-assisted bioprinting. *Methods Cell Biol*, 119, 159–74. https://doi.org/10.1016/B978-0-12-416742-1.00009-3

Dzobo, K., Motaung, K.S.C.M., & Adesida, A. (2019). Recent trends in decellularized extracellular matrix bioinks for 3D printing: An updated review. *Int J Mol Sci*, 20(18), 4628. https://doi.org/10.3390/ijms20184628

Feng, X., Ma, L., Liang, H., Liu, X., Lei, J., Li, W., Wang, K., Song, Y., Wang, B., Li, G., Li, S., & Yang, C. (2020). Osteointegration of 3D-printed fully porous polyetheretherketone scaffolds with different pore sizes. *ACS Omega*, 5(41), 26655–26666. https://doi.org/10.1021/acsomega.0c03489

Fina, F., Goyanes, A., Gaisford, S., & Basit, A.W. (2017). Selective laser sintering (SLS) 3D printing of medicines. *Int J Pharm*, 529(1–2), 285–293. https://doi.org/10.1016/j.ijpharm.2017.06.082

Gaebel, R., Ma, N., Liu, J., Guan, J., Koch, L., Klopsch, C., Gruene, M., Toelk, A., Wang, W., Mark, P., Wang, F., Chichkov, B., Li, W., & Steinhoff, G. (2011). Patterning human stem cells and endothelial cells with laser printing for cardiac regeneration. *Biomaterials*, 32(35), 9218–30. https://doi.org/10.1016/j.biomaterials.2011.08.071

Gauvin, R., Ahsan, T., Larouche, D., Lévesque, P., Dubé, J., Auger, F.A., Nerem, R.M., & Germain, L. (2010). A novel single-step self-assembly approach for the fabrication of tissue-engineered vascular constructs. *Tissue Eng Part A*, 16(5), 1737–47. https://doi.org/10.1089/ten.TEA.2009.0313

Griffith, L.G., & Naughton, G. (2002). Tissue engineering--current challenges and expanding opportunities. *Science*, 295(5557), 1009–1014.

Guillotin, B., Souquet, A., Catros, S., Duocastella, M., Pippenger, B., Bellance, S., Bareille, R., Rémy, M., Bordenave, L., Amédée, J., & Guillemot, F. (2010). Laser assisted bioprinting of engineered tissue with high cell density and microscale organization. *Biomaterials*, 31(28), 7250–56. https://doi.org/10.1016/j.biomaterials.2010.05.055

He, F., Qian, G., Ren, W., Li, J., Fan, P., Shi, H., Shi, X., Deng, X., Wu, S., & Ye, J. (2017). Fabrication of β-tricalcium phosphate composite ceramic sphere-based scaffolds with hierarchical pore structure for bone regeneration. *Biofabrication*, 9(2), 025005. https://doi.org/10.1088/1758-5090/aa6a62

Hollister, S.J. (2005). Porous scaffold design for tissue engineering. *Nat Mater*, (7):518–24. https://doi.org/10.1038/nmat1421. Erratum in: *Nat Mater*, 5(7), 590.

Hoque, M.E., Chuan, Y.L.,& Pashby, I. (2012). Extrusion based rapid prototyping technique: An advanced platform for tissue engineering scaffold fabrication. *Biopolymers*, 97(2), 83–93. https://doi.org/10.1002/bip.21701

Horch, R.E., Weigand, A., Wajant, H., Groll, J., Boccaccini, A.R., & Arkudas, A. (2018). Biofabrication: New approaches for tissue regeneration. *Handchir Mikrochir Plast Chir*, 50(2), 93–100. German. https://doi.org/10.1055/s-0043-124674

Jacob, S., Nair, A.B., Patel, V., & Shah, J. (2020). 3D printing technologies: Recent development and emerging applications in various drug delivery systems. *AAPS PharmSciTech*, 21(6), 220. https://doi.org/10.1208/s12249-020-01771-4

Kim, J., Kong, J.S., Han, W., Kim, B.S., & Cho, D.W. (2020). 3D cell printing of tissue/organ-mimicking constructs for therapeutic and drug testing applications. *Int J Mol Sci*, 21(20), 7757. https://doi.org/10.3390/ijms21207757

Kim, Y.B., Lee, H., & Kim, G.H. (2016). Strategy to achieve highly porous/biocompatible macroscale cell blocks, using a collagen/genipin-bioink and an optimal 3D printing process. *ACS Appl Mater Interfaces*, 8(47),32230–32240. https://doi.org/10.1021/acsami.6b11669

Kimlin, L.C., Casagrande, G., & Virador, V.M. (2013). In vitro three-dimensional (3D) models in cancer research: an update. *Mol Carcinog*, 52(3), 167–82. https://doi.org/10.1002/mc.21844

Koch, L., Gruene, M., Unger, C., & Chichkov, B. (2013). Laser assisted cell printing. *Curr Pharm Biotechnol*, 14(1), 91–7.

Krawiec, J.T., Liao, H.T., Kwan, L.L., D'Amore, A., Weinbaum, J.S., Rubin, J.P., Wagner, W.R., & Vorp, D.A. (2017). Evaluation of the stromal vascular fraction of adipose tissue as the basis for a stem cell-based tissue-engineered vascular graft. *J Vasc Surg*, 66(3), 883–890.e1. https://doi.org/10.1016/j.jvs.2016.09.034

Kuo, A.P., Bhattacharjee, N., Lee, Y.S., Castro, K., Kim, Y.T., & Folch, A. (2019). High-precision stereolithography of biomicrofluidic devices. *Adv Mater Technol*, 4(6), 1800395. https://doi.org/10.1002/admt.201800395

Liu, Z., Ramakrishna, S., & Liu, X. (2020). Electrospinning and emerging healthcare and medicine possibilities. *APL Bioeng*, 4(3), 030901. https://doi.org/10.1063/5.0012309

Mai, H.N., Hyun, D.C., Park, J.H., Kim, D.Y., Lee, S.M., & Lee, D.H. (2020). Antibacterial drug-release polydimethylsiloxane coating for 3d-printing dental polymer: Surface alterations and antimicrobial effects. *Pharmaceuticals*, 13(10), 304. https://doi.org/10.3390/ph13100304

Mandrycky, C., Wang, Z., Kim, K., & Kim, D.H. (2016). 3D bioprinting for engineering complex tissues. *Biotechnol Adv*, 34(4), 422–434. https://doi.org/10.1016/j.biotechadv.2015.12.011

Martin, I., Miot, S., Barbero, A., Jakob, M., & Wendt, D. (2007). Osteochondral tissue engineering. *J Biomech*, 40(4), 750–65. https://doi.org/10.1016/j.jbiomech.2006.03.008

Melchels, F.P., Feijen, J., & Grijpma, D.W. (2010). A review on stereolithography and its applications in biomedical engineering. *Biomaterials*, 31(24), 6121–30. https://doi.org/10.1016/j.biomaterials.2010.04.050

Mi, S., Du, Z., Xu, Y., & Sun, W. (2018). The crossing and integration between microfluidic technology and 3D printing for organ-on-chips. *J Mater Chem B*, 6(39), 6191–6206. https://doi.org/10.1039/c8tb01661e

Nakamura, M., Iwanaga, S., Henmi, C., Arai, K., & Nishiyama, Y. (2010). Biomatrices and biomaterials for future developments of bioprinting and biofabrication. *Biofabrication*, 2(1), 014110. https://doi.org/10.1088/1758-5082/2/1/014110

Norman, J., Madurawe, R.D., Moore, C.M., Khan, M.A., & Khairuzzaman, A. (2017). A new chapter in pharmaceutical manufacturing: 3D-printed drug products. *Adv Drug Deliv Rev*, 108, 39–50. https://doi.org/10.1016/j.addr.2016.03.001

Ohgushi, H. (2014). Osteogenically differentiated mesenchymal stem cells and ceramics for bone tissue engineering. *Expert Opin Biol Ther*, 14(2), 197–208. https://doi.org/10.151 7/14712598.2014.866086

Orringer, J.S., Shaw, W.W., Borud, L.J., Freymiller, E.G., Wang, S.A., & Markowitz, B.L. (1999). Total mandibular and lower lip reconstruction with a prefabricated osteocutaneous free flap. *Plast Reconstr Surg*, 104(3), 793–797.

Ozbolat, I.T., & Yu, Y. (2013). Bioprinting toward organ fabrication: Challenges and future trends. *IEEE Trans Biomed Eng*, 60(3), 691–99. https://doi.org/10.1109/TBME. 2013.2243912

Palo, M., Holländer, J., Suominen, J., Yliruusi, J., & Sandler, N. (2017). 3D printed drug delivery devices: Perspectives and technical challenges. *Expert Rev Med Devices*, 14(9), 685–696. https://doi.org/10.1080/17434440.2017.1363647

Parveen, S., Krishnakumar, K., & Sahoo, S. (2006). Nouvelle ère dans les soins de santé: Génie tissulaire. *J Stem Cells Reg Med*, 1(1), 8–24.

Perez-Puyana, V., Jiménez-Rosado, M., Romero, A., & Guerrero, A. (2020). Polymer-based scaffolds for soft-tissue engineering. *Polymers*, 12(7), 1566. https://doi.org/10.3390/ polym12071566

Ringeisen, B.R., Kim, H., Barron, J.A., Krizman, D.B., Chrisey, D.B., Jackman, S., Auyeung, R.Y., & Spargo, B.J. (2004). Laser printing of pluripotent embryonal carcinoma cells. *Tissue Eng*, 10(3–4), 483–91. https://doi.org/10.1089/107632704323061843

Ringeisen, B.R., Wu, P.K., Kim, H., Piqué, A., Auyeung, R.Y., Young, H.D., Chrisey, D.B., & Krizman, D.B. (2002). Picoliter-scale protein microarrays by laser direct write. *Biotechnol Prog*, 18(5), 1126–29. https://doi.org/10.1021/bp015516g

Santoro, M., Shah, S.R., Walker, J.L., & Mikos, A.G. (2016). Poly(lactic acid) nanofibrous scaffolds for tissue engineering. *Adv Drug Deliv Rev* 107, 206–212. https://doi. org/10.1016/j.addr.2016.04.019

Schiele, N.R., Corr, D.T., Huang, Y., Raof, N.A., Xie, Y., & Chrisey, D.B. (2010). Laser-based direct-write techniques for cell printing. *Biofabrication*, 2(3), 032001

Sill, T.J., & Von Recum, H.A. (2008). Electrospinning: Applications in drug delivery and tissue engineering. *Biomaterials*, 29(13), 1989–2006. https://doi.org/10.1016/j.biomaterials. 2008.01.011.

Sodian, R., Sperling, J.S., Martin, D.P., Egozy, A., Stock, U., Mayer, J.E.Jr, & Vacanti, J.P. (2000). Fabrication of a trileaflet heart valve scaffold from a polyhydroxyalkanoate biopolyester for use in tissue engineering. *Tissue Eng*, 6(2), 183–88. https://doi.org/ 10.1089/107632700320793

Sorkio, A., Koch, L., Koivusalo, L., Deiwick, A., Miettinen, S., Chichkov, B., & Skottman, H. (2018). Human stem cell based corneal tissue mimicking structures using laser-assisted 3D bioprinting and functional bioinks. *Biomaterials*, 171, 57–71. https://doi. org/10.1016/j.biomaterials.2018.04.034

Souto, E.B., Campos, J.C., Filho, S.C., Teixeira, M.C., Martins-Gomes, C., Zielinska, A., Carbone, C., & Silva, A.M. (2019). 3D printing in the design of pharmaceutical dosage forms. *Pharm Dev Technol*, 24(8), 1044–1053. https://doi.org/10.1080/10837450.2019 .1630426

Tondreau, M.Y., Laterreur, V., Vallières, K., Gauvin, R., Bourget, J.M., Tremblay, C., Lacroix, D., Germain, L., Ruel, J., & Auger, F.A. (2016). In vivo remodeling of fibroblast-derived vascular scaffolds implanted for 6 months in rats. *Biomed Res Int*, 2016, 3762484. https://doi.org/10.1155/2016/3762484

Tong, Y., Kaplan, D.J., Spivak, J.M., & Bendo, J.A. (2020). Three-dimensional printing in spine surgery: A review of current applications. *Spine*, 20(6), 833–846. https://doi.org/10.1016/j.spinee.2019.11.004

Visconti, R.P., Kasyanov, V., Gentile, C., Zhang, J., Markwald, R.R., & Mironov, V. (2010). Towards organ printing: Engineering an intra-organ branched vascular tree. *Expert Opin Biol Ther*, (3), 409–20. https://doi.org/10.1517/14712590903563352

Warsi, M.H., Yusuf, M., Al Robaian, M., Khan, M., Muheem, A., & Khan S. (2018). 3D printing methods for pharmaceutical manufacturing: Opportunity and challenges. *Curr Pharm Des*, 24(42), 4949–4956. https://doi.org/10.2174/1381612825666181206121701

Wendt, D., Jakob, M., & Martin, I. (2005). Bioreactor-based engineering of osteochondral grafts: From model systems to tissue manufacturing. *J Biosci Bioeng*, 100(5), 489–94. https://doi.org/10.1263/jbb.100.489

Xing, F., Xiang, Z., Rommens, P.M., & Ritz, U. (2020). 3D bioprinting for vascularized tissue-engineered bone fabrication. *Materials*, 13(10), 2278. https://doi.org/10.3390/ma13102278

Xu, T., Petridou, S., Lee, E.H., Roth, E.A., Vyavahare, N.R., Hickman, J.J., & Boland, T. (2004). Construction of high-density bacterial colony arrays and patterns by the ink-jet method. *Biotechnol Bioeng*, 85(1), 29–33. https://doi.org/10.1002/bit.10768

Xu, T., Zhao, W., Zhu, J.M., Albanna, M.Z., Yoo, J.J., & Atala, A. (2013). Complex heterogeneous tissue constructs containing multiple cell types prepared by inkjet printing technology. *Biomaterials*, 34(1), 130–39. https://doi.org/10.1016/j.biomaterials.2012.09.035

Yi. H.G., Lee, H., & Cho, D.W. (2017). 3D printing of organs-on-chips. *Bioengineering*, 4(1), 10. https://doi.org/10.3390/bioengineering4010010

Zeng, Z., Deng, X., Cui, J., Jiang, H., Yan, S., & Peng, B. (2019). Improvement on selective laser sintering and post-processing of polystyrene. *Polymers*, 11(6), 956. https://doi.org/10.3390/polym11060956

Zhang, J., Vo, A.Q., Feng, X., Bandari, S., & Repka, M.A. (2018). Pharmaceutical additive manufacturing: A novel tool for complex and personalized drug delivery systems. *AAPS PharmSciTech*, 19(8), 3388–3402. https://doi.org/10.1208/s12249-018-1097-x

Zhang, Y.S., Yue, K., Aleman, J., Moghaddam, K.M., Bakht, S.M., Yang, J., Jia, W., Del'Erba, V., Assawes, P., Shin, S.R., Dokmeci, M.R., Oklu, R., & Khademhosseini, A. (2017). 3D bioprinting for tissue and organ fabrication. *Ann Biomed Eng*, 45(1), 148–163. https://doi.org/10.1007/s10439-016-1612-8

17 Applications of Artificial Intelligence and Machine Learning Using Additive Manufacturing Techniques

Raj Kumar
Punjab Engineering College (Deemed to Be University),
Chandigarh, India

Harish Kumar Banga
National Institute of Fashion Technology, Mumbai, India

Parveen Kalra and R. M. Belokar
Punjab Engineering College (Deemed to Be University),
Chandigarh, India

Rajesh Kumar
UIET, Panjab University, Chandigarh, India

Rajender Kumar
Manav Rachna International Institute of Research & Studies,
Faridabad, India

Ganesh S. Jadhav
Dr VK MIT World Peace University, Pune, India

CONTENTS

DOI: 10.1201/9781003301066-17

17.1   INTRODUCTION

Additive manufacturing (AM) is a popular advance manufacturing technology which accelerates the progress of the modernisation and digitalisation of manufacturing industries [1]. AM is a computer-oriented process in which an object can be directly manufactured from 3D data, using layer by layer deposition of material [2]. AM begins with a design, made in computer-aided design (CAD) software, from which the basic information is taken. Then this design file is converted into a stereolithography (STL) file. The drawing is prepared in CAD software and then sliced, each slice containing the information of each layer that is to be made in the later steps to get the final product. AM is advantageous over conventional manufacturing processes as AM enables the fabrication of low-volume and low-cost customised objects with complicated shapes and specific material properties, in a time-efficient manner [3]. AM technology is mainly categorised into seven sub-categories: stereolithography (STL), powder bed fusion, 3D printing, material jetting, laminated object manufacturing (LOM), fuse deposition modelling (FDM) and laser engineered net shaping, as shown in Figure 17.1. These technologies can be effectively used to make metallic objects for automobiles, aerospace, agricultural, defence and biomedical applications, and are defined as follows:

- **Stereolithography (STL):** Stereolithography is a liquid-based method that works based on the principle of photo-polymerisation, in which the monomers or polymers get solidified using ultraviolet laser light as a catalyst of the reaction. The basic procedure of the process is similar to that of rapid prototype technology. Initially, the design is made in CAD, followed by conversion to an STL file; then slicing occurs; and finally, layer by layer, a three-dimensional object is created using a stereolithography machine.

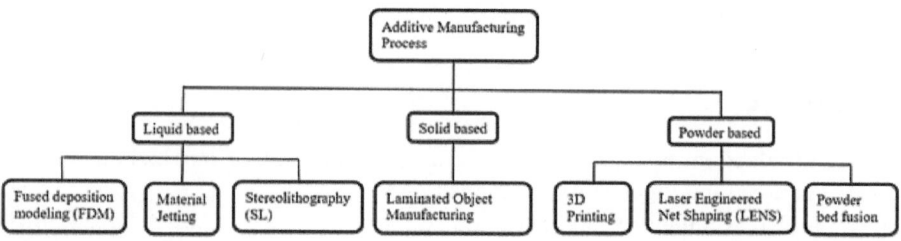

FIGURE 17.1   Types of AM process.

- **Powder bed fusion:** The process utilises an electron or laser beam to melt and fuse material powder, simultaneously. This method comprises printing techniques such as electron beam melting (EBM) and selective laser sintering (SLS). In EBM technology, the beam of laser electrons is used to melt the powder in the vacuum container to prevent oxidation. In this process, a high voltage (30 to 60 kV) electron laser beam is used. Further, the SLS method is used to sinter the powder by using CO_2 laser light. The melting point of the container is kept lower than the specific powder's melting point. The laser sinters the powder at specific locations according to the required design, and the loosely bonded powder particles are consolidated using a piston in this technique.
- **Material jetting:** This method can be used to make products in the same manner as prepared in a 2D inkjet printer. The material jet is deposited on the build surface using a drop on demand technique or continuous approach. The material solidifies on the build surface, and then the model is constructed layer by layer, the material being deposited from the nozzle moving horizontally throughout the surface. The layers of material can be cured by using UV light.
- **3D printing:** In this technique, the water-based binder is injected onto the powder to glue the powder particles according to the desired design. A variety of polymers can be processed using this technique.
- **Laminated object manufacturing (LOM):** The LOM process is based on additive and subtractive techniques. In this process, the material sheets are bonded together using pressure, high temperature and thermal adhesives. Then, the material is cut according to the shape of each layer using a carbon dioxide laser. Each layer is cut according to the CAD design and the information given in an STL file.
- **Fused deposition modelling (FDM):** FDM is a method in which a thin filament of plastic materials is fed into the machine in which a print head is provided for melting the material and extruding the material (thickness ~ 0.25mm). The plastic materials can be polycarbonate, acrylonitrile butadiene styrene, polyphenylsulfone, etc. In this technology, the support material and build material is delivered to the machine simultaneously through different channels.
- **Laser engineered net shaping (LENS):** This method uses the high-powered laser beam to melt powder injected to a specific location in an argon-filled closed chamber. This method includes the usage of a wide variety of metallic materials and the combination of them.

Despite the continuous growth of AM in the industrial sector, there are still challenges to getting a consistent quality of objects and process reliability in AM [3]. The main reasons for these challenges are the geometry and material properties of an object to be formed during the AM process. This process comprises various complex variables to be monitored and controlled during processing to achieve the desired accuracy in printing. The products of AM have a complex design, specific materials and process integrations over the course of an intricate multi-step method that involves five key steps – i.e., designing, process planning, building, post-processing, and inspection [4]. It is difficult to effectively execute these steps in a controlled and precise manner for making a quality product. Further, the barriers such as extreme time utilisation, lack of instantaneous monitoring, security risk and transformation of bulk production to bulk customisation hinder the growth of AM in this modern era.

Artificial intelligence is widely adopted in various sectors, including aerospace, computer science, finance, transportation, maintenance, education, production and healthcare. Artificial intelligence has numerous algorithms, methods and theories that enable it to transmute the conventional manufacturing processes under the state of continuously expanded data storage. Machine learning is a subset of artificial intelligence that helps machines understand and improve separately. Machine learning is used to process the useful data from present systems to provide a basic frame of the predictions for operating the machines with future decisions. Further, artificial intelligence is focused on developing intelligent agents such as software or hardware which may execute rational activities in dynamic situations. In software, the human-machine interface (HMI) can be utilised to deliver inputs and generate outputs in accordance with the instructions of humans. The data is communicated through instructions, files, proposals or other information. The hardware includes sensors which are used as input devices. These input devices can be image sensors, the Global Positioning System (GPS), audio sensors, etc. The interaction between the inputs and outputs includes events to formulate the problems and provide the solutions to formulated problems. These events are based on structured and unstructured information, including the actual model, expert opinion and historical statistics. Artificial intelligence and machine learning are not limited to being used on the production floor, but can also be used in AM and other sectors.

Artificial intelligence has recent applications in the AM for establishing intelligent, cost-effective, complex, service-oriented production processes for the industry. Further, machine learning has recently been used in conventional AM in generative design and testing in the prefabrication stage; this helps improve printing efficiency and reduce expenses. The concept of artificial intelligence can be used in AM at the factory level by preparing the machines to be more understandable than the preceding processes. The use of artificial intelligence in AM helps identify process parameters and inspect objects, improve safety characteristics and automatic post-product processing, enhance the quality of products, etc.

This chapter explores the current applications of artificial intelligence and machine learning in AM. These applications are printability checker, slicing acceleration, optimisation of nozzle path, cloud service-oriented platform, service assessment and protection against and detection of cyber-attacks.

17.2   ARTIFICIAL INTELLIGENCE APPLICATIONS IN AM

Artificial intelligence is explained as specified intelligence executed by machines, particularly focusing on making machines capable of building intelligent systems to understand and solve problems similarly to how this is done by human thinking [5]. Like many disciplines, artificial intelligence is categorised into numerous subsets, communicating a necessary approach to resolve the problems but implemented in various sectors such as from gaming to specialist systems, from machine learning to neural networks (NN) and genetic algorithms (GA) [6]. Thus, machine learning is a subset of artificial intelligence which permits the machines to understand and learn from available data without being programmed explicitly. In this section, various artificial intelligence methods and applications throughout different stages of AM are discussed for further research.

17.2.1 Printability Checker

Printability can effectively replicate a three-dimensional model using a 3D printer to print 3D objects with a 3D-printing technique. The exposure of conventional 3D printing is still limited because of time consumption, certain requirements of material and geometrical characteristics. Further, a printability checker scheme was introduced to check whether a product is able to be 3D printed or not. This helps reduce the complexity and ensures that the 3D model will be prepared optimally.

In a printability checker scheme, the printability of a model can be checked, but it is still difficult to use practically because of a lack of feasibility and smart visions to cover the actual image of the product. Then, scale-invariant feature transformations (SIFTs), in conjunction with a vector of locally collected descriptors, are implemented for encoding that image into a digital form. The encoding approach was used, over an NN-based interpretation, because of its strong rotation as well as scale invariances. After implementing the algorithm, the support vector machine (SVM) was used to categorise the several representations into various material systems, with a significant improvement in accuracy, i.e., 95 per cent.

Thus, the machine learning method was implemented into automatic rule adjustment to verify printability. Apart from this process, the model is trained to estimate printability using SVM rather than predefining the rules. This helps obtain the optimal decision function for additional classifications utilising similar parameters. By using this process, the feature extraction time of three-dimensional models is also significantly reduced without impacting the product accuracy and precision.

Further, the printability estimation depends on a single factor as well as on a combination of several factors like cost, extent, time, geometry and raw material. To test and determine the effect of a single factor or multiple factors, a problem should be formulated as an optimisation problem that can be resolved by implementing GA and a genetics-based machine learning approach. This approach helps get an optimal effect proportion of each factor with minimal complexity value. Herein, a few assumptions need to be made for constructing the objective functions. To simplify the 3D printing, the research can be further aimed at optimising the printing process to reduce the complexity under a multi-factor scenario.

17.2.2 Prefabrication

In this competitive era, the optimisation of computational prefabrication becomes a critical factor in 3D printing, due to the demand for complicated designed objects [7].

Several researchers have proposed different solutions for accelerating prefabrication. Some approaches were proposed for accelerating the slicing process [8,9]. Further, Zhou et al. proposed a hybrid slicing approach by combining laser-based vector imaging and mask projection [9,10]. Moreover, Fok et al. presented a trajectory optimiser to explore the optimum printing path [11].

17.2.2.1 Slicing Acceleration

The layer data is taken out from the triangular mesh by utilising the slicing algorithm for converting the sliced three-dimensional model into slicing planes in z-coordinates [12]. A slicing algorithm proposed by Wang et al. comprises three modules, i.e., ray-triangle intersection, trunk sorting and layer extraction. The ray-triangle intersection helps the slicing algorithm estimate the intersection points in-between upright rays on two-dimensional image pixel centres and triangle meshes in STL format. Further, the same kind of technique is used by [13,14] in which the plane triangle intersection is used for measuring the intersection points. Trunk sorting is used for sorting the intersection points in the defined manner. Furthermore, layer extraction is used to measure the binary value associated with every pixel and produce the layer images for printing, according to the position of the point and height of the layer [15].

Although the slicing algorithm develops successive layer-based additive manufacturing, it is still difficult and complex to implement parallel computing. In the present world of big data, parallel computing has enormous capability to effectively improve the computational desires of artificial intelligence in view of image processing, fabrication processes, logic mechanisation, data analysing and cleaning. The graphics processing unit (GPU) schemes were presented for accelerating the prefabrication processes with the assistance of pixel-wise parallel slicing and fully parallel slicing approaches. This helps develop the parallelism of the three modules of the slicing algorithm. Wang et al. introduced a pixel-wise parallel slicing approach, in which for every single pixel ray, one specific thread is assigned, and all the pixel-ray operations are implemented by the thread [15]. The pixel-wise parallel slicing approach is shown in Figure 17.2.

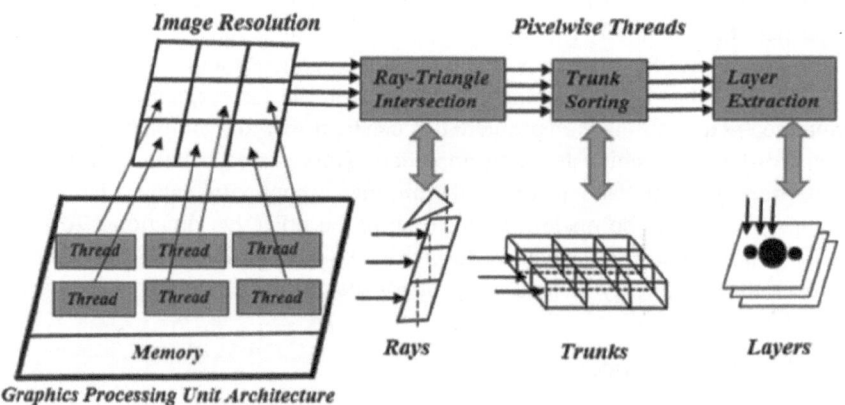

FIGURE 17.2 Pixel-wise parallel slicing approach.

17.2.2.2   Path Optimisation

The optimum printing path guides the nozzle to make specific shapes and also helps to reduce the printing and computational time. The nozzle primarily spends time traversing the print segment and transition segment during printing. Thus, there is an immense need to obtain an optimal path with shortened traversing time or distance. Fok et al. presented a 3D-printing trajectory optimiser method for computing the traversing period of the printing nozzle. The travelling salesman problem (TSP) formulates the path optimisation problem by comparing every single print segment to a town and obtaining the quickest route for visiting the entire nation. In every single layer, the optimisation is implemented at the inter-partition level, i.e. print area, and the intra-partition level, i.e. blank area, according to the borders of the areas. Between every inter-partition, TSP is able to compute the route manner and begin the route for visiting every single area. Further, a Christofides algorithm is implemented for getting the shortest visiting time period. At the intra-partition level, the transition segment is the link between the two closest endpoints situated in two neighbouring print areas.

It has been observed that parallel slicing acceleration and path optimisation can provide an effective process. The combination of printability checking, slicing and path optimisation offers a more reliable process for accelerating the prefabrication.

17.2.3   Service Platform and Evaluation

Service-oriented architecture (SOA) is a fundamental element of the computing paradigm, providing services and techniques to satisfy customer demands efficiently. The optimum SOA can smartly understand the high flexibility, customisation, and integration of 3D printing [16]. The service-oriented cloud production has serval effects and applications in AM. For example, Wu presented the 3D-printing approach in a cloud-based production system [17] and Y. Wu et al. introduced the 3D-printing cloud service-oriented platform and a service assessment model based on the cloud-oriented service system [18].

The cloud platform is a desired processing model consisting an individual computer hardware and software assets. The cloud platform provides on-request access to customers to share the collection of assets, and the shared information and capabilities of the system are integrated into a virtualised asset pool [19]. The contribution of service assessment and demand meeting algorithm provides a stage to smartly create a comprehensive estimation of terminal printers and provide the optimum allocation of assets based on printing accuracy, cost, time and quality. Further, the asset allocation algorithms were proposed to construct adaptable collective scheduling and planning of assets. The machine learning method was used to introduce an evaluation method for evaluating and selecting printers' services. A service evaluation model was proposed by using the major indexes comprising cost, trust, time and quality. The quality of the service is measured so that the service selection can be improved accordingly. Likewise, Dong et al. proposed a similar service quality acquisition approach and a trust assessment model for cloud services by employing GA [20].

17.2.4 SECURITY

In recent decades, security issues have become more important in the industrial sector. Cyber-attacks, and exposure to cyber-manufacturing techniques involving AM, can cause numerous defects in the objects, such as changes in design dimensions, infilling of voids, high temperature, nozzle travelling time and speed etc. [21]. A person-in-the-middle can attack the manufacturing process by replacing the original file in STL format with a malicious design STL file, and the attacker can disturb the user-server communication, as shown in Figure 17.3 when an attacker created a malicious infill cavity defect which cannot be noticed by seeing the product' surface so the product can be made without observing any defects. The workers cannot see the changes between the original and malevolent design due to the implication of the malicious design; the malicious STL file is sent to the 3-D printer and a defective product will be manufactured. Then this defective product will be delivered to the market.

A machine learning method was proposed by Wu et al. for real-time detection of malicious cyber-attacks in 3D-printing methods. Herein, each defected layer-based picture will be transformed into the greyscale plot. The characteristics of greyscale mean standard derivation and pixels greater than the defined maximum value are all taken out in accordance with the value distribution of greyscale. According to the extracted characteristics, the machine learning algorithms provide real-time detection in the defected areas and activate alerts to the administrative system about the defects. The irregularity detection is performed to detect strange outliers which do not adopt the predefined or recognised behaviours, i.e. increase in mean value, standard derivation, and pixels greater than the defined maximum value. In the cyber-physical structure, the unsupervised learning approach is used to detect irregularities with a low false rate by applying a recurrent neural network and cumulative sum method [22]. The random forest can not only categorise the abnormalities with the estimation of the subsequent distribution of every single image layer and also construct process-based patterns for detection based on the images.

Several of the case findings are mentioned here, including the examination of patients and the AM products chosen for diagnosis. Firstly, Banga et al. (2020) introduced a customised design of ankle foot orthosis (AFO) prepared by AM processes like 3D printing. This advanced design increases the comfort for foot drop patients.

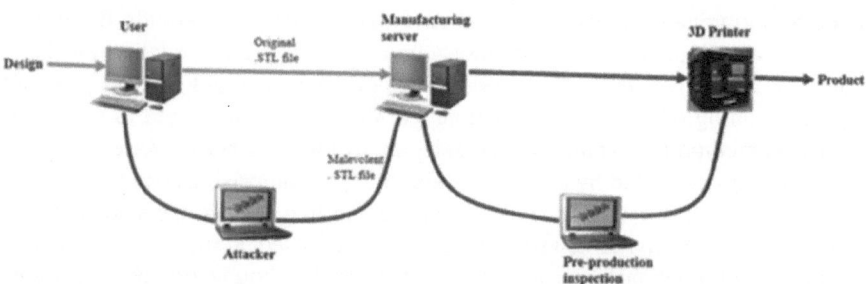

FIGURE 17.3 A person-in-the-middle attacks the server-based manufacturing process.

Moreover, the structuring of the proposed design is fabricated using AM and further investigated on ANSYS software. This customised design of AFOs has become an excellent alternative for fulfilling the needs of the patients by providing adequate comfort [23]. Kumar et al. (2020) performed a study to evaluate the AFOs on the lower limbs of physically disabled persons during their walking by utilising OpenSim software. Further, some foot drop patients were examined to perform gait analysis using a motion analysis system. The collected data is used to develop a biomechanics simulated model for measuring joint motion and angles. This study found that the use of the AFO is a legitimate effort for foot drop patients [24]. Banga et al. (2021) conducted a study to evaluate the use of AM in orthotics and prosthetic objects. This study found that AM improves the structure and progression of products by reducing the wastage of material. Further, AM improves the accuracy and steady environment of the structure, which directly enhances the performance by providing an inventive structure using various materials [25].

17.3 CONCLUSION

This chapter represents the various artificial intelligence applications in AM, including several algorithms for designing the secure, qualified and service-oriented platform for manufacturing. The recent challenges in AM are also discussed, including process acceleration, real-time monitoring, cyber-attack detection and parallel computing, for mass customization in AM. Although it is found that AM can act as an extraordinary mode of manufacturing, additional advances in artificial intelligence are also essential in AM to accelerate the realisation of this prospect. There are many AM applications which are advancing from machine learning techniques. However, some more areas are still unexplored. Like, the deep learning techniques can also be applied in AM designs to train on 3D CAD models to improve the designs for AM.

REFERENCES

1. Berman, B. (2012). "3-D printing: The new industrial revolution", *Business Horizons*, vol. 55, no. 2, pp. 155–162.
2. Tofail, S.A., Koumoulos, E.P., Bandyopadhyay, A., Bose, S., O'Donoghue, L., and Charitidis, C. (2018). "Additive manufacturing: Scientific and technological challenges, market uptake and opportunities", *Materialstoday*, vol. 21, no. 1, pp. 22–37.
3. Gao, W., Zhang, Y., Ramanujan, D., Ramani, K., Chen, Y., Williams, C. B., Wang, C. C. L., Shin, Y. C., Zhang, S., and Zavattieri, P. D. (2015). "The status, challenges, and future of additive manufacturing in engineering", *Computer-Aided Design*, vol. 69, pp. 65–89.
4. Kim, D. B., Witherell, P., Lipman, R., and Feng, S. C. (2015). "Streamlining the additive manufacturing digital spectrum: A systems approach", *Additive Manufacturing*, vol. 5, pp. 20–30.
5. Brooks, R. (1991). "Intelligence without reason", *Artificial Intelligence*, vol. 47, no. 1–3, pp. 139–159.
6. Luger, G. F., (2005), "Artificial intelligence: Structures and strategies for complex problem solving", *Pearson Education*, vol. 5, pp. 20–31.
7. Kulkarni, P., Marsan, A., and Dutta, D. (2000). "A review of process planning techniques in layered manufacturing", *Rapid Prototyping Journal*, vol. 6, no. 1, pp. 18–35.

8. Alkadi, F., Lee, K.-C., Bashiri, A. H., and Choi, J.-W. (2020). "Conformal additive manufacturing using a direct-print process", *Additive Manufacturing*, vol. 532, p. 100975.

9. Vatani, M., Rahimi, A., and Brazandeh, F. (2009). "An enhanced slicing algorithm using nearest distance analysis for layer manufacturing", *Proceedings of World Academy of Science, Engineering and Technology*, vol. 3, no. 25, pp. 721–726.

10. Zhou, C., Ye, H., and Zhang, F. (2015). "A novel low-cost stereolithography process based on vector scanning and mask projection for high-accuracy, high-speed, high-throughput, and large-area fabrication", *Journal of Computing and Information Science in Engineering*, vol. 15, no. 1, 011003.

11. Fok, K., Cheng, C., Tse, C. K., and Ganganath, N. (2016). "A Relaxation Scheme for TSP-based 3D Printing Path Optimizer", *2016 International Conference on Cyber-Enabled Distributed Computing and Knowledge Discovery (CyberC)*, Chengdu, 2016, pp. 382–385.

12. Zhou, C., Chen, Y., Yang, Z., and Khoshnevis, B. (2013). "Digital material fabrication using mask-image-projection-based stereolithography", *Rapid Prototyping Journal*, vol. 19, no. 3, pp. 153–165.

13. Minetto, R., Volpato, N., Stolfi, J., Gregori, R. M. M. H., and Silva, M. V. G. (2015). "An optimal algorithm for 3D triangle mesh slicing and loop-closure", *Computer-Aided Design*, vol. 92, pp. 1–31.

14. Gregori, R. M. M. H., Volpato, N., Minetto, R. and Silva, M. V. G. D. (2014). "Slicing triangle meshes: A asymptotically optimal algorithm", *14th International Conference on Computational Science and Its Applications*, Guimaraes, Portugal, pp. 252–255.

15. Wang, A., Zhou, C., Jin, Z., and Xu, W. (2017). "Towards Scalable and Efficient GPU-Enabled Slicing Acceleration in Continuous 3D Printing", *2017 22nd Asia and South Pacific Design Automation Conference (ASP-DAC)*, Chiba, pp. 623–628.

16. Da Silveira, G., Borenstein, D., and Fogliatto, H. S. (2001). "Mass customization: Literature review and research directions", *International Journal of Production Economics*, vol. 72, no. 49, pp. 1–13.

17. Wu, D., Thames, J. L., Rosen, D. W., and Schaefer, D. (2013). "Enhancing the product realization process with cloud-based design and manufacturing systems", *Journal of Computing and Information Science in Engineering*, vol. 13, no. 4, p. 41004.

18. Wu, Y., Peng, G., Chen, L., and Zhang, H. (2016) "Service Architecture and evaluation model of distributed 3D printing based on cloud manufacturing", *2016 IEEE International Conference on Systems, Man, and Cybernetics (SMC)*, Budapest, pp. 002762–002767.

19. Li, B.H., Zhang, L., Wang, S. L., et al. (2010). "Cloud manufacturing: A new service-oriented networked manufacturing model", *Computer Integrated Manufacturing Systems*, vol. 16, no. 1, pp. 1–7.

20. Dong, Y. F., and Gang, G. (2014). "Evaluation and selection approach for cloud manufacturing service based on template and global trust degree", *Computer Integrated Manufacturing Systems*, vol. 20, no. 1, pp. 207–214.

21. Wu, M., Song, Z., and Moon, Y. B. (2019). "Detecting cyber-physical attacks in Cyber Manufacturing systems with machine learning methods", *Journal of Intelligent Manufacturing*, vol. 30, pp. 1111–1123.

22. Goh, J., Adepu, S., Tan, M., and Lee, Z. S. (2017) "Anomaly Detection in Cyber Physical Systems Using Recurrent Neural Networks", *2017 IEEE 18th International Symposium on High Assurance Systems Engineering (HASE)*, Singapore, pp. 140–145.

23. Banga, H. K., Kalra, P., Belokar, R. M., and Kumar, R. (2020). "Customized design and additive manufacturing of kids' ankle foot orthosis", *Rapid Prototyping Journal*, vol. 26, no. 10, pp. 1677–1685.

24. Kumar, P., Sharma, P., Banga, H. K., Kalra, P., and Kumar, R. (2021). "Performance evaluation of ankle foot orthosis on lower extremity disabled persons while walking using OpenSim". In *Operations Management and Systems Engineering* (pp. 299–310). Springer, Singapore.
25. Banga, H. K., Kumar, P., and Kumar, H. (2021). Utilization of additive manufacturing in orthotics and prosthetic devices development. *IOP Conference Series: Materials Science and Engineering*, vol. 1033, no. 1, p. 012083). IOP Publishing.

Index

Page numbers in **Bold** indicate tables and page numbers in *Italics* indicate figures.

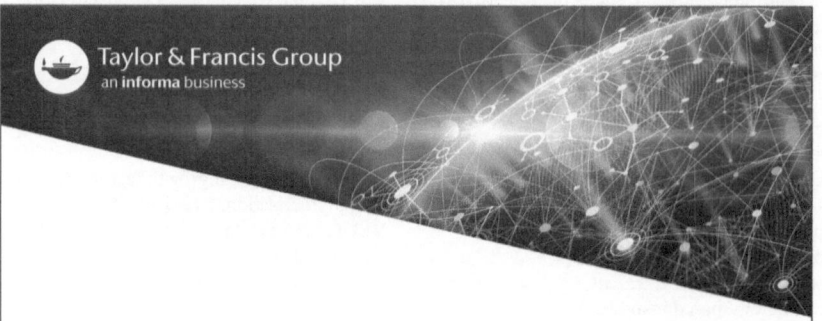
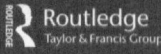
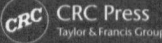